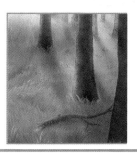

Nature Therapy

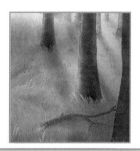

Nature Therapy

Edited by

Yonatan Kaplan, M.D.
Petros Levounis, M.D., M.A.

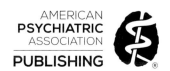

AMERICAN
PSYCHIATRIC
ASSOCIATION
PUBLISHING

If you wish to buy 50 or more copies of the same title, please go to www.appi.org/specialdiscounts for more information.

Copyright © 2025 American Psychiatric Association Publishing
ALL RIGHTS RESERVED
First Edition

Manufactured in the United States of America on acid-free paper
28 27 26 25 24   5 4 3 2 1

American Psychiatric Association Publishing
800 Maine Avenue SW, Suite 900
Washington, DC 20024-2812
www.appi.org

Library of Congress Cataloging-in-Publication Data
Names: Kaplan, Yonatan (Psychiatrist) editor. | Levounis, Petros, editor. |
American Psychiatric Association Publishing, publisher.
Title: Nature therapy / edited by Yonatan Kaplan, Petros Levounis.
Description: First edition. | Washington, D.C. : American Psychiatric
Association Publishing, [2024] | Includes bibliographical references and
index.
Identifiers: LCCN 2024011498 (print) | LCCN 2024011499 (ebook) | ISBN
9781615374571 (paperback ; alk. paper) | ISBN 9781615374588 (ebook)
Subjects: MESH: Relaxation Therapy--methods | Nature
Classification: LCC RC489.A38 (print) | LCC RC489.A38 (ebook) | NLM WM
425.5.R3 | DDC 616.89/165--dc23/eng/20240506
LC record available at https://lccn.loc.gov/2024011498
LC ebook record available at https://lccn.loc.gov/2024011499

British Library Cataloguing in Publication Data
A CIP record is available from the British Library.

CONTENTS

Contributors

Muhammad Aadil, M.D.
Assistant Professor, Albert Einstein College of Medicine/Jacobi Medical Center, Bronx, New York

Rijul Asri, M.D.
Resident Physician, Department of Psychiatry, Rutgers New Jersey Medical School, Newark, New Jersey

Sezai Ustun Aydin, M.D.
Physician, Department of Psychiatry, Rutgers New Jersey Medical School, Newark, New Jersey

Alexis Bocian-Reperowitz, M.D.
Psychiatry Resident, The Warren Alpert Medical School, Providence, Rhode Island

Leia Chemmacheril, M.D., M.B.A.
Resident, Psychiatry Department, Rutgers New Jersey Medical School, Newark, New Jersey

Diego L. Coira, M.D.
Psychiatrist, Coira Institute, Oakland, New Jersey

Rafael Coira, M.D., J.D.
Child, Adolescent, and Adult Psychiatrist, Coira Institute, Oakland, New Jersey

Ann-Marie Edwards, B.Sc. (Hons)
M.Sc. Student, Health Department, University of Essex Online, Colchester, Essex, United Kingdom

Elizabeth Fam Filtes, M.D.
Addiction Psychiatry Fellow, New York University Grossman School of Medicine, New York, New York

Andrew M. Fukuda, M.D., Ph.D.
Assistant Professor, Department of Psychiatry and Human Behavior, Brown University, Providence, Rhode Island; Associate Director, Butler Hospital TMS Clinic and Neuromodulation Research Facility, Providence, Rhode Island; Associate Director of TMS Research, McLean Hospital Psychiatric Neurotherapeutics Program, Division of Depression and Anxiety, Belmont, Massachusetts; Instructor, Harvard University, Belmont, Massachusetts

Diego Garces Grosse, M.D.
Clinical Assistant Professor, Department of Psychiatry, NYU Grossman School of Medicine, New York, New York

Ryan Behmer Hansen, M.D.
Resident, Ohio State University College of Medicine, Columbus, Ohio

Mary-Anne E. Hennen, M.D.
Consultation-Liaison Fellow, Icahn School of Medicine at Mount Sinai, New York, New York

Abby Jaroslow, M.S., HTR, CH
Horticultural Therapist, The Alice and Herbert Sachs Therapeutic Conservatory, Jefferson Moss-Magee Rehabilitation, Elkins Park, Pennsylvania

Yonatan Kaplan, M.D.
Assistant Clinical Professor, Department of Psychiatry, Icahn School of Medicine at Mount Sinai, New York, New York

Katherine G. Kennedy, M.D.
Clinical Professor of Psychiatry, Yale University School of Medicine, New Haven, Connecticut

Yasuhiro Kotera, Ph.D.
Associate Professor in Mental Health, Faculty of Medicine and Health Sciences, University of Nottingham, Nottingham, United Kingdom

Eugenia Frances Kronenberg, Sc.B.
Research Coordinator, Butler Hospital TMS Clinic and Neuromodulation Research Facility, Providence, Rhode Island

Petros Levounis, M.D., M.A.
Professor and Chair, Department of Psychiatry, and Associate Dean, Rutgers New Jersey Medical School, Newark, New Jersey; Chief of Service, University Hospital, Newark, New Jersey; President, American Psychiatric Association

Celena Q. Ma, M.D.
Resident, Rutgers New Jersey Medical School, Newark, New Jersey

Kirsten McEwan, Ph.D.
Associate Professor of Health and Wellbeing, College of Health, Psychology and Social Care, University of Derby, Derby, United Kingdom

Anne Meore, LMSW, HTR
Horticultural Therapist, New York Botanical Garden, Bronx, New York; Horticultural Therapist, Good Samaritan Hospital, Suffern, New York; Principal, Planthropy LLC, Tuxedo, New York

H. Steven Moffic, M.D.
Private Pro Bono Community Psychiatrist, Milwaukee, Wisconsin

Aitzaz Munir, M.D.
Clinical Assistant Professor and Associate Program Director, Addiction Medicine Fellowship Program, Department of Psychiatry, Rutgers New Jersey Medical School, Newark, New Jersey

Chaden Noureddine, M.D.
Resident, Icahn School of Medicine at Mount Sinai, Beth Israel, New York

Grace S. Ro, M.D.
Resident, Psychiatry Department, University of Rochester Medical Center, Rochester, New York

Stephanie Ruthberg, M.D., M.S.
Psychiatry Resident (PGY4 2024–2025), Rutgers New Jersey Medical School, Newark, New Jersey

Kishan Shah, M.D.
Assistant Program Director, Residency Training Program; Professor, Department of Psychiatry, Jersey Shore University Medical Center, Neptune, New Jersey

Freya Tsuda-McCaie, M.A., PGDip
Trainee Clinical Psychologist, University of Exeter, Exeter, United Kingdom

DISCLOSURE OF COMPETING INTERESTS

The following contributors have indicated that they have no financial interests or other affiliations that represent or could appear to represent a competing interest with their contributions to this book:

Muhammad Aadil, M.D.
Rijul Asri, M.D.
Sezai Ustun Aydin, M.D.
Alexis Bocian-Reperowitz, M.D.
Leia Chemmacheril, M.D., M.B.A.
Diego L. Coira, M.D.
Rafael Coira, M.D., J.D.
Ann-Marie Edwards, B.Sc. (Hons)
Elizabeth Fam Filtes, M.D.
Andrew M. Fukuda, M.D., Ph.D.
Diego Garces Grosse, M.D.
Ryan Behmer Hansen, M.D.
Mary-Anne E. Hennen, M.D.
Abby Jaroslow, M.S., HTR, CH
Yonatan Kaplan, M.D.
Yasuhiro Kotera, Ph.D.
Eugenia Frances Kronenberg, Sc.B.
Petros Levounis, M.D., M.A.
Celena Q. Ma, M.D.
Kirsten McEwan, Ph.D.
Anne Meore, LMSW, HTR
H. Steven Moffic, M.D.
Aitzaz Munir, M.D.
Chaden Noureddine, M.D.

Grace S. Ro, M.D.
Stephanie Ruthberg, M.D., M.S.
Kishan Shah, M.D.
Freya Tsuda-McCaie, M.A., PGDip

Foreword

This fascinating jewel of a book, beautifully written and expertly curated, unfolds the mysteries of nature-based treatments and makes a compelling argument for deeper nature engagement. With 12 richly annotated chapters, *Nature Therapy* offers a way to remember what the mental health field has forgotten: how nature can augment traditional medical treatments to restore, heal, and even prevent potential illness. Each chapter focuses on a particular aspect of nature's healing qualities and contains abundant reservoirs of robust academic research, as well as useful clinical applications and recommendations. Every chapter has key points and questions to contextualize the powerful evidence base.

Inside this expansive and multifaceted guide, you will discover that the World Health Organization has declared nature to be the greatest source of health and well-being, that access to nature is a social determinant of health, that the American Academy of Pediatrics endorses "nature prescriptions" for children, and that patients recovering from surgery heal more quickly when they are in a room with a window. You will learn that although we spend about 90% of our time indoors, having at least 10 trees on an urban block can lower anxiety. As you delve deeper into what psychiatry has ignored for the past century, your view of the benefits of nature and nature therapy may become one of curiosity and awe.

As humans, we have learned to keep nature separate, perhaps as an expression of our sense of human exceptionalism. In so doing, we may have forgotten that we are a part of nature. Our addiction to screens distances us even further from feeling connected to our natural environment. This book may actually open you up to a deeper connection with nature. As an environmental activist, ardent recycler, and someone who gave my guests 3-inch-high trees to plant as wedding favors, I had believed that I was already well engaged with nature.

But I found that reading this book has helped me connect even more deeply with my personal experiences of nature. For example, during the first summer of the coronavirus pandemic, I watched a robin build a nest outside my kitchen window. The robin had cleverly perched the nest atop a drainpipe under the eaves, and when I washed the dishes, I could see the robin sitting, its plump breast held in by a cradle of twigs. Within a few weeks, I spied three tiny heads peeking over the nest's edge. Soon after, I'd see the robin swoop in, a fat worm held firmly in its beak, and be met by a frantic chorus of seesawing, scrawny necks. Then the robin would cram its beak into one of the bobbing throats before flying off to collect another worm.

I was mesmerized.

For weeks, our family watched their family. We marveled at the robin family's habits, discussing whether one of the babies was bullying its sibs and how quickly they were growing.

One morning, I noticed one of the baby birds standing upright, teetering slightly, and gripping the edge of the nest with its claws. I called out to my family—my spouse and adult children who were back at home during the pandemic—and everyone hurried in to watch the second baby bird clamber up to the edge of the nest as the first shimmied out along the drainpipe. The third bird seemed satisfied to linger in the nest. We waited, ignoring our morning tasks, hoping to see the birds fledge, but after a couple of hours little had changed, with two baby birds standing on the drainpipe and the tiniest one sitting in the nest.

Finally, we all left the kitchen to take our Zoom calls.

An hour later, I returned. The nest was empty. All three birds had gone. Worried that the littlest one had fallen, I ran outside and searched the grass. No bird lay broken winged. All three birds had flown the nest. We had missed seeing them leave and had never said goodbye. I suddenly felt a deep pang of loss. Their transition had happened so fast.

The baby birds and the mother robin never returned to the nest. I was surprised that my heart felt so heavy. As I cleaned the morning dishes, I'd look out of the window at the empty nest and feel a wash of sadness. The nest, so full of potential, lay unused. I longed for the activity of the babies thronging together, the mother swooping in. I realized, with a laugh, that I was experiencing a true empty-nest syndrome. I soon pushed the event out of my consciousness.

However, reading this book has allowed me to reflect more deeply on my experience, instead of being ashamed of my feelings. I considered the many meanings that this encounter held for me. Most obviously, it reflected my challenge with my children transitioning into adults and the importance of acknowledging my longing to continue to be there for every step of their life journey; I needed to accept that it was no longer my place to witness every one of their future developmental steps. Less obvious was my recognition that the singular moment of passage—the birds flying away—held particular significance for me: my parents had died suddenly, and I had missed being by both of their sides when they passed away. Missing those moments was still a painful memory for me.

This book encouraged me to consider more intentionally bringing nature not only into my life but also into my clinical work. Instead of isolating nature as an entity that exists outside of human experience, today, in my deeper psychotherapy work with patients, I listen more carefully for references to nature and offer more nature-related analogies. In my more supportive clinical work, I suggest ways to engage more frequently with nature, in the same breath as I suggest good sleep hygiene and moderate exercise.

So here's my nature prescription for you: pick up this book, go outside, and read it.

Anywhere outside. A park bench. A beach blanket. A hammock. Some place where you can soak in the sun, be touched by a breeze, or swat at a gnat.

If you can't go outside, then sit by a window, preferably with a view of something green.

Every once in a while, pause. Look around. Breathe deeply. Spot a nearby bird. Whether it is a pigeon, a seagull, or a crow, chances are you will see a bird.

Reflect on the shape of a cloud. Move your eye from the horizon to the more deeply hued crown of the sky. What floats through your mind?

I hope that you will find this book as eye-opening, indispensable, and enlightening as I have.

Katherine G. Kennedy, M.D.
Clinical Professor of Psychiatry
Yale University School of Medicine
New Haven, Connecticut

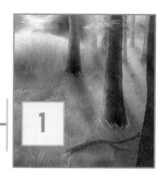

The Wise Outdoors

ON THE ORIGINS, CURRENT STATE, AND FUTURE DIRECTION OF NATURE THERAPY

Yonatan Kaplan, M.D.

And I firmly believe that nature brings solace in all troubles.
—Anne Frank (1997), Diary Entry, February 17, 1944[1]

---

[1]©ANNE FRANK FONDS, Basel, Switzerland.

Nature is brimming with emotion. Sunshine, fresh air, and the open sky convey the serene cheerfulness of an idyllic weekend getaway. The horror genre stock phrase "a dark and stormy night" poetically conjures anxious anticipation with an impending feeling of doom. Atmosphere as a literary device is effective in establishing tone because human emotional states are sensitive to nature.

Poets, philosophers, and religious leaders throughout history have written extensively about the psychological and spiritual benefits nature offers. Before the invention of psychotherapy and psychiatric medications, nature was one of the only remedies that physicians could offer for mental illness. Mental health hospitals of the eighteenth century were built with an architectural philosophy that natural settings were inherently therapeutic.

Contemporary research is producing a growing body of empirical evidence supporting the poetic sentiment of nature's benefits. Specific sensory stimuli found in nature such as aesthetics, acoustics, textures, and scents have been found to measurably reduce physiological markers of stress. Several examples explored in this book include birdsong, fractal patterns of branching trees, and even the scent of a pine forest.

Nature's sensory landscape is fading from daily life. Societal pressure and urban development are moving people indoors and replacing verdant paradises with paved parking lots. Rapid environmental transformation comes at a cost. Although the challenges of urban living, such as air pollution, noise, and overcrowding, are well documented, the full consequences of losing our connection to nature are not fully understood.

Nature's function in the psychiatrist's toolbox has evolved over the years. In this chapter, I define terms and explore how scientific and cultural advances have influenced our appreciation of nature's role in mental health. The chapter ends with a practical guide to exploring a patient's relationship with nature.

DEFINING NATURE

This book uses the following definition of *nature*:

> Elements and phenomena of Earth's lands, waters, and biodiversity, across spatial scales and degrees of human influence, from a potted plant or a small urban creek or park to expansive, "pristine" wilderness with its dynamics of fire, weather, geology, and other forces. (Bratman et al. 2019, p. 2)

"Pristine" wilderness imagines a prehuman world untouched by any "degree of human influence." The first humans to arrive to the pristine wilderness as modest troops of hunter-gatherers can easily be understood as a part of nature (Watkins 2005). Subsequent generations exerted greater control over the environment through technological advancements that distanced them from the ecological conditions experienced by their forebears. Nature therapy recognizes that contemporary lifestyles are far removed from the natural conditions that our hunter-gatherer ancestors experienced. Because such natural conditions are what our minds and bodies are adapted to, a growing body of evidence supports the health benefits of reconnecting with elements of the pristine wilderness.

The subsequent chapters describe the consequences of the societal shift away from pristine wilderness and the remedies to reintroduce lost nature into daily life.

NATURE THERAPY

Contemporary Definitions

As of 2023, no single organization is universally recognized as an authoritative institution on *nature therapy*. Scholars, researchers, individual therapists, and journalists infer their own definitions and use the term interchangeably with related phrases such as *ecotherapy*, *ecopsychology*, and *green therapy* (Summers and Vivian 2018).

Yoshifumi Miyazaki, Ph.D., of Chiba University in Japan researches the physiological effects of spending time in forests. His widely cited studies, discussed in further detail in Chapter 3, "Forest Bathing," propose the following definition for *nature therapy*:

> A set of practices aimed at achieving "preventive medical effects" through exposure to natural stimuli that render a state of physiological relaxation and boost the weakened immune functions to prevent diseases. (Song et al. 2016, p. 2)

Ronen Berger, Ph.D., director of the Nature Therapy program at Tel Aviv University in Israel, developed his own therapeutic framework for Nature Therapy. His framework incorporates elements from transpersonal and gestalt psychology, art and drama therapies, mind-body and shamanistic practices, and the adventure and wilderness therapies described in Chapter 7, "The Wild Outdoors." Berger distinguishes ecopsychology and other therapeutic uses of nature from his own Nature Therapy framework, defined as follows: "Nature therapy is an innovative, experiential, therapeutic framework that takes place in nature. It seeks to broaden the static, constantly controlled natural environment of 'therapy' to create a dynamic therapeutic environment (setting) that is a partner in shaping the process" (Berger 2008, p. 47).

Despite a lack of consensus definition, nature therapy is broadly understood by the public as intentional interactions with ecological resources to promote psychological and physical well-being. Public spaces such as parks, beaches, and the general outdoors are examples of ecological resources discussed in Chapter 4, "Urban Green Spaces." Nature's ready availability encourages self-administration free from the gatekeeping of professional prescription. Although a layperson's nature therapy may enhance their quality of life, it is not a replacement for standard-of-care treatments for diagnosed illness (Summers and Vivian 2018).

Nature Therapy
From Romanticism to the New Deal

No eighteenth-century philosopher popularized nature as body of wonderment more than German naturalist, explorer, and scientist Alexander von Humboldt. Although the prevailing scientific views at the time emphasized the categorization and division of natural phenomena into distinct taxonomies, Humboldt focused on comprehending the interconnectedness of seemingly disparate fields. Humboldt meticulously documented his observations of natural phenomena. He also emphasized the importance of examining the relationships between living organisms and their physical environments, such as climate, soil, and vegetation. One of his most significant observations was that human activities can significantly affect the environment and cause climate change. Humboldt's pioneering work laid the foundation for the modern study of ecology and helped to shape a more holistic and interdisciplinary understanding of nature in the nineteenth and twentieth centuries (Wulf 2015).

Humboldt not only studied nature but also was deeply moved by it. Never the detached observer, he documented his personal emotional responses in tandem with quantitative measurements. He referred to his theory of ecological unity as *Naturgemälde*, a poetic term that translates to "a painting of nature." His publications bridged the gap between the analytical world of Enlightenment empiricism and the countercultural European Romanticism, which emphasized a spiritual and emotional connection between people and nature (Dettelbach 2001).

Nature's soothing effects were lauded by the European Romanticism movement of the nineteenth century. Poets such as William Wordsworth wrote about nature as a source of beauty and inspiration, a refuge from the stresses of modern life, and a powerful force that could heal and restore the human spirit. The romanticists saw nature as a reflection of divinity and believed that connecting with the natural world was essential for human happiness and fulfillment (Aretoulakis 2014).

Nature's therapeutic power was more commonly explored by poets than physicians during this period. Although the psychiatric treatments of the time, such as moral and asylum treatments, incorporated nature, as discussed in Chapter 5, "Horticultural Therapy," they tended to emphasize the therapeutic value of humanizing relationships rather than the healing potential of nature itself. Chapter 5 also provides a brief chronology of the professional application of nature therapy in clinical practice (Marks 2017).

The first permutation of the term *nature therapy* in the medical literature appeared in an abstract presented at the 1865 annual meeting of the Illinois State Medical Society. The submission, titled "Report on Orthopedic Surgery," juxtaposed surgical intervention on a fracture with the bone's subsequent ossification and remodeling, or "nature's therapy" (Prince 1865). In this case, *nature* refers to an initial biological state limited in scope to the human body rather than an inclusive scale of cosmic elements and phenomena. By the end of the nineteenth century, the medical community used *nature's therapy* to describe the body's inherent homeostatic mechanisms and immune system (Ulrich 1898).

In 1934, *nature therapy* appeared in a new context in an article published in the *Common Law League Journal*. South Dakota lawyer Harry Robinson (1934) wrote, "We believe in Nature Therapy for our depressions," referring to nature as the environmental forces relevant to agriculture and using *depressions* as a double entendre for economic downturn and the resulting emotional devastation. He elaborated that the American government should develop ecologically minded agricultural policies to avoid overexploiting farmland. Although his article advocated economic policy rather than ecologically oriented psychotherapy, he was the first to publish the term *nature therapy* as relating the environment to emotional well-being (Robinson 1934, p. 191).

Robinson's use of the term *nature therapy* was probably influenced by the implementation of the Civilian Conservation Corps (CCC) as part of President Franklin D. Roosevelt's New Deal program. The New Deal was a series of economic reforms and programs aimed at reviving the American economy during the Great Depression. The CCC was a work relief program that operated from 1933 to 1942, employing young men and focusing on conservation projects such as planting trees, building trails, and developing parks. The program aimed to invigorate the young men and build character by combining manual labor and the outdoors (Maher 2008).

The CCC projects increased the accessibility of wilderness spaces, inviting Americans to experience the country's natural beauty. The CCC in Robinson's home state of South Dakota employed 30,000 men from 1933 to 1937. The CCC's success in creating jobs and completing community-based projects shifted public opinion toward nature conservation as a source of national pride and economic prosperity (Derschied 2016).

The popular attitude toward the salutary effects of national parks was not lost on the medical establishment. During World War II, the U.S. Navy established a hospital in Yosemite National Park for combat veterans, hoping that the park's sublime location would aid in their recovery. Despite the abundant outdoor recreation and hot springs for balneotherapy, as discussed in Chapter 8, "The Wet Outdoors," the isolated atmosphere proved counterproductive. The hospital shifted its treatment focus away from austere contemplation and toward social reintegration through activities such as family visits, guided hikes, and live entertainment (Kittredge 1946; Yosemite National Park 1946).

Psychiatric and Environmental Revolution

As the twentieth century brought attitudes toward nature into contact with professional health care, psychiatry underwent a series of significant advances. Sigmund Freud introduced the field to psychoanalysis, which stressed the importance of the unconscious mind in shaping human behavior. Carl Jung expanded on Freud's ideas by developing the concept of the collective unconscious. Jung's (2002) theory proposed a shared, innate reservoir of knowledge and experience that transcends individual consciousness, echoing the shared spiritual world of animism.

In 1943, humanist psychologist Abraham Maslow proposed his theory of motivation. Maslow's hierarchy of needs is a framework that categorizes the five fundamental human needs in hierarchical order, starting from physiological needs such as food and shelter to self-actualization needs such as personal growth and fulfillment. According to this theory, people must fulfill their lower-level needs before they can move toward higher-level needs (Maslow 1943).

Psychoanalytic theories emphasized internal factors driving behavior, whereas the American behavioral psychologists John Watson and B.F. Skinner investigated the effect of external stimuli. Their experiments demonstrated how environmental factors can shape and control behavior (Horowitz 1992).

From a behaviorism perspective, Homo sapiens' evolutionary course was an iterative adaptation over millions of years to a complex, though relatively stable, ecosystem of rewards and punishments. The invention of agriculture led people to radically alter the landscape, resulting in a novel environment distinct from the Pleistocene conditions that incubated them. Anthropogenic environmental modification outpaced humans' genetic ability to adapt. This concept of *nature deficit disorder*, further discussed in Chapter 2, "Theoretical Framework," is rooted in the idea that deprivation of stimuli present in the natural environment where human neurobiology evolved is detrimental to emotional well-being (Louv 2008).

Although psychoanalytic theory predominated psychiatric practice in the first half of the twentieth century, psychiatrists experimented with a variety of interventions for more immediate results. Neurosyphilis was the first psychiatric illness discovered to have a biological basis and a cure. Austrian psychiatrist Julius Wagner-Jauregg won the Nobel Prize in Medicine in 1927 for his malarial treatment of neurosyphilis, then known as "general paralysis of the insane." The treatment involved infecting a patient with malaria to induce high fevers that killed the syphilitic spirochetes. Although malarial treatment was later replaced by penicillin, it provided an example of a physical intervention that could rapidly resolve a chronic psychiatric disease (Harrington 2019).

With a few exceptions, a biological basis for psychopathology remained elusive. Contemporary hindsight harshly judges interventions such as insulin comas, ice wraps, and, most infamously, lobotomies, which were administered without a concrete understanding of the etiology of the symptoms they purported to treat. The physical psychiatric interventions had more success sedating and controlling patients than alleviating symptoms and restoring function. The same spirit of innovation also led to empirically validated treatment such as electroconvulsive therapy. Experimentation in physical psychiatry fell out of favor with the advent of medications that achieved the same behavioral control through less invasive means. In 1952, the same year that the *Diagnostic and Statistical Manual of Mental Disorders* was first published (American Psychiatric Association 1952), chlorpromazine was approved for treating schizophrenia, marking the beginning of psychiatry's age of psychopharmacology. Over the next few decades, psychiatric practice shifted away from psychoanalytic and psychotherapeutic approaches and toward prescribing medications (Harrington 2019).

The 1950s were a crossroads in psychiatric treatments as diverse treatment modalities were tested for institutionalized patients. In this historical context, Westboro State Hospital in Massachusetts hosted a nature club as an optional group for its psychiatric inpatients. The club was the brainchild of Frances Gillotti, an educator at the Massachusetts Audubon Society. The club consisted of visual presentations on a nature topic followed by a guided group discussion. Gillotti engaged patients with the use of multimedia, bringing in specimens, natural materials, and live animals. The program, which ran throughout 1951, was well received, and Gillotti wrote about the experience in the 1953 issue of *The Science Counselor*. Her article is the earliest published example of the term *nature therapy* as a psychiatric treatment (Gillotti 1953).

Despite the program's positive reception, *nature therapy* disappeared from published psychiatric discourse until the 1990s. Over the next several decades, psychiatric practice and diagnostics underwent several upheavals, driven in part by the proliferation of psychopharmaceuticals. Experiential therapies either fell out of vogue or were ceded to associated professional fields such as psychology and occupational therapy. Fresh air and sunshine were blown out of the psychiatric playbook by the god of thunder marketed under the trade name Thorazine. No bucolic stroll compared with carefree chlordiazepoxide's anxiolytic potency (Cosgrove and Vaswani 2019; Harrington 2019).

Although medications offered symptomatic relief, they were not curative. Psychiatric diagnostics were criticized for their subjective element when compared with biologically based empirical testing in other medical specialties. Psychopathology did not conform to the prevailing biomedical model of the time, which viewed illness as a quantitative deviation from a physiological norm leading to functional impairment. Psychiatrists at a crossroads contended with whether the social determinants of mental health should be included in the scope of medical practice. Prescribing medications allowed psychiatrists to mirror the practice of other medical professions more closely. However, overemphasis on pharmacotherapy at the expense of psychosocial factors risked neglecting relational aspects of treatment (Karter and Kamens 2019).

In 1977, American psychiatrist George Engel proposed a biopsychosocial model for medicine that accounted for the social determinants of health. The biopsychosocial model expanded the definition of disease to account for how variation in human experience affects functional prognosis. By centering on the patient experience, empirical quantification of biomarkers became supportive evidence of disease rather than absolutely diagnostic. Under this new definition, psychiatric diagnoses, which were almost entirely defined by patient experience, were indisputably covered under the medical umbrella (Dowling 2005; Engel 1977).

Cited nearly 19,000 times since its publication, the biopsychosocial model supplanted the strictly biomedical model as the guiding philosophy of modern medicine. Engel's model took an ecological approach to human health. The biopsychosocial model recognizes that the health of an individual human body is linked to a greater system of interdependent relationships, ranging in scale from microscopic biochemistry to macroscopic social and environmental factors. This model encourages physicians to treat illness with consideration of the patient's systemic context rather than as an isolated set of parts (Borrell-Carrió et al. 2004).

The biopsychosocial model's ecological approach to health reframed nature as an environmental determinant of health. As the medical establishment incorporated evaluation of environmental factors into its standard of care, the American public was confronted with its own effect on the health of the environment. North America's natural heritage, once a cornucopia of sublime landscapes, majestic wildlife, and bountiful waters, had been despoiled by decades of unabated industrial degradation. The assault on America's wilderness spaces was multifold. Species-rich habitats were replaced by residential, manufacturing, or agricultural development. Travel infrastructure crisscrossed once-continuous biomes into a shrunken oblivion. Toxic by-products from chemical plants poisoned the groundwater. Most notoriously, indiscriminate use of the miracle insecticide dichlorodiphenyltrichloroethane (DDT), responsible for controlling malarial outbreaks in the postwar United States, wreaked havoc on the bird population, nearly driving the bald eagle to extinction (Davis 2022).

The overexploitation of natural resources not only was detrimental to plant and animal life but also directly harmed people. Although those who lived in direct proximity to sources of toxic by-products, pesticides, and herbicides were most acutely affected, people who lived far away were exposed through ingestion of contaminated produce and tap water. American biologist, science writer, and conservationist Rachel Carson (1962) wrote about the dangers of indiscriminate pesticide use in her book *Silent Spring*. *Silent Spring* was an immediate sensation, galvanizing an outraged public into lobbying for government oversight of industrial polluters. The Environmental Protection Agency, signed into being by the Nixon administration in 1970, and the eventual agricultural ban of DDT were the direct result of activism inspired by *Silent Spring*. Although Carson was not the first to write about the dangers of pesticides and herbicides, her comprehensive and accessible presentation of the issue had wide appeal (Davis 2022).

Silent Spring is credited with launching the modern environmental movement. The book frames its persuasive argument in terms of peer-reviewed economic and physical health statistics, but its immediate effect and enduring legacy derive from its emotional appeal. The title *Silent Spring* alludes to a dystopian future devoid of the pastoral soundscape associated with the season of renewal. The uncanny silence is marked by the lack of birdsong and buzzing insects. Recognizing that human negligence is responsible for their extinction evokes regret, grief, or even rage. The title suggests that the consequences of environmental degradation are not just physical or economic but also emotional and psychological (Davis 2022).

Postmodern Roots of Nature Therapy

Spurred by increasing environmental consciousness and greater interest in social determinants of health, thought leaders in the last decades of the twentieth century more closely examined the relationship between people and nature. Despite their pertinence to emotional well-being, the investigation into nature's psychological effects occurred outside clinical psychotherapy's professional sphere.

Environmental psychology emerged as a multidisciplinary synthesis of behavioral psychology and architecture, landscape, and design in the late 1960s. Environmental psychology specifically concerned itself with understanding how elements of the physical environment influence human behavior. Stephen Kaplan and Rachel Kaplan were a husband-and-wife environmental psychologist duo who investigated the cognitive aspect of nature exposure with their attention restoration theory (ART; Kaplan and Kaplan 1989). Roger S. Ulrich (1981), with a background in architecture and environmental design, researched how nature contact modulated the physiological stress response with his stress reduction theory (SRT). Entomologist Edward O. Wilson postulated an evolutionary origin of human's interest in nature in his biophilia hypothesis (Wilson 1984). Taken together, ART, SRT, and the biophilia hypothesis formed the scientific basis on which future investigations into nature therapy were built (Sundstrom et al. 1996; Weir 2020).

Table 1–1 summarizes the three seminal theories in nature therapy, which recur throughout this book and are discussed in greater detail in Chapter 5.

Although environmental psychology described the cognitive and behavioral effects of nature interactions, it did not explore the psychodynamics of the human-nature relationship. Developments of the late twentieth century such as the discovery of a hole in the ozone layer, growing awareness of anthropogenic climate change, and the Chernobyl nuclear disaster of 1986 accentuated humanity's strained relationship with nature (Berger 2010).

American cultural historian Theodore Roszak was another nonclinician who advocated for a multidisciplinary study of the human-nature relationship. In his 1992 book *Voice of the Earth*, he coined the term *ecopsychology* to describe the study of human and nature interdependence. Roszak (1992) believed that the ongoing environmental crisis represents

Table 1–1.   Three seminal theories in nature therapy

Theory	Summary
Stress reduction theory (Ulrich 1981)	Exposure to nature encourages relaxation in stressed people.
Biophilia hypothesis (Wilson 1984)	Homo sapiens feel instinctual connection with other living organisms.
Attention restoration theory (Kaplan and Kaplan 1989)	Natural environments are inherently fascinating and can hold attention without causing mental fatigue.

a self-destructive psychopathology rooted in human alienation from the natural environment.

Ecopsychology views the human-nature dyad in developmental terms. Planet Earth, representing nature, is the secure base to which the human species forms an analogous parental bond. Roszak suggested that urbanization, overreliance on technology, and pollution of hospitable outdoor spaces disrupt the formation of secure attachment to the earth. The insecure attachment manifests as alienation from and loss of empathy toward the natural environment. Degradation of the environment continues despite its negative consequences for human health. By Roszak's formulation, the apparent disregard for human impact on the environment reflects a collective suicidal inclination. Ecopsychology advocates for repairing the human-nature relationship by cultivating a sense of ethical responsibility for the environment and replacing destructive practices with sustainable ones on individual and industrial scales (Jordan 2009; Lertzman 2004).

Shortly after ecopsychology's debut in *Voice of the Earth*, Howard Clinebell (1996), a pastoral counselor, published his own book, *Ecotherapy: Healing Ourselves, Healing the Earth*, in 1996. Clinebell envisioned ecotherapy as a practice that assumes that fostering the human-nature relationship can facilitate therapeutic change. Drawing on personal experience and incorporating ART, SRT, and the biophilia hypothesis, Clinebell believed that nature interactions improve mental health and emotional well-being. He encouraged therapists to incorporate nature-based activities into their practices (Clinebell 2013).

Nature-related modalities such as horticultural therapy, animal-assisted therapy, and wilderness therapy were well established by the 1990s. Although these therapies used nonhuman elements as tools to facilitate specific therapeutic goals, they did not directly examine the patient's relationship with nature (Nebbe 1995).

Having completed his doctoral studies at Columbia University and undergone psychotherapeutic training at the William Alanson White Institute in New York City, Clinebell brings a clinical perspective to nature's therapeutic potential. Ecotherapy posits that patients experience despair stemming from an unconscious desire to reconnect with the earth. The ecotherapist helps patients access their environmental conscience through psychodynamically informed counseling and nature-based activities. A key component of ecotherapy's treatment plan involves patients engaging in environmental activities to restore the earth, which aims to instill hope, foster a connection with nature, and provide a sense of purpose (Clinebell 2013).

Clinebell also included a spiritual aspect of the human-nature connection. He acknowledged that the transformative potential of the human-nature relationship that he described in westernized language had long been a part of the ancestral practice of many Indigenous peoples of the Americas. Although Clinebell valued spiritual wisdom, he recognized that the scientifically minded mental health professionals might be skeptical of nonvalidated methods. He cautioned readers that the evidence presented in his book was anecdotal and invited collaborators to conduct more thorough research to explore the salutary effects of nature on mental health (Clinebell 2013).

Enter the Twenty-First Century

In the decades since Roszak's call to action and Clinebell's invitation to research, a slew of writers, clinicians, and scientists have answered in kind. Research and publications on the intersection of nature and well-being have grown exponentially. A growing body of experimentally derived and statistically significant evidence has supported what ancestral knowledge had already supposed. Miyazaki's Shinrin-yoku (forest bathing) experiments demonstrated stress reduction in both physiological and psychological measures (Miyazaki et al. 2015). In 2004, the *American Journal of Public Health* published a study from the University of Illinois at Urbana-Champaign conducted by Frances E. Kuo and Andrea F. Taylor that suggested that activity in outdoor green spaces reduced ADHD symptoms (Kuo and Taylor 2004). The new wave of scientific inquiry did not focus on the psychodynamics of the nature experience but rather investigated various forms of nature exposure as potential treatments for a wide range of human ailments, from reducing cancer pain to modulating trauma responses in PTSD (Kuo and Taylor 2004; Miyazaki et al. 2015; Summers and Vivian 2018).

The spotlight on the benefits of contact with a healthy environment brought the consequences of environmental degradation into focus.

Limited access to high-quality green spaces in densely populated urban areas was found to disproportionately affect socioeconomically disadvantaged groups and people of color. A 2022 working paper from the National Bureau of Economic Research outlining a large-scale study from 2003 to 2010 reported that air pollution was an independent risk factor for suicide (Jennings et al. 2017; Persico and Marcotte 2022).

Technological advances in the twenty-first century brought more opportunities to disengage from the outdoors. The proliferation of personal electronic devices, diversification of online entertainment options, and widespread adoption of social media meant that people spent more time indoors glued to their screens than going outside. Richard Louv, an American writer and journalist, expressed concern about the potential effect on children growing up without regular exposure to nature. In his book *Last Child in the Woods: Saving Our Children From Nature-Deficit Disorder*, Louv (2008) synthesized research on the benefits of nature contact and warned of the opportunity cost for children who missed out. Louv (2008) advocated for a concerted effort by parents, educators, policymakers, and medical professionals to get children outside.

In 2010, when Louv presented his message as keynote speaker to the American Academy of Pediatrics, Robert Zarr, M.D., listened. Inspired to help patients and their families benefit from what nature could offer, Zarr partnered with the National Recreation and Park Association and the National Park Service in 2013 to develop ParkRx (or Park Prescription). ParkRx is a national coalition of clinicians, community health organizations, and park departments directed through the Institute at the Golden Gate. The coalition develops programs and educational resources promoting park activities as part of a healthy lifestyle. Physicians are encouraged to write literal nature prescriptions specifying the frequency and duration of activity to their patients (James et al. 2019). In 2022, the American Academy of Pediatrics published a press release outlining recommendations for parents to bring their children outside.

Nature prescriptions caught on internationally. Japanese doctors have been prescribing forest bathing since the 1980s, and New Zealand has had a Green Prescription program for outdoor activity since the 1990s. The nature prescription practice was picked up by South Korea, Finland, and Canada. In 2020, as part of its coronavirus disease 2019 (COVID-19) recovery plan, the U.K. government allocated £4 million ($5.2 million) to fund a 2-year green prescription pilot program (Broom 2022).

Nature prescriptions for children not only increased physical activity and psychological well-being but also fostered positive early interactions with nature. Louv echoed Roszak's concern that nature was imperiled by human indifference to ecological harmony. Louv argued that the antidote to the unabated destruction of the environment was to ensure that the coming generation was invested in its preservation. Louv's hunch is supported by a cross-sectional study from Universidade Estadual de Santa Cruz, which found that pro-environmental behavior in adults was associated with formative nature experiences during childhood (Fyfe-Johnson et al. 2021; Rosa et al. 2018).

Environmental health concerns extend beyond access to municipal parks. Breathable air, potable water, stable shelter, and nutritious food are the physiological basis of Maslow's hierarchy of needs and are inextricably linked to planetary environmental health. The COVID-19 pandemic, which claimed the lives of more than 6 million people between 2020 and 2023, highlights the extreme consequences of disregarding ecological interdependencies. Shrinking wildlife habitats and the black market bushmeat trade have led to increased conflict between wildlife and people. Endangered animal populations that are concentrated in certain areas can harbor zoonotic illnesses that can be transmitted to humans through contact with poachers who bring infected animals to market. Like HIV, Ebola, and severe acute respiratory syndrome before it, COVID-19 is believed to have a zoonotic origin. The tragic toll of the pandemic has spurred the international community to examine the systemic failures that enabled its spread (World Health Organization 2020).

In 2020, the World Health Organization (WHO) declared nature as the greatest source of health and well-being. The first item of their six-point manifesto for a healthy recovery from COVID-19 was to "[p]rotect and preserve the source of human health: nature" (World Health Organization 2020, p. 4).

This declaration lent institutional weight to Clinebell's hypothesis that people who participate in preservation of the environment are also contributing to their own health and well-being.

The scope of nature therapy is as vast and diverse as nature itself. It can be practiced through formal sessions or integrated into daily life as spontaneous activities. Nature therapy encompasses cognitive exercises that reduce stress and restore attention through sensory exploration of natural elements. Some may practice nature therapy as a means of ensuring a sustainable future for nature, allowing future generations to derive their own benefits. The WHO declaration acknowledges the importance of nature to human health and well-being, but it does not guarantee the execution of conservation plans. The future of nature depends on motivated people who understand the significance of preserving nature and advocate for its protection. As Dr. Seuss's (1971, p. 58) mythical Lorax once said, "Unless someone like you cares a whole awful lot, nothing is going to get better. It's not."

LIMITATIONS

Although a growing body of evidence supports the psychological benefits of nature-based interventions, limitations to the evidence prevent nature therapy's adoption into conventional medical practice.

One limitation is the high amount of variability in the methods of nature delivery, which makes direct comparisons between studies nearly impossible. Additionally, most studies on nature therapy are cross-sectional, survey based, or case control in design. Although these types of studies are useful in generating hypotheses and identifying potential associations, they cannot definitively prove causation by nature therapy for improved health outcomes.

A few cohort studies have been done on nature therapy, but they have limited statistical power because of the small number of participants. Randomized controlled trials (RCTs) are the gold standard of evidence-based treatments. RCTs can compare experimental treatments, such as nature therapy, with care as usual to assess for comparative efficacy. To date, one RCT has investigated the application of nature therapy for a psychiatric condition.

Researchers from the University of Copenhagen, Denmark, compared nature-based therapy with a specialized form of cognitive-behavioral therapy (CBT). Inclusion criteria required patients to have a functionally impairing diagnosis of adjustment disorder or acute stress reaction. The primary outcome was the mean aggregate score on the Psychological General Well-Being Index. The study found no statistically significant differences between the treatment groups. Several drawbacks to the study design may have affected the results. As with the cohort studies, the number of participants was low, with 39 randomly assigned to the nature-based therapy group and 37 to the CBT group. Additionally, bias may have been introduced by the inability to blind participants to the type of therapy they were receiving. Nature-based therapy involved 3 hours of therapy per session with three different therapists, and CBT involved 1 hour of therapy per session with one therapist (Stigsdotter et al. 2018).

Another limitation of the evidence base for nature therapy is that many studies use measures of "wellness" rather than clinical psychiatric symptom scales. This validation measure probably reflects the choice to study how nature affects mental well-being in a generally healthy population rather than treating a diagnosed psychiatric disorder.

Although measures of wellness can provide valuable insights into the subjective experiences of participants, their results may not be generalizable to improvements in psychiatric illness. Nature's effects on patients, much like psychiatric symptoms, are phenomenological, meaning that they are based on subjective experiences and perceptions. Review papers and meta-analyses examining the available literature suggest that although observational studies indicate a small to moderate effect size, more powerful and rigorous studies using standardized clinical psychiatric symptom scales are needed to assess nature therapy's applicability to psychiatric treatment (Annerstedt and Währborg 2011; Bonham-Corcoran et al. 2022).

Clinical research on nature therapy is conspicuously absent from psychiatric literature, with most articles on the subject appearing in journals of environmental psychology, landscape and architectural design, and tourism. Although researching novel therapeutic modalities is not explicitly discouraged in psychiatry, receiving support for such experiments can be difficult. Large-scale clinical trials are funded by private industry, which expects a return on investment. Pharmaceutical companies can patent and market their medications, but no equivalent market incentive is available to promote greater use of nature, which is freely available to the public.

Not-for-profit research, such as in academics, often relies on obtaining grants, primarily through the National Institutes of Health. However, the grant approval process is highly competitive, with only a 20% approval rate. Grants are more likely to be awarded to proposals that conform to currently trending topics of interest rather than unconventional or unproven hypotheses.

Academic psychiatrists also may feel pressure to rapidly produce a high volume of publications for professional advancement, which can be easier to accomplish by continuing work in an established line of research rather than constructing a new experimental paradigm from scratch (Lilienfeld 2017).

At the time of this writing, one large 5-year RCT is underway through Kaiser Permanente investigating health outcomes of the ParkRx nature prescription program. The study is expected to be completed by 2025. More RCTs with larger sample sizes and standardized measures of psychiatric symptoms are needed to definitively establish the efficacy of nature therapy and identify which populations and conditions are most likely to benefit from this approach (Zarr et al. 2022).

GUIDELINES

Even without the backing of large-scale, double-blind RCTs, the available evidence suggests that nature has a positive effect on overall well-being. The following chapters discuss a variety of therapeutic nature interactions that vary in breadth, intensity, and scale. Although there is some overlap, the various nature therapies each carry their own sets of risks and benefits. Nature therapies are typically nonpharmaceutical, noninvasive, and highly customizable to meet individual patient needs.

Identifying patients who could benefit from nature therapy and selecting the best approach to recommend relies on various patient factors, such as their attitudes toward nature, mobility level, and access to nature. Physicians can perform a comprehensive nature history as part of the biopsychosocial evaluation to determine these factors. The following suggested questions can investigate the patient's relationship with nature.

- How would you describe your relationship with nature?
- How much time do you spend inside?
- When inside, how often are you near an uncovered window? What is the view from the window?
- Are there any images of nature (pictures, paintings, or posters) in your indoor areas?
- Are there any plants or animals in your indoor areas?
- What sounds, sights, and smells are most common in your indoor areas?
- Are there any nearby public natural settings such as parks or gardens that you feel comfortable visiting?
- What are your preferred types of natural environments?
- Do you engage in any outdoor activities, such as hiking or gardening?
- Are there any specific natural environments that you find particularly calming or rejuvenating?
- Have you ever experienced any positive or negative emotional responses to nature?
- How do you typically feel after spending time in nature?
- Have you ever used nature as a coping mechanism during a difficult time in your life?
- Do you have any concerns or barriers that prevent you from spending time in nature?
- How accessible is nature for you? Do you have transportation or mobility issues that may affect your ability to access natural environments?
- Do you have any physical limitations that may affect your ability to participate in nature therapy activities?
- Do you feel comfortable spending time in nature alone, or do you prefer to be with others?
- Have you ever had a negative experience in nature? If so, can you describe it?

- Have you ever tried any nature-based therapies before? If so, what was your experience like?
- Is there anything else you would like to share about your relationship with nature?

KEY POINTS

- Nature is an umbrella term that describes Earth's environment, geology, and inhabitants, including people, and the forces that govern their interactions.

- Experiences in nature have been valued for their profound spiritual and emotional effect across cultures since the earliest recorded history.

- Parallel revolutions in psychiatric medicine and environmentalism converged in the late twentieth century to inspire scientific examination of nature's phenomenology.

- A growing body of observational and correlational studies suggest significant mental health implications of nature interactions, but higher-powered and more specific clinical trials are needed to test applicability to clinical populations.

- Nature is a finite resource vulnerable to depletion by human activity. Measures for nature conservation can be incentivized by recognizing the long-term benefits at both the individual and the population levels.

QUESTIONS

1. Which of the following activities most aligns with Clinebell's principles of ecotherapy?

    A. A family trip to the zoo.
    B. Watching birds through the window.
    C. Sunbathing at the beach.
    D. Buying flowers.
    E. Planting a tree.

Correct answer: E. Planting a tree.

Clinebell's ecotherapy emphasizes a reciprocal relationship between people and nature. Of the available options, planting a tree is the only activity that involves participating in environmental conservation or restoration.

2. After reading Rachel Carson's *Silent Spring*, a gardener continues to spray insecticides on their crops. Which theory considers this activity a pathological response?

   A. Maslow's hierarchy of needs.
   B. Humboldt's Naturgemälde.
   C. Roszak's ecopsychology.
   D. Wilson's biophilia hypothesis.
   E. Bowlby and Ainsworth's attachment theory.

Correct answer: C. Roszak's ecopsychology.

The gardener continues using toxic pesticides even after reading about how they harm people and the environment in *Silent Spring*. Ecopsychology sees environmental destruction as counter to human interest and survival and reflects a self-destructive societal psychopathology. Maslow's hierarchy of needs (A) is a theory of human motivation. Humboldt's Naturgemälde (B) recognizes the interconnectedness of the planetary ecology. Wilson's biophilia hypothesis (D) theorizes that people evolved to be interested in other living organisms. Bowlby and Ainsworth's attachment theory (E) describes the infant-parent bond.

3. According to the World Health Organization manifesto on global recovery from the coronavirus disease 2019 (COVID-19) pandemic, what is the most important source of human health?

   A. Nature.
   B. Pharmaceuticals.
   C. Clean air and water.
   D. Medical education.
   E. Nutrition.

Correct answer: A. Nature.

In 2020, the World Health Organization declared nature as the greatest source of health and well-being. The first item of their six-point manifesto for a healthy recovery from COVID-19 was to "[p]rotect and preserve the source of human health: nature" (World Health Organization 2020, p. 4).

REFERENCES

American Academy of Pediatrics: AAP offers tips for keeping kids active, healthy through outdoor play. May 11, 2022. Available at: https://www.aap.org/en/news-room/news-releases/health--safety-tips/aap-offers-tips-for-keeping-kids-active-healthy-through-outdoor-play. Accessed March 31, 2024.

American Psychiatric Association: Diagnostic and Statistical Manual: Mental Disorders. Washington, DC, American Psychiatric Association, 1952

Annerstedt M, Währborg P: Nature-assisted therapy: systematic review of controlled and observational studies. Scand J Public Health 39(4):371–388, 2011 21273226

Aretoulakis E: Towards a posthumanist ecology: nature without humanity in Wordsworth and Shelley. European Journal of English Studies 18(2):172–190, 2014

Berger R: Developing an ethical code for the growing nature therapy profession. Australian Journal of Outdoor Education 12(2):47–52, 2008. Available at: https://go.gale.com/ps/i.do?id=GALE%7CA191189517&sid=googleScholar&v=2.1&it=r&linkaccess=abs&issn=13241486&p=AONE&sw=w&userGroupName=nysl_oweb&isGeoAuthType=true&aty=geo. Accessed March 29, 2024.

Berger EM: The Chernobyl disaster, concern about the environment, and life satisfaction. Kyklos 63:1–8, 2010

Bonham-Corcoran M, Armstrong A, O'Briain A, et al: The benefits of nature-based therapy for the individual and the environment: an integrative review. Irish Journal of Occupational Therapy 50(1):16–27, 2022

Borrell-Carrió F, Suchman AL, Epstein RM: The biopsychosocial model 25 years later: principles, practice, and scientific inquiry. Ann Fam Med 2(6):576–582, 2004 15576544

Bratman GN, Anderson CB, Berman MG, et al: Nature and mental health: an ecosystem service perspective. Sci Adv 5(7):eaax0903, 2019

Broom D: Health: what are green prescriptions and which countries offer them? World Economic Forum, February 21, 2022. Available at: https://www.weforum.org/agenda/2022/02/green-prescriptions-health-wellbeing. Accessed March 31, 2024.

Carson R: Silent Spring. Boston, MA, Houghton Mifflin, 1962

Clinebell H: Ecotherapy: Healing Ourselves, Healing the Earth. New York, Haworth, 1996

Clinebell H: Ecotherapy: Healing Ourselves, Healing the Earth. London, Taylor & Francis, 2013

Cosgrove L, Vaswani A: The influence of pharmaceutical companies and restoring integrity to psychiatric research and practice, in Critical Psychiatry. Edited by Steingard S. Cham, Switzerland, Springer, 2019, pp 71–96

Davis JE: The Bald Eagle: The Improbable Journey of America's Bird. New York, Liveright, 2022

Derschied LA: The What and Who of the CCC. South Dakota CCC Museum, January 13, 2016. Available at: https://southdakotaccc.org/post.php?read-about=what-and-who. Accessed March 31, 2024.

Dettelbach M: Alexander von Humboldt between Enlightenment and Romanticism. Northeastern Naturalist 8:9–20, 2001. Available at: http://www.jstor.org/stable/4130723. Accessed March 31, 2024.

Dowling AS: George Engel, M.D. (1913–1999). Am J Psychiatry 162(11):2039, 2005 16263840

Dr. Seuss: The Lorax. New York, Random House, 1971

Engel GL: The need for a new medical model: a challenge for biomedicine. Science 196(4286):129–136, 1977 847460

Frank A: The Diary of a Young Girl: Anne Frank. Edited by Pressler M. New York, Bantam Books, 1997

Fyfe-Johnson AL, Hazlehurst MF, Perrins SP, et al: Nature and children's health: a systematic review. Pediatrics 148(4):e2020049155, 2021 34588297

Gillotti FJ: An experience in nature therapy, in The Science Counselor. Pittsburgh, PA, Duquesne University Press, June 1, 1953. Available at: https://archive.org/details/sim_duquesne-science-counselor-for-better-science-training_1953-06_16_2/page/n1/mode/2up. Accessed March 29, 2024.

Harrington A: Mind Fixers: Psychiatry's Troubled Search for the Biology of Mental Illness. New York, WW Norton, 2019

Horowitz FD: John B. Watson's legacy: learning and environment. Dev Psychol 28(3):360–367, 1992

James JJ, Christiana RW, Battista RA: A historical and critical analysis of park prescriptions. J Leisure Res 50(4):311–329, 2019

Jennings V, Floyd MF, Shanahan D, et al: Emerging issues in urban ecology: implications for research, social justice, human health, and well-being. Popul Environ 39:69–86, 2017

Jordan M: Nature and self—an ambivalent attachment? Ecopsychology 1(1):26–31, 2009

Jung CG: The Earth Has a Soul: CG Jung on Nature, Technology and Modern Life. Berkeley, CA, North Atlantic, 2002

Kaplan R, Kaplan S: The Experience of Nature: A Psychological Perspective. Cambridge, UK, Cambridge University Press, 1989

Karter JM, Kamens SR: Toward conceptual competence in psychiatric diagnosis: an ecological model for critiques of the DSM, in Critical Psychiatry. Edited by Steingard S. Cham, Switzerland, Springer, 2019, pp 17–69

Kittredge FA: Yosemite during the war years. Yosemite Nature Notes 25(5):73–77, 1946

Kuo FE, Taylor AF: A potential natural treatment for attention-deficit/hyperactivity disorder: evidence from a national study. Am J Public Health 94(9):1580–1586, 2004 15333318

Lertzman R: Ecopsychological theory and critical intervention: review of ecopsychological theory and critical intervention. Organ Environ 17(3):396–401, 2004

Lilienfeld SO: Psychology's replication crisis and the grant culture: righting the ship. Perspect Psychol Sci 12(4):660–664, 2017 28727961

Louv R: Last Child in the Woods: Saving Our Children From Nature-Deficit Disorder. Chapel Hill, NC, Algonquin, 2008

Maher NM: Nature's New Deal: The Civilian Conservation Corps and the Roots of the American Environmental Movement. New York, Oxford University Press, 2008

Marks S: Psychotherapy in historical perspective. Hist Human Sci 30(2):3–16, 2017 28690369

Maslow AH: A theory of human motivation. Psychol Rev 50(4):370–396, 1943

Miyazaki Y, Song C, Ikei H: Preventive medical effects of nature therapy and their individual differences. Jpn J Physiol Anthropol 20:19–32, 2015

Nebbe LL: Nature as a Guide: Nature in Counseling, Therapy, and Education. Franklin, TN, Educational Media, 1995

Persico C, Marcotte DE: Air Quality and Suicide (No w30626). Cambridge, MA, National Bureau of Economic Research, 2022

Prince D: Report on orthopedic surgery for the Annual Meeting of the Illinois State Medical Society, held in Bloomington, May 2, 1865. Chic Med Exam (1860–1871) 6(8):449, 1865

Robinson HA: Nature and the New Deal. Comm Law League J 39:184, 1934

Rosa CD, Profice CC, Collado S: Nature experiences and adults' self-reported pro-environmental behaviors: the role of connectedness to nature and childhood nature experiences. Front Psychol 9:1055, 2018 30013494

Roszak T: The Voice of the Earth. New York, Simon & Schuster, 1992

Song C, Ikei H, Miyazaki Y: Physiological effects of nature therapy: a review of the research in Japan. Int J Environ Res Public Health 13(8):781, 2016 27527193

Stigsdotter UK, Corazon SS, Sidenius U, et al: Efficacy of nature-based therapy for individuals with stress-related illnesses: randomised controlled trial. Br J Psychiatry 213(1):404–411, 2018 29793588

Summers JK, Vivian DN: Ecotherapy—a forgotten ecosystem service: a review. Front Psychol 9:1389, 2018 30123275

Sundstrom E, Bell PA, Busby PL, et al: Environmental psychology 1989–1994. Annu Rev Psychol 47(1):485–512, 1996 8624141

Ulrich CF: Physiatrics, or nature's therapy. JAMA 31(27):1553–1556, 1898

Ulrich RS: Natural versus urban scenes: some psychophysiological effects. Environ Behav 13(5):523–556, 1981

Watkins T: The Neolithic revolution and the emergence of humanity: a cognitive approach to the first comprehensive world-view, in Archaeological Perspectives on the Transmission and Transformation of Culture in the Eastern Mediterranean. Edited by Clarke J. Oxford, UK, Oxbow, 2005, pp 84–88

Weir K: Nurtured by nature. Monitor on Psychology 51(3):50, 2020. Available at: https://www.apa.org/monitor/2020/04/nurtured-nature. Accessed March 31, 2024.

Wilson EO: Biophilia. Cambridge, MA, Harvard University Press, 1984

World Health Organization: WHO Manifesto for a healthy recovery from COVID-19: prescriptions for a healthy and green recovery from COVID-19. World Health Organization, May 26, 2020. Available at: https://www.who.int/news-room/feature-stories/detail/who-manifesto-for-a-healthy-recovery-from-covid-19. Accessed August 13, 2022.

Wulf A: The Invention of Nature: The Adventures of Alexander von Humboldt, the Lost Hero of Science. London, John Murray, 2015

Yosemite National Park: History of the United States Naval Special Hospital. Yosemite, CA, Yosemite Park and Curry Company, 1946

Zarr R, Han B, Estrada E, et al: The Park Rx trial to increase physical activity among low-income youth. Contemp Clin Trials 122:106930, 2022 36184966

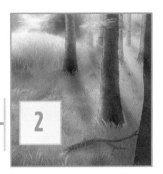

Theoretical Framework

THE MECHANISMS UNDERLYING NATURE THERAPY

Eugenia Frances Kronenberg, Sc.B.
Andrew M. Fukuda, M.D., Ph.D.

Just living is not enough.
One must have sunshine, freedom, and a little flower.
—Hans Christian Andersen, author of *Hans Andersen's Fairy Tales*
(Andersen et al. 1916)

In this chapter, we address some hypothesized theories for why nature therapy (i.e., interaction with nature as a method to improve well-being) is effective from a neurobiological, physiological, and psychosocial perspective. We define *nature* as a broad category as defined by Bratman et al. (2019) in Chapter 1, "The Wise Outdoors."

For example, a garden falls under this definition of nature, even though a human is usually responsible for growing and caring for this piece of nature. By contrast, geological formations such as cliffs, waterfalls, and canyons created with little human influence also fall under this definition of nature. More examples of nature include biodiversity, wilderness, weather, parks, oceans, lakes, and rivers. Human-made structures lacking natural elements, "indoors," and urban environments fall outside our definition of nature. Interaction with nature in the context of nature therapy is a mindful experience with nature through any mode of human perception (i.e., some combination of visual, auditory, olfactory, and somatosensory experience).

Interaction with nature has long been recognized as an important aspect of our well-being. Roszak et al. (1995) developed the ecopsychology theory, the idea that our outer world influences our internal world. Thus, they argued that the concept of nature therapy inevitably follows because just as some environments may be detrimental to our internal state, some environments may be healing (Louv 2005).

Correlational evidence consistently shows the benefits of living in environments with more nature available and the detriments of living in urban environments. Urban populations experience significantly more mental illness, including mood disorders, anxiety disorders, and schizophrenia, compared with rural populations, even when confounding variables are controlled for (Maas et al. 2009; Nutsford et al. 2013; Peen et al. 2010). A positive relationship is also seen between time growing up in an urban environment and risk of developing schizophrenia, suggesting that increasing exposure to nature in childhood may reduce the risk of developing schizophrenia later in life (Engemann et al. 2018; Pedersen and Mortensen 2001). A study of 400,000 U.K. residents reported that those who spent more hours in outdoor light had lower chances of lifetime major depressive disorder or antidepressant use; lower chances of reporting anhedonia, low mood, neuroticism, and sleep problems; and greater reported happiness, after correction for demographic factors, lifestyle, and employment status (Burns et al. 2021). Thus, access to green space and outdoor light may mediate the mental health risks associated with living in an urban environment (Beyer et al. 2014; Nutsford et al. 2013). Beyond the psychiatric context, the prevalence of and mortality from many illnesses are negatively correlated with access to nearby nature (Kuo 2015). For example, those with more access to nature have a lower prevalence of acute urinary tract infections (Maas et al. 2009). Evidence indicates that those with more nature in their residential areas have a lower prevalence of allergies and asthma, although results are mixed (Fuertes et al. 2014; Hanski et al. 2012; Kuo 2015; Lovasi et al. 2008; Maas et al. 2009). Surrounding nature also may influence birth outcomes, being positively associated with higher birth weights (Markevych et al. 2014). Those living in rural areas or areas with more surrounding nature also have lower blood pressure and lower prevalence of and mortality from cardiovascular disease (Maas et al. 2009; Mitchell and Popham 2008; Pereira et al. 2012; Tamosiunas et al. 2014; Villeneuve et al. 2012). Both type 1 and type 2 diabetes mellitus are less prevalent in those living near more nature (Astell-Burt et al. 2014; Maas et al. 2009). A study examining U.S. residents found that those living near more forests, pastures, and water had higher overall life expectancies, even when confounding variables were controlled for (Poudyal et al. 2009).

Although this correlational evidence is useful in establishing the positive relationship between exposure to nature and well-being, the bulk of this chapter explores the experimental psychological, physiological, and neurobiological evidence supporting the potential cause-and-effect relationships and some of the theoretical frameworks behind nature's positive effects on human health.

ATTENTION RESTORATION THEORY

One major theory that attempts to explain the mechanism by which nature improves well-being, especially psychological well-being, was developed by a couple (Rachel and Stephen Kaplan) in the 1980s. Attention restoration theory (ART) posits that interaction with nature restores a resource called *directed/voluntary attention*. This resource is limited and thought to be depleted by attentionally demanding tasks. Nature therapy replenishes this resource through the activation of a more primitive, less conscious type of attention. Neurological evidence indicates a distinction between these two types of attention, with directed attention being a top-down attentional process and unconscious attention being a bottom-up attentional process (Fan et al. 2005). ART hypothesizes that nature scenes capture bottom-up attention automatically through four separate features—being away, extent, soft fascination, and compatibility—that allow the directed attention resource to recover (Kaplan and Kaplan 1989).

1. *Being away* describes a combination of the feeling of being physically distanced from daily life and the feeling of being mentally distanced from daily responsibilities. Thus, the idea of being away assumes that

one's daily life is not immersed in nature. Given the extent of urbanization today, this assumption is reasonable for most U.S. residents.

2. *Extent* describes the content of a landscape such that the scope and connectedness of the landscape may provide sufficient and pleasing stimuli to occupy one's mind.

3. *Soft fascination*, designated by the Kaplans as the most important of the four features, describes the involuntary attentional draw to the landscape and is the main mechanism by which directed attention is restored.

4. *Compatibility* refers to whether the types of interactions a person can have with a landscape are accessible and meaningful given the person's needs and the landscape's needs. As an example, someone who has difficulty walking would find the most compatible landscapes those that they can view and interact with while seated, such as bird-watching from an outdoor deck (Herzog et al. 2003; Kaplan and Kaplan 1989).

Directed attention as described by the Kaplans has been associated with activation of the prefrontal cortex and assessed by tasks of working memory and executive function. Working memory tasks test our ability to hold and manipulate information in our mind. A comprehensive systematic review of 31 studies that examined the effect of being in a natural versus a nonnatural environment on attention tasks showed that the Digit Span Forward, Digit Span Backward, and Trail Making Test B resulted in significant and consistent improvement after interaction with nature relative to interaction with an urban environment (Ohly et al. 2016). Another meta-analysis expanded on the previous results and examined the effects of interacting with nature across eight cognitive domains while also controlling for baseline differences between groups and found that interaction with nature improved performance across three cognitive domains: working memory, attentional control, and cognitive flexibility (Stevenson et al. 2018). Furthermore, working memory tasks showed significantly more improvement in studies that tested subjects who were attentionally fatigued (as a result of either pretest activities that drained mental energy or a diagnosis that impairs attention such as ADHD). In a randomized study of women with recent diagnoses of breast cancer, women who were randomly assigned to the group incorporating at least 2 hours of nature activities per week performed significantly better on cognitive tasks than did the nonintervention group (Cimprich and Ronis 2003).

The studies included in Ohly et al. (2016) and Stevenson et al. (2018) had some limitations, such as the fact that most of these studies cannot blind subjects to the environment. Nevertheless, the fact that the improvements in these tasks after exposure to nature were consistent, even across different studies and different experimental conditions, suggests that interaction with nature has a positive effect on attention and executive function in a way that interaction with urban environments does not.

Correlational evidence in both children and adults corroborates ART. Girls who lived in an apartment that looked at a more natural view performed significantly better on self-discipline tasks, such as a delayed gratification task, than girls whose apartment looked over a less natural view (Faber Taylor et al. 2002). The same result was not found in boys, but Faber Taylor et al. (2001, 2002) explained this discrepancy by citing evidence that boys typically play farther from home, and boys' attentional function is possibly related to the amount of nature in their play space rather than the amount of nature directly around the home. Children who moved to areas with more nature around had better attentional function than those who moved to areas with less nature around (Wells 2000). Faber Taylor et al. (2001) also found that children with attention-deficit disorder (as it was characterized by DSM-IV in 2001; American Psychiatric Association 1994) had reduced symptoms after activities in green space, as reported by parents (Faber Taylor et al. 2001). Kuo (2001) studied 145 inner-city public housing residents who were randomly assigned to apartments. They found that those assigned to buildings with more nearby nature reported less procrastination and believed that their personal challenges were less severe compared with those assigned to buildings with less nature nearby. Levels of violence and aggression were lower in residential areas with more green space available (Kuo and Sullivan 2001). Those who were attentionally fatigued before nature exposure had lower levels of provoked aggression after exposure to nature (Wang et al. 2018), and participants reported less anger and aggression during nature exposure relative to urban exposure (Oh et al. 2017; Ulrich et al. 1991).

In addition, some physiological benefits of time spent in nature may be indirectly improved by restored directed attention. For example, executive function is inversely correlated with impulsivity, propensity for risky behaviors, and "unhealthy" habits such as snacking on sugary foods (Dohle et al. 2018; Reynolds et al. 2019). Improved eating habits could explain the lower risk of obesity, type 2 diabetes mellitus, and cardiovascular disease seen in those who spend more time in nature (Aljadani et al. 2015; Pan et al. 2018; Sami et al. 2017). In fact, evidence suggests that more interaction with nature is associated with a better diet (Milliron et al. 2022). However, many of the physiological benefits, such as improved immune function, may not be fully explained by this theory.

STRESS REDUCTION THEORY

Alongside ART, Roger Ulrich, a prolific researcher, developed a similar but distinct theory named stress reduction theory (SRT). SRT is based on the idea that humans are biologically predisposed to interpret natural scenes, given the fact that the great majority of our ancestral evolution has occurred in a natural environment (Ulrich 1983; Ulrich et al. 1991). However, contrary to ART's description of the restorative aspect of nature as a result of its properties that capture a "soft fascination," Ulrich noted that many natural environments capture involuntary attention without being restorative. For example, a snake image will pull your attention toward it; however, this situation may not elicit the sense of relief and awe suggested by ART. Instead, SRT suggests that only natural scenes that humans interpret as biologically fit, such as scenes with an open green field and flowing water, are restorative. The theory suggests that we are biologically predisposed to feel calmer and happier in response to a scene that contains elements that we once needed to survive.

Furthermore, the theory posits that we respond positively to these natural scenes because they elicit positive emotions and reduce arousal. Specifically, they increase parasympathetic activity and decrease sympathetic activity. Thus, in the process of spending time in nature, we can reduce the negative effects of stress and hyperarousal.

Ulrich et al. (1991) found that participants watching nature videos had lower systolic blood pressure, lower skin conductance, and less tension in the frontalis muscle than those watching a video of an urban environment. Participants in the nature video group also endorsed less anger and aggression, less fear, and greater positive affect compared with the urban video group. Richardson et al. (2016) conducted a meta-analysis across 13 studies and 871 participants comparing heart rate variability (HRV) data in response to nature exposure versus urban exposure. Increased high-frequency power HRV is associated with increased parasympathetic activity, and low-frequency power HRV is associated with sympathetic activity. High total HRV is associated with balanced sympathetic-parasympathetic activity, whereas low total HRV is associated with unbalanced autonomic activity and worse health outcomes (Carney et al. 2005; Thayer et al. 2010). This meta-analysis found that exposure to natural environments significantly increased parasympathetic activity, with a medium effect size, and significantly decreased sympathetic activity, with a small effect size, when compared with exposure to urban environments. The investigators suggested that the small effect size in the sympathetic response may be due to some feeling higher arousal emotions with a positive valence in response to nature, which would activate the sympathetic nervous system in conjunction with a feeling such as excitement. These results suggest that nature does have a significant effect on our autonomic responses, and this autonomic regulation may in turn regulate our stress response.

Functional MRI studies have shown some support for the idea that a natural environment supports stress regulation. Researchers found that healthy participants had reduced amygdala activity (fear and anxiety in response to threats) after a nature walk, but not after a walk in an urban environment, when presented with stress-inducing tasks including the Fearful Faces Task and the Montreal Imaging Stress Task (Sudimac et al. 2022). Those currently living in an urban environment had more amygdala activity than those living in a more natural environment when presented with stress-inducing tasks (Lederbogen et al. 2011). These investigators also found that those who were raised in an urban environment had more activity in the perigenual anterior cingulate, a region of the brain highly associated with the amygdala, during the stress-inducing task.

Some studies suggest that nature therapy, even something as minimal as sitting in front of a window view of nature, may play a role in stress regulation. Surgery and major diagnoses can lead to acute and chronic stress. In one study, Ulrich (1984) found that simply being in a hospital room with a window view of nature (compared with a view of a building) improved recovery rates after cholecystectomy surgery, as evidenced by shorter hospital stays, fewer prescribed potent analgesics, and fewer negative evaluations in medical record notes. Another study found that lack of exposure to natural light at the workplace was associated with higher cortisol levels at night, higher melatonin levels in the morning, and lower melatonin levels at night. The higher cortisol levels were associated with depressive symptoms, and lower melatonin levels at night were associated with insomnia symptoms (Harb et al. 2015).

Oh et al. (2017) conducted a systematic review examining the health benefits of forest therapy through six randomized trials. Two studies examined blood pressure and found that blood pressure decreased significantly during forest exposure compared with urban exposure. In one of the studies, they also found that forest exposure decreased levels of hypertension biomarkers, including endothelin-1, homocysteine, angiotensinogen, and angiotensin. One of the studies examining cortisol levels found lower serum cortisol levels after forest exposure compared with urban exposure. Evidence also showed that mood improves as a result of forest exposure compared with a control. Three studies found significantly improved results on questionnaires examining anger and hostility, tension and anxiety, depression, fatigue, and confusion after forest therapy. In a small (N=12) randomized study examining the effects of forest therapy, those who spent time in a forest had significantly less prefrontal cortical activity as measured by blood flow. They also had lower salivary cortisol levels (an indicator of current stress level) compared with those who spent time in the city (Park et al. 2007). In a study of 115 adults randomly assigned to a nature walk group or an urban walk group, Hartig et al. (2003) found lower systolic blood pressure during a nature walk than during an urban walk. They also found that self-reported positive affect increased and anger decreased as a result of the nature walk relative to the urban walk.

Based on the extensive literature, interaction with nature has a clear effect on our stress levels. Chronic stress has been implicated in multiple illnesses such as cardiovascular disease, obesity, type 2 diabetes mellitus, and major depressive disorder (Chu and Chu 2021; Hammen et al. 2009; Matheson et al. 2006; Sharma and Singh 2020; Steptoe and Kivimaki 2012). Thus, nature's ability to reduce stress has far-reaching health benefits that probably play a role in the lower prevalence of and mortality from diseases in those with more access to nature.

ADDITIONAL THEORIES

Some researchers have suggested other theories explaining the mechanism behind nature's health benefits. Kuo (2015) theorized that the most likely "central pathway" behind nature therapy is nature's regulation of the immune system. The benefits of time in nature affect a wide array of bodily systems beyond our brains. For example, greener residential areas do not consistently predict increased physical activity (Lachowycz and Jones 2011); however, they do consistently predict lower rates of obesity (Bell et al. 2008; Huang et al. 2020; Liu et al. 2007). More time in nature has also been associated with fewer acute urinary tract infections, improved birth outcomes, fewer musculoskeletal complaints, lower risk of diabetes mellitus, and lower risk of cardiovascular disease (Kuo 2015; Maas et al. 2009). In an experimental study, blood tests after a walk in nature showed higher dehydroepiandrosterone (DHEA), adiponectin, and natural killer cell levels relative to a walk in an urban environment (Kuo 2015; Li et al. 2011). Serum DHEA levels decrease with age; lower levels of DHEA are associated with chronic disease in men, such as coronary artery disease, and chronic smoking decreases levels of DHEA (Bjornerem et al. 2004). Thus, higher levels of

DHEA correlate with better health. Higher levels of adiponectin are associated with a lower risk of coronary artery disease, type 2 diabetes mellitus, and dyslipidemia as well as reduced inflammatory markers (Hotta et al. 2000; Lara-Castro et al. 2006; Simpson and Singh 2008; Vilarrasa et al. 2005). Natural killer cells are involved in fighting viral infections and cancer and are thus integral to immune function (Kuo 2015; Orange and Ballas 2006). In addition, higher cytotoxic activity of natural killer cells has been associated with about 40% lower incidence of cancer (Imai et al. 2000; Kuo 2015). A forest walk has also been shown to lower inflammatory cytokines relative to an urban walk (Kuo 2015; Mao et al. 2012). Inflammatory cytokines have been implicated in a wide array of chronic illnesses, such as depression, diabetes, and cardiovascular disease (Cesari et al. 2003; Dowlati et al. 2010; Kuo 2015; Wellen and Hotamisligil 2005). In the systematic review by Oh et al. (2017), four studies reported improved immune function after forest therapy relative to control subjects. Results indicated decreased perforin and granzyme B, two markers associated with worsening chronic obstructive pulmonary disease, after 1 day in the forest but not after 1 day in an urban environment. Another study in those with chronic obstructive pulmonary disease found that the proinflammatory cytokines interferon gamma, interleukin-6, interleukin-8, and interleukin-1β were significantly lower after forest exposure but not after urban exposure. A study in patients with essential hypertension also found decreased interleukin-6 after forest exposure but not after urban exposure. Three studies found that C-reactive protein was significantly lower after forest exposure but not after urban exposure. Thus, considerable evidence indicates that the immune system is significantly improved by exposure to nature, even after as little as 1 day.

Similarities are also found between the neurological effects of nature therapy and those of mindfulness, suggesting that they may be effective for similar reasons. For example, Bratman et al. (2015) found that a nature walk reduces rumination and activity in the subgenual prefrontal cortex, as measured by arterial spin labeling MRI to monitor cerebral blood flow, whereas a walk in an urban environment does not. Subgenual prefrontal cortex activity has been associated with rumination and self-referential thought linked to depression (Berman et al. 2011). The ventral medial prefrontal cortex, a region that contains the subgenual prefrontal cortex, also has been shown to be active during self-referential thought (Frith and Frith 2003; Gusnard and Raichle 2001; Northoff and Bermpohl 2004). Similarly, medial prefrontal cortex activity has been shown to be lower in experienced meditators (Brewer et al. 2011; Farb et al. 2007; Hasenkamp and Barsalou 2012).

Clinical Translation: Case Example

Mr. G, a 43-year-old man, has a long history of recurrent major depressive disorder and opioid use disorder. He rents a room at a boarding house in a large city and works in retail. He is in treatment at an academic outpatient clinic, where his psychiatrist provides weekly therapy and medication management. Despite trials of multiple antidepressant medications, including escitalopram, venlafaxine, and one treatment of intranasal ketamine, he remains symptomatic. His current medications are sertraline and buprenorphine/naltrexone for his opioid use disorder. Although he reports some response to the sertraline, he continues to report distressing symptoms, including chronic dysphoric mood, insomnia, and poor appetite. His symptom progress is tracked periodically through the Montgomery-Åsberg Depression Rating Scale.

Although he works a steady job, he reports living paycheck to paycheck and is unhappy with his living situation. He is on edge in his boarding room because of the confined space and lack of privacy. He often feels overwhelmed and struggles to maintain motivation, so he is worried that he will lose his job, become homeless, and relapse on heroin. As part of a supportive framework, the therapist and Mr. G strategize how to find a designated space that is comfortable and allows relaxation. The therapist explores Mr. G's attitude toward nature and the outdoors. Mr. G identifies a park in his neighborhood that he has often walked past on his way to work but has never gone into. He is open to making an effort to enter the park and practice breathing relaxation exercises.

He returns the next week with a positive account of his park experience. He remarks feeling surprised by how much he enjoyed his visit and regrets that he "missed out" by not visiting the park sooner. Although he did not practice the breathing techniques, he sat on a bench and felt his body decompress. He comments on the tranquil aesthetics of the foliage, the sounds of rustling leaves, and the sense of escape from the urban landscape just beyond the park boundary. He returned several times that week, sat for 1–2 hours, and felt refreshed when he left.

Mr. G continued his regular park visits over the next several months. Although his job and living situation have not changed, he feels better able to think beyond his immediate stressors. His Montgomery-Åsberg Depression Rating Scale scores declined from persistent moderate scores to sustained mild depression. He is more motivated to increase his social engagement and has received positive feedback at work and even started dating again.

LIMITATIONS AND FUTURE DIRECTIONS

Although research to date provides clear and consistent evidence that nature is beneficial to our psychological and physical well-being, two areas of health that are intimately connected, we still cannot pinpoint the exact mechanism by which nature improves well-being. The studies examined in this chapter demonstrate that certain natural scenes improve attentional performance and reduce the physiological and psychological experience of stress, two results that support ART and SRT, respectively. These theories may indirectly explain some of the other health benefits observed as a result of time in nature; however, the extent of benefits observed is too great to be fully accounted for by ART and SRT alone. Thus, future research should examine other mechanisms by which interaction with nature can benefit our health. We may find that nature therapy, in fact, improves our health through a multitude of mechanisms that work together to improve our overall well-being.

KEY POINTS

- Correlational evidence supports the idea that those who are consistently exposed to natural environments have significantly better health outcomes than those who are not exposed to nature very frequently.

- Evidence suggests that exposure to nature improves attention. The prevailing theory behind this attentional improvement is called attention restoration theory (ART). However, this theory may not fully explain all of the benefits seen in those who spend more time in nature.

- Evidence indicates that interaction with nature reduces stress. Stress reduction theory (SRT) suggests that the health benefits observed after exposure to nature result from stress mediation through decreased sympathetic activity and increased parasympathetic activity. SRT specifies that this benefit would be observed only in natural environments that humans deem beneficial to survival.

- ART and SRT may not fully explain the extensive health benefits observed in persons who spend more time in nature.

- Nature may regulate the immune system, which has major effects on the entire body, and evidence indicates that nature therapy induces a neurological response similar to that of mindfulness therapy.

- We still have a great deal to learn about the exact mechanisms behind nature's effect on human health; however, research provides clear and consistent evi-

dence that interaction with nature improves psychological and physiological well-being.

QUESTIONS

1. What are the four elements of a nature scene that make it restorative
   according to attention restoration theory (ART)?

    A. Soft fascination, awe, excitement, and calmness.
    B. Extent, soft fascination, compatibility, and being away.
    C. Trees, water, open space, and daylight.
    D. Greens, browns, reds, and yellows.
    E. Running water, pleasant weather, daylight, and a calm envi-
       ronment.

**Correct answer: B. Extent, soft fascination, compatibility, and being
away.**

ART suggests that extent (the components of a nature scene that
make it interesting and pleasing), soft fascination (ability of a nature scene to capture one's involuntary attention), compatibility
(when interactions with a natural environment fit with a person's
needs), and being away (the feeling of being mentally and physically distanced from the stressors of daily life) are the qualities
of a natural environment that make it restorative. Although some
research studies have determined that certain elements of a natural scene, such as water (Ulrich 1981) and daylight (Cheon et al.
2019), are more impactful than others, ART, as described by the
Kaplans, focuses on the four qualities described above.

2. How is stress reduction theory (SRT) distinct from ART?

    A. SRT suggests that the benefits observed during and after in-
       teraction with nature are a result of the idea that natural
       scenes humans deem useful to survival reduce stress by in-
       creasing parasympathetic activity and decreasing sympa-
       thetic activity. ART suggests that the benefits of interacting
       with nature are due to restoring directed attention.
    B. SRT suggests that interaction with a natural environment will
       not affect scores on attentional tasks.

C. SRT suggests that natural scenes reduce cortisol levels, which improves immune function, and ART suggests that natural scenes improve attentional function.

D. ART suggests that all natural scenes are beneficial, whereas SRT suggests that only natural scenes that humans deem necessary for survival are beneficial.

E. ART suggests that interaction with a natural environment will not improve measures of stress.

Correct answer: A. SRT suggests that the benefits observed during and after interaction with nature are a result of the idea that natural scenes humans deem useful to survival reduce stress by increasing parasympathetic activity and decreasing sympathetic activity. ART suggests that the benefits of interacting with nature are due to restoring directed attention.

SRT does not rule out improvement in attentional tasks, and ART does not rule out improvement in measures of stress. These theories differ mostly on the mechanism behind these improvements. Each respective theory suggests that there will be more significant improvement in measures relevant to their respective mechanism; however, improving attentional function may indirectly lead to reduced stress measures, and reduced stress may indirectly improve scores on attentional tasks. Thus, answers (B) and (E) are incorrect. SRT does not mention immune function, so (C) is incorrect. ART does not suggest that all natural scenes are beneficial; rather, it suggests that scenes that have qualities of extent, soft fascination, compatibility, and being away are restorative. Thus, (D) is also incorrect.

3. What physiological and neurological changes have been observed in response to nature therapy?

A. Decreased salivary cortisol levels, increased systolic blood pressure, decreased electroencephalographic alpha wave power, decreased inflammatory cytokines, and increased C-reactive protein.

B. Increased blood pressure and increased inflammatory markers.

C. Decreased cortical activity, decreased blood pressure, decreased muscle tension, and decreased immune function.

D. Decreased cortisol levels, decreased blood pressure, decreased amygdala and subgenual prefrontal cortex activity, decreased inflammatory cytokines, and decreased C-reactive protein.

E. Decreased muscle tension, pupil dilation, and decreased natural killer cells.

Correct answer: D. Decreased cortisol levels, decreased blood pressure, decreased amygdala and subgenual prefrontal cortex activity, decreased inflammatory cytokines, and decreased C-reactive protein.

Studies have shown that interaction with nature decreases stress markers such as cortisol levels and blood pressure; activity in the amygdala and subgenual prefrontal cortex associated with fear or negative emotions and self-referential thought or rumination, respectively; and inflammatory markers, such as inflammatory cytokines and C-reactive protein.

REFERENCES

Aljadani H, Patterson A, Sibbritt D, et al: Diet quality and weight change in adults over time: a systematic review of cohort studies. Curr Nutr Rep 4:88–101, 2015

American Psychiatric Association: Diagnostic and Statistical Manual of Mental Disorders, 4th Edition. Washington, DC, American Psychiatric Association, 1994

Andersen HC, Paulsen VE, Winter M: Hans Andersen's Fairy Tales. Chicago, IL, Rand McNally, 1916

Astell-Burt T, Feng X, Kolt GS: Is neighborhood green space associated with a lower risk of type 2 diabetes? Evidence from 267,072 Australians. Diabetes Care 37(1):197–201, 2014 24026544

Bell JF, Wilson JS, Liu GC: Neighborhood greenness and 2-year changes in body mass index of children and youth. Am J Prev Med 35(6):547–553, 2008 19000844

Berman MG, Peltier S, Nee DE, et al: Depression, rumination and the default network. Soc Cogn Affect Neurosci 6(5):548–555, 2011 20855296

Beyer KM, Kaltenbach A, Szabo A, et al: Exposure to neighborhood green space and mental health: evidence from the survey of the health of Wisconsin. Int J Environ Res Public Health 11(3):3453–3472, 2014 24662966

Bjornerem A, Straume B, Midtby M, et al: Endogenous sex hormones in relation to age, sex, lifestyle factors, and chronic diseases in a general population: the Tromso Study. J Clin Endocrinol Metab 89(12):6039–6047, 2004 15579756

Bratman GN, Hamilton JP, Hahn KS, et al: Nature experience reduces rumination and subgenual prefrontal cortex activation. Proc Natl Acad Sci U S A 112(28):8567–8572, 2015 26124129

Bratman GN, Anderson CB, Berman MG, et al: Nature and mental health: an ecosystem service perspective. Sci Adv 5(7):eaax0903, 2019

Brewer JA, Worhunsky PD, Gray JR, et al: Meditation experience is associated with differences in default mode network activity and connectivity. Proc Natl Acad Sci U S A 108(50):20254–20259, 2011 22114193

Burns AC, Saxena R, Vetter C, et al: Time spent in outdoor light is associated with mood, sleep, and circadian rhythm-related outcomes: a cross-sectional and longitudinal study in over 400,000 UK Biobank participants. J Affect Disord 295:347–352, 2021 34488088

Carney RM, Blumenthal JA, Freedland KE, et al: Low heart rate variability and the effect of depression on post-myocardial infarction mortality. Arch Intern Med 165(13):1486–1491, 2005 16009863

Cesari M, Penninx BWJH, Newman AB, et al: Inflammatory markers and onset of cardiovascular events: results from the Health ABC study. Circulation 108(19):2317–2322, 2003 14568895

Cheon S, Soyoung H, Kim M, et al: Comparison between daytime and nighttime scenery focusing on restorative and recovery effect. Sustainability 11(12):3326, 2019

Chu WW, Chu NF: Adverse childhood experiences and development of obesity and diabetes in adulthood—a mini review. Obes Res Clin Pract 15(2):101–105, 2021 33518485

Cimprich B, Ronis DL: An environmental intervention to restore attention in women with newly diagnosed breast cancer. Cancer Nurs 26(4):284–294, 2003 12886119

Dohle S, Diel K, Hofmann W: Executive functions and the self-regulation of eating behavior: a review. Appetite 124:4–9, 2018 28551113

Dowlati Y, Herrmann N, Swardfager W, et al: A meta-analysis of cytokines in major depression. Biol Psychiatry 67(5):446–457, 2010 20015486

Engemann K, Pedersen CB, Arge L, et al: Childhood exposure to green space—a novel risk-decreasing mechanism for schizophrenia? Schizophr Res 199:142–148, 2018 29573946

Faber Taylor A, Kuo FE, Sullivan WC: Coping with ADD: the surprising connection to green play settings. Environ Behav 33:54–77, 2001

Faber Taylor A, Kuo FE, Sullivan WC: Views of nature and self-discipline: evidence from inner city children. J Environ Psychol 22:49–63, 2002

Fan J, McCandliss BD, Fossella J, et al: The activation of attentional networks. Neuroimage 26(2):471–479, 2005 15907304

Farb NA, Segal ZV, Mayberg H, et al: Attending to the present: mindfulness meditation reveals distinct neural modes of self-reference. Soc Cogn Affect Neurosci 2(4):313–322, 2007 18985137

Frith U, Frith CD: Development and neurophysiology of mentalizing. Philos Trans R Soc Lond B Biol Sci 358(1431):459–473, 2003 12689373

Fuertes E, Markevych I, von Berg A, et al: Greenness and allergies: evidence of differential associations in two areas in Germany. J Epidemiol Community Health 68(8):787–790, 2014 24862831

Gusnard DA, Raichle ME: Searching for a baseline: functional imaging and the resting human brain. Nat Rev Neurosci 2(10):685–694, 2001 11584306

Hammen C, Kim EY, Eberhart NK, et al: Chronic and acute stress and the prediction of major depression in women. Depress Anxiety 26(8):718–723, 2009 19496077

Hanski I, von Hertzen L, Fyhrquist N, et al: Environmental biodiversity, human microbiota, and allergy are interrelated. Proc Natl Acad Sci U S A 109(21):8334–8339, 2012 22566627

Harb F, Hidalgo MP, Martau B: Lack of exposure to natural light in the workspace is associated with physiological, sleep and depressive symptoms. Chronobiol Int 32(3):368–375, 2015 25424517

Hartig T, Evans GW, Jamner LD, et al: Tracking restoration in natural and urban field settings. J Environ Psychol 23:109–123, 2003

Hasenkamp W, Barsalou LW: Effects of meditation experience on functional connectivity of distributed brain networks. Front Hum Neurosci 6:38, 2012 22403536

Herzog TR, Maguire CP, Nebel MB: Assessing the restorative components of environments. J Environ Psychol 23:159–170, 2003

Hotta K, Funahashi T, Arita Y, et al: Plasma concentrations of a novel, adipose-specific protein, adiponectin, in type 2 diabetic patients. Arterioscler Thromb Vasc Biol 20(6):1595–1599, 2000 10845877

Huang WZ, Yang BY, Yu HY, et al: Association between community greenness and obesity in urban-dwelling Chinese adults. Sci Total Environ 702:135040, 2020 31726339

Imai K, Matsuyama S, Miyake S, et al: Natural cytotoxic activity of peripheral-blood lymphocytes and cancer incidence: an 11-year follow-up study of a general population. Lancet 356(9244):1795–1799, 2000 11117911

Kaplan R, Kaplan S: The Experience of Nature: A Psychological Perspective. New York, Cambridge University Press, 1989

Kuo FE: Coping with poverty: impacts of environment and attention in the inner city. Environ Behav 33(1):5–34, 2001

Kuo FE, Sullivan WC: Aggression and violence in the inner city: effects of environment via mental fatigue. Environ Behav 33(4):543–571, 2001

Kuo M: How might contact with nature promote human health? Promising mechanisms and a possible central pathway. Front Psychol 6:1093, 2015 26379564

Lachowycz K, Jones AP: Greenspace and obesity: a systematic review of the evidence. Obes Rev 12(5):e183–189, 2011 21348919

Lara-Castro C, Luo N, Wallace P, et al: Adiponectin multimeric complexes and the metabolic syndrome trait cluster. Diabetes 55(1):249–259, 2006 16380500

Lederbogen F, Kirsch P, Haddad L, et al: City living and urban upbringing affect neural social stress processing in humans. Nature 474(7352):498–501, 2011 21697947

Li Q, Otsuka T, Kobayashi M, et al: Acute effects of walking in forest environments on cardiovascular and metabolic parameters. Eur J Appl Physiol 111(11):2845–2853, 2011 21431424

Liu GC, Wilson JS, Qi R, et al: Green neighborhoods, food retail and childhood overweight: differences by population density. Am J Health Promot 21(4 Suppl):317–325, 2007 17465177

Louv R: Last Child in the Woods: Saving Our Children From Nature-Deficit Disorder. Chapel Hill, NC, Algonquin Books, 2005

Lovasi GS, Quinn JW, Neckerman KM, et al: Children living in areas with more street trees have lower prevalence of asthma. J Epidemiol Community Health 62(7):647–649, 2008 18450765

Maas J, Verheij RA, de Vries S, et al: Morbidity is related to a green living environment. J Epidemiol Community Health 63(12): 967–973, 2009 19833605

Mao GX, Cao YB, Lan XG, et al: Therapeutic effect of forest bathing on human hypertension in the elderly. J Cardiol 60(6):495–502, 2012 22948092

Markevych I, Fuertes E, Tiesler CMT, et al: Surrounding greenness and birth weight: results from the GINIplus and LISAplus birth cohorts in Munich. Health Place 26:39–46, 2014 24361636

Matheson FI, Moineddin R, Dunn JR, et al: Urban neighborhoods, chronic stress, gender and depression. Soc Sci Med 63(10):2604–2616, 2006 16920241

Milliron BJ, Ward D, Granche J, et al: Nature relatedness is positively associated with dietary diversity and fruit and vegetable intake in an urban population. Am J Health Promot 36(6):1019–1024, 2022 35382562

Mitchell R, Popham F: Effect of exposure to natural environment on health inequalities: an observational population study. Lancet 372(9650):1655–1660, 2008 18994663

Northoff G, Bermpohl F: Cortical midline structures and the self. Trends Cogn Sci 8(3):102–107, 2004

Nutsford D, Pearson AL, Kingham S: An ecological study investigating the association between access to urban green space and mental health. Public Health 127(11):1005–1011, 2013 24262442

Oh B, Lee KJ, Zaslawski C, et al: Health and well-being benefits of spending time in forests: systematic review. Environ Health Prev Med 22(1):71, 2017 29165173

Ohly H, White MP, Wheeler BW, et al: Attention Restoration Theory: a systematic review of the attention restoration potential of exposure to natural environments. J Toxicol Environ Health B Crit Rev 19(7):305–343, 2016 27668460

Orange JS, Ballas ZK: Natural killer cells in human health and disease. Clin Immunol 118(1):1–10, 2006 16337194

Pan A, Lin X, Hemler E, et al: Diet and cardiovascular disease: advances and challenges in population-based studies. Cell Metab 27(3):489–496, 2018 29514062

Park BJ, Tsunetsugu Y, Kasetani T, et al: Physiological effects of Shinrin-yoku (taking in the atmosphere of the forest)—using salivary cortisol and cerebral activity as indicators. J Physiol Anthropol 26(2):123–128, 2007 17435354

Pedersen CB, Mortensen PB: Evidence of a dose-response relationship between urbanicity during upbringing and schizophrenia risk. Arch Gen Psychiatry 58(11):1039–1046, 2001 11695950

Peen J, Schoevers RA, Beekman AT, et al: The current status of urban-rural differences in psychiatric disorders. Acta Psychiatr Scand 121(2):84–93, 2010 19624573

Pereira G, Foster S, Martin K, et al: The association between neighborhood greenness and cardiovascular disease: an observational study. BMC Public Health 12:466, 2012 22720780

Poudyal NC, Hodges DG, Bowker JM, et al: Evaluating natural resource amenities in a human life expectancy production function. Forest Policies and Economics 11(4):253–259, 2009

Reynolds BW, Basso MR, Miller AK, et al: Executive function, impulsivity, and risky behaviors in young adults. Neuropsychology 33(2):212–221, 2019 30589284

Richardson M, McEwan K, Maratos F, et al: Joy and calm: how an evolutionary functional model of affect regulation informs positive emotions in nature. Evol Psychol Sci 2(4):308–320, 2016

Roszak T, Gomes ME, Kanner AD (eds): Ecopsychology: Restoring the Earth, Healing the Mind. San Francisco, CA, Sierra Club Books, 1995

Sami W, Ansari T, Butt NS, et al: Effect of diet on type 2 diabetes mellitus: a review. Int J Health Sci (Qassim) 11(2):65–71, 2017 28539866

Sharma VK, Singh TG: Chronic stress and diabetes mellitus: interwoven pathologies. Curr Diabetes Rev 16(6):546–556, 2020 31713487

Simpson KA, Singh MA: Effects of exercise on adiponectin: a systematic review. Obesity (Silver Spring) 16(2):241–256, 2008 18239630

Steptoe A, Kivimaki M: Stress and cardiovascular disease. Nat Rev Cardiol 9(6):360–370, 2012 22473079

Stevenson MP, Schilhab T, Bentsen P: Attention Restoration Theory II: a systematic review to clarify attention processes affected by exposure to natural environments. J Toxicol Environ Health B Crit Rev 21(4):227–268, 2018 30130463

Sudimac S, Sale V, Kuhn S: How nature nurtures: amygdala activity decreases as the result of a one-hour walk in nature. Mol Psychiatry 27(11):4446–4452, 2022 36059042

Tamosiunas A, Grazuleviciene R, Luksiene D, et al: Accessibility and use of urban green spaces, and cardiovascular health: findings from a Kaunas cohort study. Environ Health 13(1):20, 2014 24645935

Thayer JF, Yamamoto SS, Brosschot JF: The relationship of autonomic imbalance, heart rate variability and cardiovascular disease risk factors. Int J Cardiol 141(2):122–131, 2010 19910061

Ulrich RS: Natural versus urban scenes: some psychophysiological effects. Environ Behav 13(5):523–556, 1981

Ulrich RS: Aesthetic and affective response to natural environment. Human Behavior and Environment 6:85–125, 1983

Ulrich RS: View through a window may influence recovery from surgery. Science 224(4647):420–421, 1984 6143402

Ulrich RS, Simons RF, Losito BD, et al: Stress recovery during exposure to natural and urban environments. J Environ Psychol 11:201–230, 1991

Vilarrasa N, Vendrell J, Maravall J, et al: Distribution and determinants of adiponectin, resistin and ghrelin in a randomly selected healthy population. Clin Endocrinol (Oxf) 63(3):329–335, 2005 16117822

Villeneuve PJ, Jerrett M, Su JG, et al: A cohort study relating urban green space with mortality in Ontario, Canada. Environ Res 115:51–58, 2012 22483437

Wang Y, She Y, Colarelli SM, et al: Exposure to nature counteracts aggression after depletion. Aggress Behav 44(1):89–97, 2018 28857239

Wellen KE, Hotamisligil GS: Inflammation, stress, and diabetes. J Clin Invest 115(5):1111–1119, 2005

Wells NM: At home with nature: effects of "greenness" on children's cognitive functioning. Environ Behav 32(6):775–795, 2000

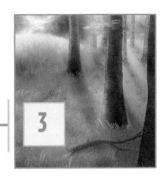

3

Forest Bathing

HISTORY, CULTURE, AND THOUGHTS FOR CLINICAL PRACTICE AND RESEARCH

Yasuhiro Kotera, Ph.D.
Freya Tsuda-McCaie, M.A., PGDip
Ann-Marie Edwards, B.Sc. (Hons)
Kirsten McEwan, Ph.D.

It would seem from this fact, that man is naturally a wild animal, and that when taken from the woods, he is never happy in his natural state, 'till he returns to them again.
—Dr. Benjamin Rush (Rush et al. 1905, p. 46)

In this chapter, we focus on forest bathing (Shinrin-yoku), a Japanese healing practice that has been attracting attention in science globally. Forest bathing was developed in 1982 to counter heightened stress at the national level, which was associated with Japan's rapid economic growth. Considering today's global mental health crisis, it is understandable why this practice now has international appeal. We 1) review the history, culture, and science (i.e., health benefits) of forest bathing; 2) offer practical guidelines for clinicians; 3) discuss areas for future research and practice; and 4) provide case examples. Although cost-effectiveness, accessibility, flexibility, and eco-friendliness are regarded as major advantages of forest bathing, more diverse samples must be evaluated to establish conclusive therapeutic efficacy (and safety) of forest bathing. Insights offered in this chapter can help health care workers, researchers, and patients identify safe and helpful ways to implement this treatment.

CULTURE, PSYCHOLOGY, AND CONTEXT OF FOREST BATHING

Perceptions of nature vary by culture (Gierlach et al. 2010), and in Japan, forests are important spaces for religion and culture. Shintō (神道), Japan's Indigenous religion, is considered a polytheistic nature religion. In Shintō, objects, places, and phenomena, including natural phenomena, are believed to be inhabited by kami (神), or spirits. For example, ancient trees, large waterfalls, winds, storms, or fires may be understood to be inhabited by kami. Shintō does not draw hard distinctions between the physical and the spiritual, and thus many natural places, such as forests, are also sacred places. Traditional Japanese art also draws attention to the beauty and interconnectedness of the natural world, including forests (Ulak 2020). For example, traditional Japanese haiku (俳)—a type of short poem—contains a seasonal, natural reference including phenomena or objects found in forests, such as the morning dew or leaves with changing colors. Paintings, screens, and ceramics also commonly depict the natural world across the seasons as, for example, the blossoming of trees or the falling of leaves (Metropolitan Museum of Art 2004). This artistic interest in the seasons and the natural world is reflected in cultural practices too, such as *hanami* (花見; flower viewing) and ikebana (生け花; flower arranging). Throughout history, Japanese culture has drawn attention to the natural world and encouraged consciously engaging with and reflecting on nature, including trees and forests. Thus, it is perhaps not surprising that Japan is described as a forest civilization (Li 2018).

Forest bathing, also known as Shinrin-yoku (森林浴), is a Japanese therapeutic practice in which participants experience nature in a forest by using their senses, aiming to harmonize with the forest (Miyazaki 2018). Often involving walking or breathing exercises, forest bathing has been practiced with various activities such as yoga, meditation, farming, and cooking (Kotera et al. 2020). In the period after World War II up until the early 1990s—commonly referred to as the Japanese Economic Miracle—Japan successfully reformed its financial system and became the third largest economy in the world. This rapid economic growth was accompanied by technological advances and large-scale migration from rural to urban areas. Accordingly, people's lifestyles changed: consumption increased, and long commutes, overworking, and disconnection from nature became more common. This period also saw the emergence of stress- and lifestyle-related illnesses in Japan (Li 2018). Indeed, the term *Karōshi* (過労死), meaning "overwork death," was coined in 1978 to describe the increasing numbers of otherwise healthy people dying from strokes, myocardial infarctions, or suicide. These deaths were seemingly connected to long working hours and intense work-related stress. The Japanese government needed to implement an effective well-being strategy to protect the health of its people.

The word *Shinrin-yoku* was coined in 1982 by Tomohide Akiyama at the Japanese Forestry Agency as an antidote to burnout from an urbanized, fast-paced, technology-oriented lifestyle and a way of preventing and remediating stress-related illness. The first appearance of the term *Shinrin-yoku* in literature was on July 29, 1982, in *Asahi Shimbun*, one of the major newspapers in Japan. The word *shinrin* means "forests" and *yoku* means "bathing," implying that you immerse yourself in a forest. Although there was no research on forest bathing back then, Akiyama suggested that individuals can improve their physical and mental health by immersing themselves in the smell of a forest. Moreover, Japan is a forest-rich country. Two-thirds of Japanese lands are forests (as opposed to other countries such as China and the United Kingdom, where only about 10% of the land is forests), and policymakers intended to capitalize on this abundant natural resource. Scientific research on forest bathing was initiated by Yoshifumi Miyazaki, a physiological anthropology professor at Chiba University, in 1990. About a decade later, Qing Li, a physician and immunologist at Nihon Medical School, advanced forest bathing research. Building on their promising findings, the Japanese government promoted forest bathing by funding research into its potential benefits, protecting forests for public use, and making it part of the country's health care program (Li 2018). Subsequently, forest bathing became a popular "social prescription" (the referral or linking of patients to nonclinical services by health care professionals with the aim of promoting patients' well-being and health) among Japanese health care professionals. Additionally, in Japan, many medical doctors are now certified in forest medicine and can provide services directly to patients (Miyazaki 2018). Forest bathing is also popular in Japan as a preventive and remedial strategy for illness: 60 official forest therapy trails are used by approximately 5 million people annually (Miyazaki 2018). In 2010, the *New York Times* featured forest bathing (O'Connor 2010), reporting on the scientific health benefits of this practice. The 2010 *New York Times* article is widely regarded as the first step for the global recognition of forest bathing. Today, forest bathing is being researched internationally because this practice has the potential to address people's health problems in an affordable and accessible way (Kotera et al. 2020).

Japanese Forests

Specific qualities of Japanese forest environments may influence the effect of forest bathing on health. Li (2010) argued that high concentrations of phytoncides or volatile organic compounds (VOCs; compounds emitted by trees and other organic matter into the air) are partially responsible for the positive effects of forest bathing on health. The dominant tree species in Japanese forests are cedar and cypress, which are both conifers. Tree composition affects the types and amounts of phytoncides, with conifer forests having higher levels of VOCs than deciduous forests, possibly influencing outcomes (Antonelli et al. 2020). Indeed, Lee et al. (2015) found that phytoncide levels varied by location and weather. However, researchers caution that although VOCs may play a role in the effects of forest bathing, visual, auditory, and social factors also contribute to the positive effects of forest bathing on health (Antonelli et al. 2020; Li 2010). Indeed, McEwan et al. (2021) found that participants in forest bathing activities reported using their visual and auditory senses more than their sense of smell.

Healing Forests of South Korea

Reports of the benefits of Shinrin-yoku crossed the ocean a long time ago, and Shinrin-yoku has been enjoyed by people in Japan's neighboring countries, such as South Korea. Through rapid urbanization and technological development, 85% of South Koreans live in cities. This development comes with significant challenges, with suicide being one of the most common causes of death (Rezaei et al. 2021). According to a recent report, 7 of 10 employees in South Korea experience burnout (Seo-Hyum 2020), resulting in high levels of stress. Furthermore, alcohol use and other psychiatric disorders have been identified as a major problem. The Korean Alcohol Research Center studied depression in 92 patients with chronic alcohol use disorder (Shin et al. 2012). The study found that forest therapy can help reduce symptoms of depression in patients with alcohol use disorder (effect size $r=0.68$). This study yielded promising evidence of the possible effect of the forest environment on depression among people with substance use disorders, a subject that has received little attention in the literature.

Forest bathing—or forest healing, as it is sometimes called in South Korea—has been receiving increased attention, and South Korea is now a leading country using forest therapy (Mao et al. 2017) as part of innovative systems that are being developed to counter the detrimental health effects of urban living. The Korea Forest Service has designed several healing forests, with the first therapeutic forest opening in 2009. By 2020, there were 32 specifically designated areas across the country (Park et al. 2021), similar to Japan's "power spots" in nature. Public interest in these therapeutic forests increased during the coronavirus disease 2019 pandemic, with stress levels motivating people to visit nature (Chae et al. 2021).

Cultures Outside Asia

Given the context of forest bathing in Japan and South Korea, the positive effects of forest bathing may be culturally specific. Japanese and Asian participants reported greater mental health benefits from forest bathing than did their Western counterparts (Kotera et al. 2020). Possibly, the positive associations with forests in Asian cultures increase forest bathing's effectiveness for these populations. Research on forest bathing is limited in non-Asian populations (Kotera et al. 2020). The preliminary evidence from outside Asia, such as the United Kingdom and Poland, is promising, with positive results for psychological conditions such as depression, anxiety, anger, rumination, emotions, and mood disturbance (e.g., Bielinis et al. 2019; McEwan et al. 2021). The U.K.-based study (McEwan et al. 2021) found that participants receiving a forest bathing intervention reported significant benefits across many psychological variables, but no difference was seen in the magnitude of effects between forest bathing and an established well-being intervention. Taken together, the positive effects of forest bathing appear to transcend culture. However, more research is needed, and outside Asia, forest bathing's effect on mental health may be similar in magnitude to other well-being interventions. Given that a person's culture and associations with forests may affect efficacy and other established well-being interventions appear to have similar benefits for psychological health, patient preference and interest (Antonelli et al. 2020) may play an important role in the appropriateness of recommending forest bathing to a given person.

HEALTH BENEFITS OF FOREST BATHING

Although research on forest bathing is still nascent, diverse and salient health benefits of this approach have been reported in the scientific literature. In the physical health domain, immersion in nature increases the number and activity of natural killer cells, leading to improved function of the immune, cardiovascular, and respiratory systems. Song et al. (2016) theorized that the underlying mechanism of forest bathing is that the restorative effect of nature reduces stress, leading to physiological relaxation and immune function recovery, which protects us from various illnesses. These relaxation and stress reduction effects have been identified through salivary cortisol levels, heart rate variability–related sympathetic and parasympathetic nervous activity, blood pressure measurements, and pulse rate.

Likewise, the mental health benefits of forest bathing have been identified. Depression, anxiety, and anger were often evaluated in forest bathing research targeting mental health outcomes by using the Profile of Mood States; overall positive effects on those outcomes have been reported. Among those three mental health outcomes (depression, anxiety, and anger), Kotera et al.'s (2020) meta-analysis identified that forest bathing reduced anxiety the most. This can be explained by the calming effects of forest bathing; however, a scientific evaluation is needed.

Moreover, forest bathing also has been shown to have psychological and physiological benefits in patients with prehypertension and hypertension. Chronically high stress levels can lead to hypertension, myocardial infarction, or stroke. In recent years, forest bathing has been adopted as a prevention strategy to reduce blood pressure and stress and induce feelings of relaxation in hypertensive patients (Mao et al. 2017), and it could be adopted by health care professionals as a complementary therapy for several other physical ailments (Yau and Loke 2020).

Along with these empirical findings, several theories have been proposed to explain how nature heals us. Attention restoration theory posits that our concentration is restored by time in nature because we pay attention to items in nature effortlessly. This state of effortless attention is thought to recover our concentration. Stress reduction theory claims that being in a natural environment lowers stress levels and strengthens physiological functions such as heart rate and blood pressure. (See Chapters 1, "The Wise Outdoors," and 5, "Horticultural Therapy," for more details on attention restoration theory and stress reduction theory.) Recently, forest bathing's positive effects on mental health were explained via the affect regulation model. The affect regulation model theorizes that spending time in nature activates our soothing system (and the parasympathetic system), which is associated with feelings of safety and compassion, leading to better mental health (Richardson et al. 2016). Recent forest bathing studies that evaluated levels of self-compassion support the positive effect of spending time in nature on our soothing system (Kotera and Fido 2021; McEwan et al. 2021).

Additionally, from a historical perspective, humans are more accustomed to being in nature than in urban environments. In 7 million years of human history, humans have spent 99.99% of their time in nature (Miyazaki 2018). This can explain why we do not feel well in urban settings compared with nature. Mortality was 12% lower among women living in nature than among those living in urban areas (James et al. 2016). The duration of time spent in nature was negatively associated with rates of depression and high blood pressure (Shanahan et al. 2016). The levels of awe and prosocial behaviors were higher among participants who viewed a towering tree for 1 minute than among those who viewed an urban building of the same height (Piff et al. 2015). Another experimental study compared 3 days of forest bathing with 3 days of walking in a city and found that the number and activity of natural killer cells were higher in the forest group than in the city group (Li 2010). Shorter exposure to nature is also reported to be effective. A 90-minute walk in nature was shown to reduce the degree of rumination (negative recurrent thoughts that are related to poor mental health) and the activities of the brain part that is associated with mental health problems (subgenual prefrontal cortex) (Bratman et al. 2015). More recently, researchers found that visits and time in nature may facilitate nature connectedness (Martin et al. 2020)—affective and cognitive connection with a natural environment (Capaldi et al. 2014).

Wen et al. (2019) summarized the health benefits of Shinrin-yoku (Table 3–1).

Although diverse health benefits of forest bathing have been reported, Miyazaki stressed that it does not cure diseases; it is a preventive practice. The mechanism suggested is that forest bathing reduces the stress we experience, which strengthens our immune system, pre-

Table 3–1.   Potential psychological and physiological health benefits of Shinrin-yoku

Psychological	Physiological
Improved emotional state	Improved cardiovascular function and hemodynamic indexes
Improved attitude toward things	Improved neuroendocrine indexes
Improved psychological and physiological recovery	Improved metabolism indexes
Improved adaptive behavior	Improved immune and inflammatory indexes
Reduced levels of anxiety and depression	Improved antioxidation indexes
	Improved electrical physiological indexes

Source.   Adapted from Wen Y, Yan Q, Pan Y, et al: "Medical Empirical Research on Forest Bathing (Shinrin-Yoku): A Systematic Review." *Environmental Health and Preventive Medicine* 24(1):1–21, 2019 31787069. This article is distributed under the terms of the Creative Commons Attribution 4.0 International License (http://creativecommons.org/licenses/by/4.0/).

venting us from getting diseases (Miyazaki 2018). Many of us today live in an environment we are not suited to, which increases our stress level, in turn increasing our susceptibility to diseases. By connecting with nature through practices such as forest bathing, we are living as we evolved to live, resulting in a reduction of stress. Therefore, researchers recommend that if forests are inaccessible (one impediment to forest bathing; Kotera et al. 2021), people can connect with nature through items such as plants or essential oils of trees, which have been reported to be effective for stress reduction too.

More rigorous forest bathing research must be conducted. Many studies in this field have methodological weaknesses such as a lack of follow-up assessments and unrepresentative sampling (Kotera et al. 2020). In forest bathing randomized controlled trials, randomization and blinding often were not maintained. Relatedly, many researchers have used a crossover design with no or short intervals and did not conduct intention-to-treat analyses. Moreover, key figures such as Miyazaki and Li were often involved. This may have meant that participants who believed in forest bathing received the intervention with high expectations, which could have exaggerated the effect. Lastly, because forest bathing can include a variety of activities such as yoga, meditation, and other recreational activities, the practice of forest bathing must be controlled in scientific research. For example, mindfulness is often used in forest bathing, but that blurs a boundary between those two; whether the positive effects were derived from forest bathing or mindfulness was left ambiguous in some cases (Clarke et al. 2021). Future research must address these weaknesses in order to advance the science and practice of forest bathing.

Below we suggest areas to focus on in future forest bathing research.

Neurodevelopmental Disorders

People with disorders such as autism can enjoy the benefits of forest bathing. The mental health of autistic persons has been receiving attention, because they experience high rates of mental health problems. What makes treatment difficult is that traditional, established approaches do not necessarily work well because autistic persons often have difficulties with social and communication skills. For example, cognitive-behavioral therapy does not work well because autistic persons often cannot verbalize their emotions well. Mindfulness is also contraindicated with this population, because autistic persons often struggle to stay focused on their internal processes. Forest bathing may be a better therapeutic fit, because autistic people can enjoy being in a forest and paying attention to external stimuli through their senses. Additionally, the most effective clinical outcome of forest bathing appears to be reducing anxiety, which is the primary emotional difficulty that autistic people encounter. This good match indicates that empirical research should be conducted to evaluate whether forest bathing will improve the well-being of autistic people by reducing their anxiety. We plan to conduct this trial.

Moreover, forest bathing is regarded as a potential treatment for ADHD, a neurodevelopmental disorder that is characterized by inattentiveness, hyperactivity, and impulsiveness and can interfere with the functioning and development of patients. First-line treatment for ADHD usually consists of prescription medication such as methylphenidate. However, although prescription medications have proven effective in the treatment of symptoms, they have unwanted side effects such as sleep problems, decreased appetite, headaches, and mood disorders. Nature therapy, in contrast, has been shown in studies to have a positive effect on ADHD symptoms (Donovan et al. 2019; Kuo and Faber Taylor 2004) and can be used as a supplemental therapy or primary treatment for ADHD.

Heart Failure in Older Adults

Emerging evidence shows the beneficial effects of forest bathing on human health, particularly in preventing heart failure in older adults. A study by Mao et al. (2017) found that forest bathing was a beneficial nature-based intervention contributing to the physical health of older adults with chronic heart failure. As shown in Figure 3–1, patients with chronic heart failure who took part in a 4-day forest bathing trip had lower levels of brain natriuretic peptide levels, a biomarker of heart failure, compared with older adults in the urban control group or the baseline level before the experiment. Such findings provide evidence of the positive effects of forest bathing in patients with heart conditions and lay the groundwork for further research into this adjunctive treatment.

Cancer Treatment Side Effects

Conventional treatments for many cancers include surgery, radiation, and chemotherapy; however, such treatments can cause some unpleasant side effects depending on the type of treatment administered. Connecting with nature can reduce treatment side effects, with improved cognition, memory, and attention, as well as improved quality of life for patients with cancer. Therefore, forest therapy could prove beneficial as an adjunct to standard cancer treatment (Kim et al. 2015).

Forest Rx

The number of clinicians practicing nature therapy is unknown. However, an increasing number of clinicians are actively prescribing nature therapy to their patients. La Puma (2019), the author of "Nature Therapy: An Essential Prescription for Health," believes that clinicians should prescribe nature therapy for people who have nature deficit. Emerging evidence suggests that nature-based activities can have a positive effect on health and well-being. Therefore, mental health charities and community groups have been working with health care professionals to actively encourage nature therapy prescriptions (Applied Research Collaboration South West Peninsula 2021).

The growing field of nature therapy is becoming more widely recognized as an alternative to traditional medicine for the treatment of a number of ailments, and it is gaining popularity among clinicians. It is already recognized as an approved clinical therapy in some countries, such as Japan, where it is available by prescription for the treatment of mental and physical health.

PRACTICAL GUIDELINES

The fact that forest bathing has no definite methods of practice is both an advantage and a disadvantage; every practitioner finds their own way to connect with nature. However, it is often helpful to pay attention

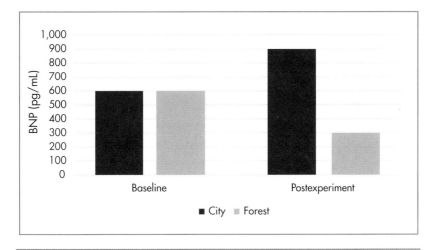

Figure 3–1. Effect of forest bathing on brain natriuretic peptide (BNP) levels in patients with chronic heart failure.

Source. Adapted from Mao G, Cao Y, Wang B, et al: "The Salutary Influence of Forest Bathing on Elderly Patients With Chronic Heart Failure." *International Journal of Environmental Research and Public Health* 14(4):368, 2017 28362327. This article is distributed under the terms of the Creative Commons Attribution 4.0 International License (http://creativecommons.org/licenses/by/4.0/).

to one's senses, particularly vision, hearing, touch, and smell. Patients often report that getting in touch with the senses is one of the most helpful aspects of this therapy because, in their busy daily lives, they are often asked to use their heads instead of noticing their senses. Indeed, noticing one's senses is helpful in stress reduction (Ahmed et al. 2017). Forest bathing supports this process.

Forest bathing can take a variety of forms, including walking, meditation, and yoga. Patients need to find their own way that makes them feel comfortable and supports their healing. If they want to see rays of light between leaves, then they can do so. If they want to hear the sounds of a river, then they can get closer to it. This inner sense of what your body wants is the central guidance in this treatment to heal from mental distress. Developing this inner sense can take time, and thus sharing common ways or activities to facilitate forest bathing is helpful to some patients, especially in the beginning. One of us (Y.K.) had a patient who was not familiar with "noticing" and "sensing," and this patient struggled with engaging in forest bathing. If Y.K. asked the patient about his feelings, the patient responded, "Nothing" or "I don't know." Y.K. decided to take a walk with the patient in the forest. As the patient walked, he started to notice more about nature (e.g., different colors of green among leaves) as well as his inner state (e.g., "feels different," "not bad," or "good"). For such a patient, this type of initial support may be effective because forest bathing is an experiential treatment. Assuming that those patients have other major duties in their lives, often 15 minutes per session of getting in touch with nature is the minimum duration needed to yield positive effects (Kotera et al. 2021), but frequency depends on the patient's lifestyle, and longitudinal assessments are needed.

This also means that the clinician's lived experience of being healed through forest bathing is certainly advantageous or necessary. Many patients find forest bathing appealing, but some do not. Clinicians need to listen to patients' concerns and advise accordingly. If a patient has had a traumatic experience being in nature (e.g., being bitten by a snake), then forest bathing cannot be recommended.

SPECIAL CONSIDERATIONS

Special considerations regarding the appropriateness of forest bathing for a given patient include assessing feelings of safety in natural spaces, such as forests. Given the proposed mechanisms underlying the positive effects of forest bathing on mental health—for example, stress reduction theory and affect regulation model—feeling safe and accepted in natural environments is probably important for efficacy. Moreover, how safe and accepted people feel in natural environments varies. For example, writers and activists have drawn attention to the exclusion of people of color from nature in the United States and the depiction of wild spaces (including forests) as populated exclusively or mostly by White, affluent people (Finney 2014). Finney argued that because of historical associations and these depictions, African American people specifically may feel excluded from or fearful of natural spaces. Additionally, people of color in the United States have recently drawn attention to their experiences of racism in natural spaces (e.g., Samayoa 2020). However, activists are reclaiming these spaces and promoting and celebrating nature-based activities among people of color.

A patient's access to forests is also important to consider. In the United States, access to nature is deeply divided along economic and racial lines (Landau et al. 2020), and similar divisions in access are found in the United Kingdom (Environment Agency 2021). Moreover, in the United States many public forests are not reachable via public transport, impeding access for non–car owners. Thus, it is important to discuss with patients the feasibility of forest bathing.

CHILDREN AND ADOLESCENTS

Initial findings suggest that children and adolescents may gain significant mental health benefits from forest bathing, but the research is currently limited. A systematic review of elementary school children found that forest-based interventions, including forest therapy, led to improvements in self-esteem and mental health and a reduction in depressive symptoms and anger, among other outcomes (Song and Bang 2017), and a study with Japanese adolescent girls found that forest bathing improved mood and increased feelings of relaxation (Hohashi and Kobayashi 2013). Given the significant percentage of children and adolescents who experience mental health problems, further research with these populations is needed.

Clinical Translation: Case Example

In a series of urban forest bathing walks, a practitioner worked with several adults who were struggling with long-term anxiety. During registration for the walks, the practitioner was alerted to patients' anxiety by patients or their caregivers. She adapted her walks to make them more accessible for this patient group. For example, she anticipated that they might feel self-conscious, so all activities were framed as suggestions, which patients could choose not to do or could adapt to suit their needs. She also anticipated that they might have particular difficulties with the slower pace of the walks; she therefore gave a prompt at the start, recognizing that it is normal to rush about in daily life and to feel pressure to achieve things and that if patients noticed any feelings of frustration about the slower pace, they could try noting this and making a conscious effort to slow down further. The practitioner also provided a psychological framework and rationale for the forest bathing walk, explaining that we spend a lot of our daily lives in either "fight or flight" or "doing and achieving." She explained that the aim of forest bathing was to help patients access "rest and digest" and engage their soothing system (i.e., parasympathetic system).

The patients engaged fully in the sensory activities, and all reported feeling very grateful for the opportunity to slow down, noting that this was the most they had ever slowed down and really noticed their surroundings. One younger woman was extremely pleased with herself for coping; normally, group activities would result in her breaking down, crying, and running away, and her caregiver noted how exceptional it was to see her so calm and coping so well. Two younger women who had entered the session avoiding all eye contact and not speaking during group discussions became more able to tolerate eye contact and had animated conversations with the practitioner about how much they loved spending time in nature and how this helped them manage their anxiety. One older woman began a session crying, stating that she was so plagued by anxiety that even coming to the walk had caused a huge increase in anxiety (e.g., worrying about being late, being able to find the meeting point, parking). She visibly calmed down during the session and was very open when it came to sharing positive experiences during the walk with other participants. After the walk, she contacted the guide and provided the following feedback: "It's now nearly 8 hours since I came home, and I'm still feeling so relaxed. My mind isn't full of 'stuff,' and I don't feel any anxiety—something I've been plagued with for nearly a year now. I'm going to be making regular trips to the park and bathing in the sights, sounds, and smells of nature." Two older men commented that normally when they walked, they marched through at a fast pace, feeling angry about life, and did not take in their surroundings at all. The walk made them stop ruminating on problems almost instantly and see their local park in a completely different way, and it helped them slow down and relax. Since the walk, one of these men has been reading about how to rekindle his connection with nature and has been practicing the activities every day in the park. In addition to collecting informal feedback about patients' experiences, the practitioner collected survey data at the start and end of the walks. She found a 54% reduction in ruminating about problems and a 34% reduction in anxiety. These are the most notable benefits patients reported from forest bathing walks, noting that the activities allowed them to put aside their usual anxious thoughts and preoccupation with progress and to-do lists.

KEY POINTS

- Forest bathing was originally developed in Japan to address the increasing stress among people as a cost-effective and environmentally friendly approach.

- Forest bathing has been found effective for reducing diverse physical (e.g., heart failure) and mental health problems (e.g., anxiety, stress, anger, depression).

- This rather freestyle approach can be conducted in a variety of forms, such as walking, meditation, or yoga. Those methods can be used to help patients access their senses, which are central to forest bathing.

- Although the research and practice of forest therapy have been increasing in recent years, many populations are still underrepresented in this domain. Future research and practice must focus on these populations to increase the inclusivity and utility of this intervention.

- Clinicians can take advantage of the flexibility of this intervention, as demonstrated in the case example, to notice patients' status sensitively and offer alternative activities to ensure patient safety and positive effects.

QUESTIONS

1. In the research conducted to date, forest bathing has been reported most effective in reducing which of the following?

    A. Anger.
    B. Depression.
    C. Anxiety.
    D. Loneliness.
    E. Irritability.

Correct answer: C. Anxiety.

> Kotera et al.'s (2020) meta-analysis reported that the Profile of Mood States is the most frequently used scale in forest bathing research, making depression, anger, and anxiety the most frequent target outcomes. Among those three outcomes, anxiety had the largest effect sizes in various study designs.

2. In the 7 million years of human history, humans have spent more than what percentage of the time in nature?

    A. 20%.
    B. 40%.
    C. 60%.
    D. 80%.
    E. 99%.

Correct answer: E. 99%.

> Miyazaki's (2018) book discusses why we feel good in nature. In this book, he introduced a historical perspective: humans have spent more than 99.99% of their history in nature. Only very recently have many people lived in urban settings. Miyazaki posited that we feel good in nature because that is where we evolved.

3. When practicing forest bathing, it is essential to do which of the following?

    A. Walk as fast as possible.
    B. Breathe as slowly as possible.
    C. Try to find a solution to your problem.
    D. Use your senses (e.g., vision, hearing, touch, and smell).
    E. Talk to others.

Correct answer: D. Use your senses (e.g., vision, hearing, touch, and smell).

One of the most helpful aspects of forest bathing is that individuals can become more in touch with their senses by immersing themselves in nature. Often in daily life, we are forced to use the cognitive aspects of our brain, missing the experiences of our senses. Forest bathing allows people to access their senses, reducing stress.

REFERENCES

Ahmed MMH, Silpasuwanchai C, Niksirat KS, et al: Understanding the role of human senses in interactive meditation. Paper presented at Conference on Human Factors in Computing Systems, Denver, CO, May 2017

Antonelli M, Donelli D, Barbieri G, et al: Forest volatile organic compounds and their effects on human health: a state-of-the-art review. Int J Environ Res Public Health 17(18):6506, 2020 32906736

Applied Research Collaboration South West Peninsula: PenARC. NIHR ARC South West Peninsula, 2021. Available at: https://arc-swp.nihr.ac.uk. Accessed April 13, 2024.

Bielinis E, Bielinis L, Krupińska-Szeluga S, et al: The effects of a short forest recreation program on physiological and psychological relaxation in young Polish adults. Forests 10:34, 2019

Bratman GN, Hamilton JP, Hahn KS, et al: Nature experience reduces rumination and subgenual prefrontal cortex activation. Proc Natl Acad Sci U S A 112(28):8567–8572, 2015 26124129

Capaldi CA, Dopko RL, Zelenski JM: The relationship between nature connectedness and happiness: a meta-analysis. Front Psychol 5:976, 2014 25249992

Chae Y, Lee S, Jo Y, et al: The effects of forest therapy on immune function. Int J Environ Res Public Health 18(16):8440, 2021 34444188

Clarke FJ, Kotera Y, McEwan K: A qualitative study comparing mindfulness and shinrin-yoku (forest bathing): practitioners' perspectives. Sustainability 13(12):6761, 2021

Donovan GH, Michael YL, Gatziolis D, et al: Association between exposure to the natural environment, rurality, and attention-deficit hyperactivity disorder in children in New Zealand: a linkage study. Lancet Planet Health 3(5):e226–e234, 2019 31128768

Environment Agency: Environmental inequality must not be ignored. July 20, 2021. Available at: https://www.gov.uk/government/news/environmental-inequality-must-not-be-ignored. Accessed April 13, 2024.

Finney C: Black Faces, White Spaces: Reimagining the Relationship of African Americans to the Great Outdoors. Chapel Hill, NC, UNC Press Books, 2014

Gierlach E, Belsher BE, Beutler LE: Cross-cultural differences in risk perceptions of disasters. Risk Anal 30(10):1539–1549, 2010 20626692

Hohashi N, Kobayashi K: The effectiveness of a forest therapy (shinrin-yoku) program for girls aged 12 to 14 years: a crossover study. Stress Sci Res 28:82–89, 2013

James P, Hart JE, Banay RF, et al: Exposure to greenness and mortality in a nationwide prospective cohort study of women. Environ Health Perspect 124(9):1344–1352, 2016 27074702

Kim BJ, Jeong H, Park S, et al: Forest adjuvant anti-cancer therapy to enhance natural cytotoxicity in urban women with breast cancer: a preliminary prospective interventional study. European Journal of Integrative Medicine 7(5):474–478, 2015

Kotera Y, Fido D: Effects of Shinrin-Yoku retreat on mental health: a pilot study in Fukushima, Japan. Int J Mental Health Addiction 2021:1–13, 2021

Kotera Y, Richardson M, Sheffield D: Effects of Shinrin-Yoku (forest bathing) and nature therapy on mental health: a systematic review and meta-analysis. Int J Mental Health Addiction 20:337–361, 2020

Kotera Y, Lyons M, Vione KC, et al: Effect of nature walks on depression and anxiety: a systematic review. Sustainability 13(7):4015, 2021

Kuo FE, Faber Taylor A: A potential natural treatment for attention-deficit/hyperactivity disorder: evidence from a national study. Am J Public Health 94(9):1580–1586, 2004 15333318

Landau VA, McClure ML, Dickson BG: Analysis of the disparities in nature loss and access to nature. Conservation Science Partners, 2020. Available at: https://www.csp-inc.org/public/CSP-CAP_Disparities_in_Nature_Loss_FINAL_Report_060120.pdf. Accessed April 13, 2024.

La Puma J: Nature therapy: an essential prescription for health. Alternative and Complementary Therapies 25(2):1–4, 2019

Lee YK, Woo JS, Choi SR, et al: Comparison of phytocide (monoterpene) concentration by type of recreational forest. J Environ Health Sci 41(4):241–248, 2015

Li Q: Effect of forest bathing trips on human immune function. Environ Health Prev Med 15(1):9–17, 2010 19568839

Li Q: Forest Bathing: How Trees Can Help You Find Health and Happiness. London, Penguin, 2018

Mao G, Cao Y, Wang B, et al: The salutary influence of forest bathing on elderly patients with chronic heart failure. Int J Environ Res Public Health 14(4):368, 2017 28362327

Martin L, White MP, Hunt A, et al: Nature contact, nature connectedness and associations with health, wellbeing and pro-environmental behaviours. J Environ Psychol 68:101389, 2020

McEwan K, Giles D, Clarke FJ, et al: A pragmatic controlled trial of forest bathing compared with compassionate mind training in the UK: impacts on self-reported wellbeing and heart rate variability. Sustainability 13(3):1380, 2021

Metropolitan Museum of Art: Seasonal Imagery in Japanese Art. New York, Department of Asian Art, Metropolitan Museum of Art, 2004. Available at: http://www.metmuseum.org/toah/hd/seim/hd_seim.htm. Accessed April 13, 2024.

Miyazaki Y: Shinrin Yoku: The Japanese Art of Forest Bathing. Portland, OR, Timber Press, 2018

O'Connor A: The claim: exposure to plants and parks can boost immunity. New York Times, July 5, 2010. Available at: https://www.nytimes.com/2010/07/06/health/06real.html. Accessed April 13, 2024.

Park S, Kim S, Kim G, et al: Evidence-based status of forest healing program in South Korea. Int J Environ Res Public Health 18(19):10368, 2021 34639668

Piff PK, Dietze P, Feinberg M, et al: Awe, the small self, and prosocial behavior. J Pers Soc Psychol 108(6):883–899, 2015 25984788

Rezaei M, Kim D, Alizadeh A, et al: Evaluating the mental-health positive impacts of agritourism; a case study from South Korea. Sustainability 13(16):8712, 2021

Richardson M, McEwan K, Maratos F, et al: Joy and calm: how an evolutionary functional model of affect regulation informs positive emotions in nature. Evol Psychol Sci 2(4):308–320, 2016

Rush B, Biddle LA, Williams HJ: A Memorial Containing Travels Through Life or Sundry Incidents in the Life of Dr. Benjamin Rush, Born December 24, 1745 (Old Style) Died April 19, 1813. Philadelphia, PA, Sign of the Ivy Leaf, 1905

Samayoa M: Racism in the great outdoors: Oregon's natural spaces feel off limits to Black people. OPB News, June 18, 2020. Available at: https://www.opb.org/news/article/oregon-northwest-racism-outdoors-nature-hiking. Accessed April 13, 2024.

Seo-Hyum S: 70% of workers in Korea are burned out, survey says. Korea Joong Daily, November 23, 2020. Available at: https://koreajoongangdaily.joins.com/2020/11/23/business/industry/stress-burnout-satisfaction/20201123200600460.html. Accessed April 13, 2024.

Shanahan DF, Bush R, Gaston KJ, et al: Health benefits from nature experiences depend on dose. Sci Rep 6(1):28551, 2016 27334040

Shin WS, Shin CS, Yeoun PS: The influence of forest therapy camp on depression in alcoholics. Environ Health Prev Med 17(1):73–76, 2012 21503628

Song C, Ikei H, Miyazaki Y: Physiological effects of nature therapy: a review of the research in Japan. Int J Environ Res Public Health 13(8):781, 2016 27527193

Song MK, Bang KS: A systematic review of forest therapy programs for elementary school students. Child Health Nursing Res 23(3):300–311, 2017

Ulak JT: Japanese art. Encyclopedia Britannica, March 24, 2020. Available at: https://www.britannica.com/art/Japanese-art. Accessed April 13, 2024.

Wen Y, Yan Q, Pan Y, et al: Medical empirical research on forest bathing (Shin-rin-yoku): a systematic review. Environ Health Prev Med 24(1):1–21, 2019 31787069

Yau KKY, Loke AY: Effects of forest bathing on pre-hypertensive and hypertensive adults: a review of the literature. Environ Health Prev Med 25(1):23, 2020 32571202

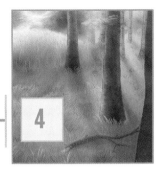

Urban Green Spaces

Sezai Ustun Aydin, M.D.
Aitzaz Munir, M.D.
Rijul Asri, M.D.

> *Anyone who believes growth can go on forever is*
> *either a madman or an economist.*
> —Attributed to economist Kenneth Boulding (Olson 1973, p. 3)

A lush, green oasis amid a concrete jungle is a welcome sight! The urban green space is a necessary product of urbanization (Anguluri and Narayanan 2017), but how this concept is translated or defined varies. Many urban green areas include natural surfaces or settings, even tree-lined streets. Others find this description too narrow and consider water elements such as ponds and shores as requisite to a true urban green space. On this matter, the European Environment Agency (2011) defines green urban areas as spaces including gardens, zoos, parks, suburban natural areas, and forests, or green areas bordered by urban areas that are managed or used for recreational purposes. The U.S. Environmental Protection Agency also includes agricultural areas to broaden the definition of an urban green space (Pickard et al. 2015). In this chapter, we delve into the implications of urbanization for mental health and the value of urban green spaces in accessing ecotherapy and promoting wellness.

Ecotherapy is based on the growing body of research that associates nature with positive physical and mental health outcomes. Connecting with nature reminds us that we are part of the ecosystem rather than separate from it (Buzzell 2009; Jones 2010). However, with each passing year, urbanization significantly transforms the environment. Beginning in the second half of the twentieth century, humankind started to shape ecosystems more widely and rapidly than ever before. These changes include the transformation of forests and grasslands into cropland, the alteration and storage of freshwater behind dams, and the loss of mangroves and coral reefs (Millennium Ecosystem Assessment 2005). More than half of the human population lives in urban settings, and that figure is projected to increase to 70% by the year 2050 (Dye 2008). The societal shift from rural to urban spaces has many benefits, such as easier access to basic services, health, education, employment, and infrastructure (United Nations 2020), but it is not without drawbacks. In moving away from nature, people have lost touch with an essential resource for mental health that was freely available. Ultimately, removing people from the natural ecosystem has negative implications for mental wellness (van den Berg et al. 2010; Ward Thompson et al. 2012).

CONSEQUENCES OF URBANIZATION

The adverse effects of urbanization on mental health attracted the attention of researchers in the early 1990s, and studies since then have characterized the mental health burden of city living. Living in an urban area was linked to a 39% higher risk of having a psychiatric disorder in a large-sample study (Peen et al. 2010). Similarly, in a study that screened for major depressive disorder, the Canadian National Population Health Survey reported a lower prevalence of major depressive disorder in rural areas than in urban areas (Wang 2004). *Urbanization* refers not only to the creation of cities but also to the loss of natural environments, the latter of which more notably affects mental health. Two large-sample surveys, one from Wisconsin and one from the Netherlands, found a significant positive correlation between the availability of nature and better mental health outcomes (Beyer et al. 2014; White et al. 2013). A more recent study echoed these results, showing that increased exposure to tree canopies decreased the incidence of psychological distress by nearly a third (Astell-Burt and Feng 2019). Furthermore, a nationwide sweep study in Denmark that canvased more than 900,000 people found that exposure to green space during childhood decreased the occurrence of psychiatric disorders during adolescence and adulthood. This study reviewed the effect of residential green areas, not natural spaces in general, on mental health and reported a 55% higher risk of depression, anxiety, and substance use disorder later in life for people without exposure to green spaces (Engemann et al. 2019).

PSYCHOLOGICAL BENEFITS OF URBAN GREEN SPACE

Studies from several nations showed a positive correlation between better mental health outcomes and access to green spaces (Alcock et al. 2014; Beyer et al. 2014; Reklaitiene et al. 2014; Sugiyama et al. 2009; van den Bosch et al. 2015; Völker and Kistemann 2015; White et al. 2013). Green spaces were associated with lower mental distress scores on the General Health Questionnaire–12 in a study conducted in England (White et al. 2013). Neighboring green spaces are a protective factor against depression, stress, and anxiety, according to a Wisconsin study that used the 42-item Depression, Anxiety, and Stress Scale (Beyer et al. 2014). Adults living closer to green areas had lower Center for Epidemiologic Studies Depression Scale scores than their peers who lived further away from parks in Lithuania. Interestingly, they reported not only fewer depressive symptoms but also better perceived general health (Reklaitiene et al. 2014). Another British study showed that older adults had better lifestyle satisfaction when they had more access to neighborhood open spaces (Sugiyama et al. 2009). Researchers in Germany who conducted open interviews with 113 participants found that urban green spaces act as therapeutic landscapes within a city (Völker and Kistemann 2015). Going beyond the static effects of green spaces, several studies determined that moving to greener spaces can also improve mental health. In two 6- and 17-year studies in Sweden and England, respectively, it was shown that after moving to a greener area, participants reported improved General Health Questionnaire–12 mental health scores (Alcock et al. 2014; van den Bosch et al. 2015). These studies underscore the value of urban green spaces in promoting mental health during an era of urbanization.

ATTENTION RESTORATION AND STRESS REDUCTION IN THE URBAN SETTING

It is evident that urbanization and nature affect mental health, but what is the underlying mechanism? Anecdotally, people often report feelings of calm and freshness after being in nature that are not replicated in an urban environment. Wirth (1938), one of the first to build a theoretical framework around this issue, suggested that urbanization produces excessive differentiation between the occupational, recreational, and institutional aspects of life, ultimately driving poor social integration and social withdrawal. However, researchers did not begin to study the effects of nature on human psychology until the late 1970s. In a series of studies, Ulrich described a net positive effect of nature on mental health. Participants described increased friendliness, affection, and joy when shown scenes of nature, and conversely, they described feelings of sadness when shown scenes of urban areas. Urban areas increased feelings of aggression, and scenes of nature reduced those feelings. Finally, participants shown videos of nature after exposure to a stressful stimulus reported a reduction in their perceived stress that was not replicated for participants who were shown videos of an urban setting (Ulrich 1979, 1981, 1983, 1986; Ulrich et al. 1991b). Wilson (1984) described an innate need for humans to affiliate with a natural environment. The therapeutic effects of nature on mental health are now well documented (Hartig 2007), and two principal theories have emerged to explain these processes:

- The psychophysiological stress reduction theory posits that contact with nature elicits a positive emotional state (Ulrich 1983). This theory identifies nature as a nonthreatening stimulus. It follows that we recognize this stimulus as relaxing, which activates the parasympathetic nervous system to slow down the body and mind.
- The attention restoration theory holds that exposure to nature improves overall cognitive performance (Kaplan and Kaplan 2011). This theory characterizes nature as full of rich stimuli that attract involuntary attention. Direct attention, which is used to complete

tasks, takes effort and exists in a fixed quantity. In contrast, involuntary attention is a passive process that allows relaxation and improves subjective well-being.

Several studies examining the neurobiological effect of nature on mental health augment this psychological schema. One posited mechanism is that exposure to nature decreases rumination (Bratman et al. 2015). Rumination is defined as the continuous preoccupation with sad, dark, or negative thoughts, and it is highly correlated with psychiatric disorders (Nolen-Hoeksema 2000). Activity in the subgenual prefrontal cortex, which has been linked to rumination, decreases after a walk in nature but does not change after a walk in an urban setting (Bratman et al. 2015). The amygdala, which plays a key role in fear-related behaviors by detecting and responding to perceived dangerous stimuli, is also implicated in the response to urban settings. Amygdalar activity is greater in people brought up or living in urban areas than in people brought up or living in rural areas (Lederbogen et al. 2011). This increased activity can lead to maladaptive stress responses and negative mood when not tied to a noxious stimulus (Diorio et al. 1993). More globally, electroencephalography studies documented relaxing and restorative brain activity when participants walked in green spaces (Aspinall et al. 2015) and increased serotonin production, which is linked to elevated mood, associated with views of nature (Ulrich et al. 1991b).

In addition to these neurobiological changes, the urban environment affects hormonal antecedents to behavior. Cortisol is central to many body functions, including the regulation of the stress response. During a stressful event, the body releases cortisol so that people can respond to the environment appropriately. Dysregulation of cortisol release, and consequently a maladaptive stress response, is linked to psychiatric disorders (Vreeburg et al. 2010). A small-scale study showed a negative correlation between access to green space and daytime cortisol levels, with participants also self-reporting decreased stress levels (Ward Thompson et al. 2012). Natural environments also reduced other objective measures of stress, including blood pressure, heart rate, and muscle tension (Ottosson and Grahn 2005; Park et al. 2007; Ulrich et al. 1991a).

CONSIDERATIONS FOR SPECIAL POPULATIONS

Although most of these studies focused on adults, emerging evidence suggests that green spaces have positive effects on pediatric mental health. Increased access to green spaces at home and school is associated with better memory and attention (Dadvand et al. 2015). Additionally, in two large-sample studies, access to nature was associated with decreased hyperactivity and inattention symptoms for children with ADHD, the most prevalent neurodevelopmental disorder of childhood that affects millions of children across the United States alone (Amoly et al. 2014; Danielson et al. 2018; Faber Taylor and Kuo 2011). Engagement with nature also benefited children with autism spectrum disorder (Faber Taylor and Kuo 2011). In a longitudinal study from Spain, researchers described the association between improved overall health and access to green spaces as independent of co-occurring physical activity, suggesting that nature alone has a notable effect on pediatric mental health (Triguero-Mas et al. 2015). In response to these data, the World Health Organization (2010) set a goal to provide each child with access to green spaces worldwide. As part of its continued efforts, the World Health Organization (2017) published a brief for action that illustrated key considerations for incorporating green spaces into urban planning through reviewing research findings and highlighting case examples. In 2023, the World Health Organization (2023) released a valuation tool to strengthen the economic argument for policymakers to invest in urban green spaces for public health.

LESSONS FROM THE COVID-19 GLOBAL PANDEMIC

The need for urban green spaces has been powerfully underscored during worldwide crises, including the coronavirus disease 2019 (COVID-19) pandemic. In one study, one-third of participants reported moderate to severe anxiety on the Depression, Anxiety, and Stress Scale after 24 hours of at-home isolation. In the setting of travel restrictions, neighboring urban forests and green areas offered access to nature that reduced the mental health burden of the pandemic (Frühauf et al. 2020). Green parks provide a haven for people living in cities to mitigate mental stressors, and several studies from around the world concluded that open green spaces are more essential for mental health than they were before the pandemic (Lopez et al. 2021; Shabi 2020; Uchiyama and Kohsaka 2020).

Access to green spaces is linked with better mental health outcomes, and the quality of the space, including amenities, aesthetics, and safety, plays a more prominent role than the number of spaces available (Francis et al. 2012). Three specific perceived aspects of urban parks are strongly linked to decreased stress (Annerstedt et al. 2012; Grahn and Stigsdotter 2010): 1) *refuge,* defined as being in a place surrounded by higher vegetation, providing a feeling of safety; 2) *nature,* defined as "being in nature"; and 3) *serenity,* defined as being in a calm, undisturbed environment. Urban planners create multiple small green spaces that meet these criteria in lieu of a singular green space. However, meeting these high-quality demands still takes priority over quantity (Madureira et al. 2018; Wood et al. 2018).

Providing adequate green spaces to meet these standards in some major cities is challenging, but they are critical to mental wellness in our increasingly urbanizing society. Green spaces could be created wherever possible, be it unused lots, blocks, rooftops, or even walls of buildings; simply adding a layer of vegetation to existing buildings still has a positive effect (Mair 2024). The Atlanta BeltLine, Brooklyn Bridge Park, Railroad Park, the High Line, and Millennium Park are all examples of successful urban green space projects in the United States. Another good example of nature-urban integration is Singapore's Gardens by the Bay (Figure 4–1), which effectively uses buildings to create abundant green spaces.

NATURE THERAPY FOR URBAN INHABITANTS

Practical examples of using urban green spaces as mental health interventions validate their therapeutic utility across ages and disease presentations. In Belgium, some schools recruited students and parents to replace their concrete outdoor areas with trees, hedges, edible plants, and bird and insect hotels in order to increase active outdoor playtime and improve social behavior (European Environment Agency 2022). A small-scale intervention for children with ADHD included taking a 20-minute walk in a city park, which improved concentration when compared with a group that walked in a strictly urban setting. In Philadelphia, Pennsylvania, 342 adults participated in another promising urban green space intervention in 2018. Participants self-reported symptoms of depression on the Kessler-6 Psychological Distress Scale before and 18 months after the intervention. Half of the group then engaged in landscaping activities, including gardening and tree planting, whereas the other half did not. The "greening intervention" group reported fewer depressive symptoms on the postintervention evaluation

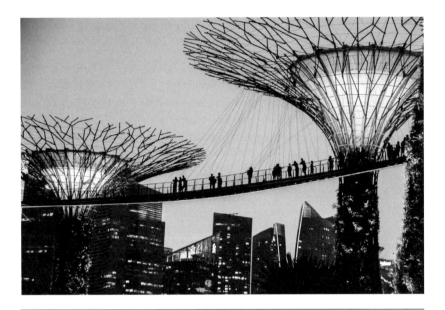

Figure 4–1. People standing on bridge at Gardens by the Bay in Singapore.
Source. Photograph by Vernon Raineil Cenzon, May 24, 2019. Reprinted under the Unsplash License. Available at: https://unsplash.com/photos/people-standing-on-bridge-RxhoczTcXbk. Accessed April 13, 2024.

than did the control group (South et al. 2018). In yet another intervention, patients with major depressive disorder managed with medication began 4 weeks of cognitive-behavioral therapy in either a forest environment or a hospital environment. Montgomery-Åsberg Depression Rating Scale scores of the forest group were significantly lower than those of the hospital group (Kim et al. 2009). Likewise, a 9-day therapy program conducted in a forest for people with alcohol use disorder and depression resulted in remission of depressive symptoms (Shin et al. 2012).

LIMITATIONS

As with any therapeutic modality, the potential risks of urban green spaces should be considered alongside their benefits. Although greenery effectively mitigates some airborne pollutants, the presence of a closed canopy near an industrial area can trap and contain carbon (Jin et al. 2014). Green spaces adjacent to heavily used roads have greater exposure to ozone, nitrogen dioxide, sulfur dioxide, and other pollutants (Carlisle 2001). Excessive and inappropriate use of pesticides and herbicides in urban parks introduces possible carcinogen exposure to humans (Guyton et al. 2015). Although evidence of a direct association between urban green areas and asthma or allergy is inconclusive (World Health Organization 2010), some studies include pollen exposure associated with urban green spaces as a self-reported trigger of asthma (Keddem et al. 2015). Any natural setting, including urban green spaces, can harbor vectors for zoonotic infections. These include diseases transmitted by ticks (e.g., Lyme disease), mosquitoes (e.g., chikungunya fever, dengue fever), and sand flies (e.g., leishmaniasis) (Medlock and Leach 2015). Domesticated and wild animal feces also may contaminate soil, increasing infection risk from agents such as *Toxocara canis* and *Toxoplasma gondii* (World Health Organization 2010). Simple precautions, such as limiting pets' access to children's play areas and encouraging pet walkers to remove their pets' excrement from the parks, can help prevent infections (Despommier 2003). Despite the countless benefits of physical activity in urban green spaces, there is a risk for accidental injuries such as falls and drowning (Kendrick et al. 2005). Most playground equipment–related injuries that occur in public urban green spaces can be reduced by the introduction of artificial, impact-absorbing surfaces (Ball 2004). Finally, excessive exposure to ultraviolet radiation by sunlight is another concern, but these negative effects can be mitigated by simple measures such as hats, clothing, and sunblock or by innovative architectural strategies to create shade (Boldemann et al. 2011).

More work remains to elucidate the complex link between nature and the mind, but it is clear that urban green spaces are beneficial for mental wellness. Mental health professionals should consider actively using nature in their treatment plan for their patients whenever possible. Given the ongoing trend of urbanization, urban green spaces will be an essential tool for people to mitigate the burden of stress, anxiety, depression, attention deficits, hyperactivity, and many other pervasive mental health problems.

Clinical Translation: Case Example

A 35-year-old White cisgender man with a history of generalized anxiety disorder and no medical problems presents with worsening anxiety to a standing virtual appointment with his psychiatrist. He lives in a one-bedroom apartment in New York City, works as a project manager from home, and spends his limited free time at his friend's apartment or at the gym. He received a diagnosis of generalized anxiety disorder 5 years before this appointment, did not benefit from sertraline, is currently taking escitalopram 15 mg/day and clonazepam 0.5 mg as needed for breakthrough anxiety, and attends weekly psychotherapy. He drinks alcohol socially and does not use tobacco products or other drugs. He reported an increase in his anxiety over the past week that he believes is associated with increased pressure at work. His schedule has not changed significantly, and he still keeps his gym schedule, but he has increased his use of clonazepam. Instead of changing his medication regimen, his psychiatrist recommended incorporating a walk in Central Park twice a week into his schedule.

One month later, the patient returned to the office and reported a decrease in his anxiety. He noted that his ruminating thoughts decreased, and he has not been using his clonazepam as frequently. He also stated that he has since purchased plants for his apartment, which have improved his mood even in the setting of increased demands at work and other life stressors.

KEY POINTS

- Having access to green spaces in cities improves mental health outcomes.

- Initially having limited access to green spaces but subsequently moving to a place with better access results in improved mental health outcomes.

- Although more extensive studies are needed, urban green areas can be used with other treatments for select patients.

- Many studies support the beneficial effects of green spaces on mental health among all age groups.

- There are many examples of inexpensive, innovative, and accessible ways of creating green spaces within cities, including building walls and rooftops.

QUESTIONS

1. A 9-year-old boy with a history of mild intermittent asthma and ADHD is brought into the clinic by his parents for shortness of breath. He was playing in a city park when he suddenly had difficulty breathing. He correctly used his albuterol inhaler as prescribed, with good effect. He is sitting comfortably and breathing without accessory muscle use. Examination shows no abnormalities. The patient shares that he feels better able to concentrate on his homework on days when he goes to the city park, but his parents are worried about his respiratory symptoms. What is the most appropriate recommendation to make at this time?

A. "Given that being in the park triggered his asthma, he should stop spending time at the park and should play indoors instead."
B. "Being outdoors in nature can worsen symptoms of ADHD, so he should stop spending time at the park and should play indoors instead."
C. "Spending time in nature is an important part of managing his ADHD symptoms, so he should keep spending time in the park, should carry his albuterol inhaler with him, and could use his inhaler before going outside if he plans to stay outside for a long time."
D. "Spending time in nature is an important part of managing his ADHD symptoms, so he should keep spending time in the park and does not need to carry his inhaler with him."
E. "Indoor physical activity is just as effective as outdoor physical activity for ADHD symptoms, so he should join a gym instead of playing outside in order to minimize his asthma triggers."

Correct answer: C. "Spending time in nature is an important part of managing his ADHD symptoms, so he should keep spending time in the park, should carry his albuterol inhaler with him, and could use his inhaler before going outside if he plans to stay outside for a long time."

Spending time in nature is associated with improved ADHD symptoms (B) so that treatment modality should be prioritized as long as it is safe for the patient. Given that his asthma symptoms were mild, responded well to his rescue inhaler, and did not cause prolonged respiratory distress, the benefits of being in nature outweigh the risks of asthma exacerbation (A). However, appropriate measures to manage his asthma should be taken, including always having a rescue inhaler and even considering pretreatment (D). Finally, spending time in nature improves ADHD symptoms in an independent and even additive way to physical activity, so indoor physical activity would not have the same beneficial effects (E).

2. A 36-year-old woman with a history of generalized anxiety disorder presents for an annual physical examination. She takes a daily multivitamin and escitalopram 10 mg/day for her anxiety, which is working well without side effects. With the medication, she noticed

an improvement in her fearlike anxiety response to new situations, but she still ruminates over minor incidents throughout her day. Her physician recommends that she go for a daily walk in her local city park. Which area of the brain is this new intervention most likely to target for this specific patient?

    A. Substantia nigra.
    B. Subgenual prefrontal cortex.
    C. Amygdala.
    D. Occipital cortex.
    E. Pons.

Correct answer: B. Subgenual prefrontal cortex.

The neurobiological basis of ecotherapy is a very active area of research, but some brain areas have already been implicated in its mechanism. This patient's main concern is rumination, which is thought to be mediated by the subgenual prefrontal cortex and can be influenced by exposure to nature. Another target of ecotherapy is the amygdala and the fear response, which is not this patient's concern (C). There is no evidence linking ecotherapy to the substantia nigra (movement regulation), occipital cortex (visual processing), or pons (brain stem reflexes) as a way to mitigate anxiety symptoms (A, D, E).

3. A city planner is working with your local health department to design a healthy city. The team has already planned to use green energy sources, to appropriately map out access to grocery stores, and to spread out hospitals and urgent care centers. The city planner is now working on parks. In order to maximize this population's mental health, what is the best recommendation to make regarding city parks?

    A. Build as many parks as possible with concrete and minimal greenery.
    B. Do not build any parks.
    C. Build as many parks as possible, with minimal greenery and high pesticide use.
    D. Build a few parks with lush greenery, some large trees, and minimal sound pollution.
    E. Do not build any parks, but plant a few trees on the outskirts of the city.

Correct answer: D. Build a few parks with lush greenery, some large trees, and minimal sound pollution.

Numerous benefits are associated with urban green spaces, including the maintenance and treatment of mental health. City parks are an effective way to introduce green spaces into a highly urban environment and should be integrated whenever possible (B, E). Although having more parks available increases access to green spaces, the beneficial effects of these parks are also heavily dependent on their quality. Key elements of urban green spaces that promote mental health include refuge, nature, and serenity, which cannot be accomplished with minimal greenery (A). Additionally, excessive pesticide use introduces physical health concerns (C). In these situations, fewer parks that meet the criteria for effectively promoting mental health would be most effective.

REFERENCES

Alcock I, White MP, Wheeler BW, et al: Longitudinal effects on mental health of moving to greener and less green urban areas. Environ Sci Technol 48(2):1247–1255, 2014 24320055

Amoly E, Dadvand P, Forns J, et al: Green and blue spaces and behavioral development in Barcelona schoolchildren: the BREATHE Project. Environ Health Perspect 122(12):1351–1358, 2014 25204008

Anguluri R, Narayanan P: Role of green space in urban planning: outlook towards smart cities. Urban for Urban Green 25:58–65, 2017

Annerstedt M, Östergren PO, Björk J, et al: Green qualities in the neighbourhood and mental health: results from a longitudinal cohort study in Southern Sweden. BMC Public Health 12(1):337, 2012 22568888

Aspinall P, Mavros P, Coyne R, et al: The urban brain: analysing outdoor physical activity with mobile EEG. Br J Sports Med 49(4):272–276, 2015 23467965

Astell-Burt T, Feng X: Association of urban green space with mental health and general health among adults in Australia. JAMA Netw Open 2(7):e198209, 2019 31348510

Ball DJ: Policy issues and risk–benefit trade-offs of "safer surfacing" for children's playgrounds. Accident Anal Prev 36(4):661–670, 2004 15094421

Beyer K, Kaltenbach A, Szabo A, et al: Exposure to neighborhood green space and mental health: evidence from the Survey of the Health of Wisconsin. Int J Environ Res Public Health 11(3):3453–3472, 2014 24662966

Boldemann C, Dal H, Martensson F, et al: Preschool outdoor play environment may combine promotion of children's physical activity and sun protection: further evidence from Southern Sweden and North Carolina. Science and Sports 4(2):72–82, 2011

Bratman GN, Hamilton JP, Hahn KS, et al: Nature experience reduces rumination and subgenual prefrontal cortex activation. Proc Natl Acad Sci U S A 112(28):8567–8572, 2015 26124129

Buzzell LCC: Ecotherapy: Healing With Nature in Mind. Edited by Chalquist C, Buzzell L. San Francisco, CA, Sierra Club Books, 2009

Carlisle AJ: Exercise and outdoor ambient air pollution. Br J Sports Med 35(4):214–222, 2001 11477012

Dadvand P, Nieuwenhuijsen MJ, Esnaola M, et al: Green spaces and cognitive development in primary schoolchildren. Proc Natl Acad Sci U S A 112(26):7937–7942, 2015 26080420

Danielson ML, Bitsko RH, Ghandour RM, et al: Prevalence of parent-reported ADHD diagnosis and associated treatment among U.S. children and adolescents, 2016. J Clin Child Adolesc Psychol 47(2):199–212, 2018 29363986

Despommier D: Toxocariasis: clinical aspects, epidemiology, medical ecology, and molecular aspects. Clin Microbiol Rev 16(2):265–272, 2003 12692098

Diorio D, Viau V, Meaney M: The role of the medial prefrontal cortex (cingulate gyrus) in the regulation of hypothalamic-pituitary-adrenal responses to stress. J Neurosci 13(9):3839–3847, 1993 8396170

Dye C: Health and urban living. Science 319(5864):766–769, 2008 18258905

Engemann K, Pedersen CB, Arge L, et al: Residential green space in childhood is associated with lower risk of psychiatric disorders from adolescence into adulthood. Proc Natl Acad Sci U S A 116(11):5188–5193, 2019 30804178

European Environment Agency: Mapping Guide for a European Urban Atlas. Copenhagen, Denmark, European Environment Agency, 2011

European Environment Agency: Green schoolyards in Flemish Brabant, Belgium. February 1, 2022. Available at: https://www.eea.europa.eu/publications/who-benefits-from-nature-in/green-schoolyards-in-flemish-brabant-belgium. Accessed April 13, 2024.

Faber Taylor A, Kuo FEM: Could exposure to everyday green spaces help treat ADHD? Evidence from children's play settings. Appl Psychol Health Well Being 3(3):281–303, 2011

Francis J, Wood LJ, Knuiman M, et al: Quality or quantity? Exploring the relationship between public open space attributes and mental health in Perth, Western Australia. Soc Sci Med 74(10):1570–1577, 2012 22464220

Frühauf A, Schnitzer M, Schobersberger W, et al: Jogging, Nordic walking and going for a walk—inter-disciplinary recommendations to keep people physically active in times of the COVID-19 lockdown in Tyrol, Austria. Current Issues in Sport Science 5:10011–10014, 2020

Grahn P, Stigsdotter UK: The relation between perceived sensory dimensions of urban green space and stress restoration. Landsc Urban Plan 94(3–4):264–275, 2010

Guyton KZ, Loomis D, Grosse Y, et al: Carcinogenicity of tetrachlorvinphos, parathion, malathion, diazinon, and glyphosate. Lancet Oncol 16(5):490–491, 2015 25801782

Hartig T: Three steps to understanding restorative environments as health resources, in Open Space: People Space. Edited by Ward Thompson C, Travlou P. Oxford, UK, Taylor & Francis, 2007, pp 163–179

Jin S, Guo J, Wheeler S, et al: Evaluation of impacts of trees on PM2.5 dispersion in urban streets. Atmos Environ 99:277–287, 2014

Jones P: Roosters, hawks and dawgs: toward an inclusive, embodied eco/feminist psychology. Fem Psychol 20(3):365–380, 2010

Kaplan R, Kaplan S: Well-being, reasonableness, and the natural environment. Appl Psychol Health Well Being 3(3):304–321, 2011

Keddem S, Barg FK, Glanz K, et al: Mapping the urban asthma experience: using qualitative GIS to understand contextual factors affecting asthma control. Soc Sci Med 140:9–17, 2015 26184704

Kendrick D, Mulvaney C, Burton P, et al: Relationships between child, family and neighbourhood characteristics and childhood injury: a cohort study. Soc Sci Med 61(9):1905–1915, 2005 15927334

Kim W, Lim SK, Chung EJ, et al: The effect of cognitive behavior therapy-based psychotherapy applied in a forest environment on physiological changes and remission of major depressive disorder. Psychiatry Investig 6(4):245–254, 2009 20140122

Lederbogen F, Kirsch P, Haddad L, et al: City living and urban upbringing affect neural social stress processing in humans. Nature 474(7352):498–501, 2011 21697947

Lopez B, Kennedy C, Field C, et al: Who benefits from urban green spaces during times of crisis? Perception and use of urban green spaces in New York City during the COVID-19 pandemic. Urban for Urban Green 65:127354, 2021

Madureira H, Nunes F, Oliveira J, et al: Preferences for urban green space characteristics: a comparative study in three Portuguese cities. Environments 5(2):23, 2018

Mair C: City life: Why are green spaces important? London, Natural History Museum. Available at: https://www.nhm.ac.uk/discover/why-we-need-green-spaces-in-cities.html. Accessed April 13, 2024.

Medlock JM, Leach SA: Effect of climate change on vector-borne disease risk in the UK. Lancet Infect Dis 15(6):721–730, 2015 25808458

Millennium Ecosystem Assessment: How have ecosystems changed?, in Scientific Facts on Ecosystem Change. Edited by Green-Facts Scientific Board. Brussels, Belgium, GreenFacts, 2005, p 3

Nolen-Hoeksema S: The role of rumination in depressive disorders and mixed anxiety/depressive symptoms. J Abnormal Psychol 109(3):504–511, 2000 11016119

Olson M: Introduction. Daedalus 102(4):1–13, 1973. Available at: http://www.jstor.org/stable/20024163. Accessed April 14, 2024.

Ottosson J, Grahn P: A comparison of leisure time spent in a garden with leisure time spent indoors: on measures of restoration in residents in geriatric care. Landsc Res 30(1):23–55, 2005

Park BJ, Tsunetsugu Y, Kasetani T, et al: Physiological effects of Shinrin-yoku (taking in the atmosphere of the forest)—using salivary cortisol and cerebral activity as indicators. J Physiol Anthropol 26(2):123–128, 2007 17435354

Peen J, Schoevers RA, Beekman AT, et al: The current status of urban-rural differences in psychiatric disorders. Acta Psychiatr Scand 121(2):84–93, 2010 19624573

Pickard BR, Daniel J, Mehaffey M, et al: EnviroAtlas: a new geospatial tool to foster ecosystem services science and resource management. Ecosyst Serv 14:45–55, 2015

Reklaitiene R, Grazuleviciene R, Dedele A, et al: The relationship of green space, depressive symptoms and perceived general health in urban population. Scand J Public Health 42(7):669–676, 2014 25118199

Shabi R: Sanctuary in the city: how urban parks saved our summer. The
    Guardian, August 9, 2020. Available at: https://www.theguardian.com/
    travel/2020/aug/09/sanctuary-in-the-city-how-urban-parks-saved-our-
    summer. Accessed April 13, 2024.
Shin WS, Shin CS, Yeoun PS: The influence of forest therapy camp on depres-
    sion in alcoholics. Environ Health Prev Med 17(1):73–76, 2012 21503628
South EC, Hohl BC, Kondo MC, et al: Effect of greening vacant land on mental
    health of community-dwelling adults. JAMA Netw Open 1(3):e180298,
    2018 30646029
Sugiyama T, Thompson CW, Alves S: Associations between neighborhood
    open space attributes and quality of life for older people in Britain. Environ
    Behav 41(1):3–21, 2009
Triguero-Mas M, Dadvand P, Cirach M, et al: Natural outdoor environments
    and mental and physical health: relationships and mechanisms. Environ
    Int 77:35–41, 2015 25638643
Uchiyama Y, Kohsaka R: Access and use of green areas during the COVID-19
    pandemic: green infrastructure management in the "new normal." Sustain-
    ability 12(23):9842, 2020
Ulrich RS: Visual landscapes and psychological well-being. Landsc Res 4(1):17–
    23, 1979
Ulrich RS: Natural versus urban scenes. Environ Behav 13(5):523–556, 1981
Ulrich RS: Aesthetic and affective response to natural environment, in Behavior
    and the Natural Environment. Edited by Altman I, Wohlwill JF. New York,
    Springer, 1983, pp 85–125
Ulrich RS: Human responses to vegetation and landscapes. Landsc Urban Plan
    13:29–44, 1986
Ulrich RS, Dimberg U, Driver BL: Psychophysiological indicators of leisure ben-
    efits, in Benefits of Leisure. Edited by Driver BL, Brown PJ, Peterson GL.
    State College, PA, Venture, 1991a, pp 154–166
Ulrich RS, Simons RF, Losito BD, et al: Stress recovery during exposure to nat-
    ural and urban environments. J Environ Psychol 11(3):201–230, 1991b
United Nations: Urbanization: expanding opportunities but deeper divides, in
    World Social Report 2020. New York, February 21, 2020. Available at:
    https://www.un.org/development/desa/en/news/social/urbanization-
    expanding-opportunities-but-deeper-
    divides.html#:~:text=Whether%20the%20process%20of%20urbanization,
    DESA's%20World%20Social%20Report%202020. Accessed April 13, 2024.
van den Berg AE, Maas J, Verheij RA, et al: Green space as a buffer between
    stressful life events and health. Soc Sci Med 70(8):1203–1210, 2010
    20163905
van den Bosch M, Östergren PO, Grahn P, et al: Moving to serene nature may
    prevent poor mental health—results from a Swedish longitudinal cohort
    study. Int J Environ Res Public Health 12(7):7974–7985, 2015 26184268
Völker S, Kistemann T: Developing the urban blue: comparative health re-
    sponses to blue and green urban open spaces in Germany. Health Place
    35:196–205, 2015 25475835
Vreeburg SA, Zitman FG, van Pelt J, et al: Salivary cortisol levels in persons with
    and without different anxiety disorders. Psychosom Med 72(4):340–347,
    2010 20190128

Wang JL: Rural-urban differences in the prevalence of major depression and associated impairment. Soc Psychiatry Psychiatr Epidemiol 39(1):19–25, 2004 15022042

Ward Thompson C, Roe J, Aspinall P, et al: More green space is linked to less stress in deprived communities: evidence from salivary cortisol patterns. Landsc Urban Plan 105(3):221–229, 2012

White MP, Alcock I, Wheeler BW, et al: Would you be happier living in a greener urban area? A fixed-effects analysis of panel data. Psychol Sci 24(6):920–928, 2013 23613211

Wilson EO: Biophilia. Cambridge, MA, Harvard University Press, 1984

Wirth L: Urbanism as a way of life. Am J Sociol 44(1):1–24, 1938

Wood E, Harsant A, Dallimer M, et al: Not all green space is created equal: biodiversity predicts psychological restorative benefits from urban green space. Front Psychol 9:2320, 2018 30538653

World Health Organization: Parma Declaration on Environment and Health, presented at Fifth Ministerial Conference on Environment and Health, "Protecting Children's Health in a Changing Environment." Copenhagen, Denmark, WHO Regional Office for Europe, March 2010

World Health Organization: Urban Green Spaces: A Brief for Action. Copenhagen, Denmark, WHO Regional Office for Europe, 2017

World Health Organization: Assessing the Value of Urban Green and Blue Spaces for Health and Well-Being (No WHO/EURO 2023-7508-47275-69347). Copenhagen, Denmark, WHO Regional Office for Europe, 2023

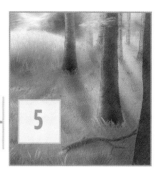

5

Horticultural Therapy

AN APPLICATION FOR WHOLE HEALTH AND HEALING

Abby Jaroslow, M.S., HTR, CH
Anne Meore, LMSW, HTR

> *In every walk with nature,*
> *one receives far more than he seeks.*
> —John Muir (1877, p. 3)

Since early civilization, the people-plant relationship has influenced many aspects of human culture. Plants have given us food, shelter, and safety and inspired us to create through art and science, and we have found respite and rejuvenation while being near them. Modern re-

The authors would like to thank Lauren Byma for her contribution of the case study of Ms. D.

search and clinical observation support the belief that people have an innate inclination to be connected with nature. Research also supports the belief that beyond spending time in nature, active engagement in caring for plants at home, in the garden, at the office or school, and even in health care settings provides physiological, psychological, and social benefits. Registered horticultural therapists (HTRs) and trained allied professionals use this knowledge to develop treatment plans by incorporating horticultural activities to support clinical healing, health, and wellness goals across a wide spectrum of individual needs, as shown in Figure 5–1.

The unique quality of horticultural therapy, setting it apart from other nature therapies, is the close relationship a person has with a plant when caring for and nurturing it (planting, grooming, watering, feeding, weeding, pruning, harvesting). Plants respond in a nonjudgmental, positive way, over time, providing an opportunity for the therapist to guide the patient in observing how aspects of the person-plant relationship are transferable to the human relationships we have with family, friends, and self. The horticultural therapist in Figure 5–2 joins hands with the patient, nurturing both the growth of the plant and the therapeutic alliance. Like a plant, a person needs attention, kindness, water, food, patience, time, and compassion to thrive and make healthy relationships. Metaphors found in nature, and with plant life, are abundant and serve as impactful tools in horticultural therapy.

In the following pages, we present an overview of horticultural therapy as a professional practice in its own right and describe the history and theoretical underpinnings of the practice. Next, we introduce therapeutic horticulture, which can be applied across a broader field of professional specialties or in collaboration with a credentialed horticultural therapist. Finally, we describe the knowledge and practical considerations needed to use horticultural therapy or therapeutic horticulture as a therapeutic modality. We address the following:

- The evolution of the relationship between health care and nature and people and plants
- The history of horticultural therapy as a professional practice for improving function across multiple functional domains by using patient engagement in horticultural activities
- The theoretical underpinnings of the practice of horticultural therapy
- An overview of early research and an introduction to current research that seeks to document clinical evidence of the efficacy of the practice
- The commonalities and differences between horticultural therapy and therapeutic horticulture as defined by the American Horticultural Therapy Association (2021)

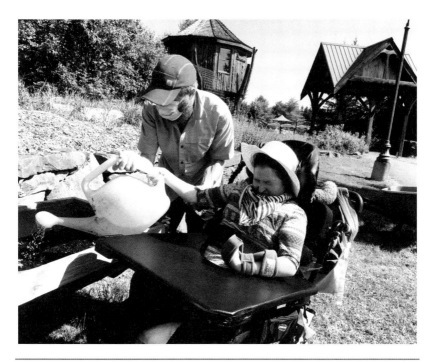

Figure 5–1.   Therapeutic healing garden at an intermediate care facility.

Source.   Photograph courtesy of A. Jaroslow.

- The practical application of therapeutic horticulture for allied professionals (psychologists, psychiatrists, physical and occupational therapists, social workers, addiction counselors, teachers, nurses) and anyone interested in understanding how human engagement with plants provides therapeutic benefit, whether guided by a therapist or when caring for plants independently

HEALTH CARE– NATURE RELATIONSHIP: A DYNAMIC PARTNERSHIP

The first recorded use of nature engagement in a formal garden for improving health, wellness, and quality of life has been traced to ancient Egypt, 3000 B.C. Supported by the Tigris, Euphrates, and Nile rivers, the fertile region fostered terraced gardens and water features (Mulligan

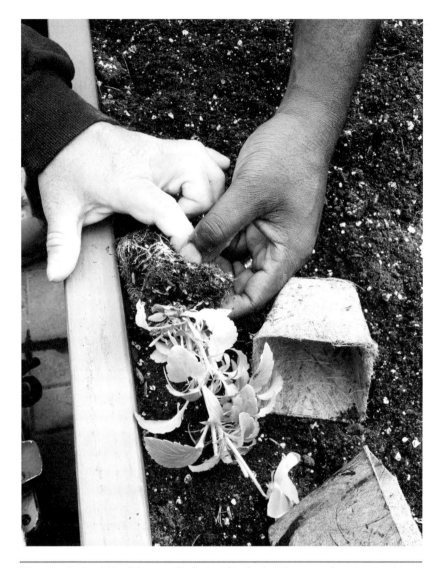

Figure 5-2. Working collaboratively in the garden to nurture plants and the people-plant relationship.
Source. Photograph courtesy of A. Meore.

1995). In these gardens, physicians used horticulture as a therapeutic treatment by prescribing walks in the garden to calm royal family members deemed to have mental illness (Lewis 1976).

According to Mulligan (1995), garden aesthetics spread from one culture to another. People, regardless of backgrounds, cultures, and class, have consistently turned to nature for relaxation and in times of celebration or misfortune. Evidence was found confirming the existence of bathhouses in Greece in the fourth century B.C., where healing rituals were performed to cleanse and rejuvenate the body with pure, fresh spring water in natural settings, lush with plants (Gesler 2003).

Monastic communities of the Middle Ages provided a safe haven to people in need because of physical or mental illness, poverty, or homelessness before hospitals, as we know them, existed. The monastic garden, surrounded by a covered cloister, may have provided herbs for remedies, but the monks were not trained in providing medical care. They could only provide comfort, food, and a warm place to sleep to those they sheltered. Nonetheless, the gardens would have provided access to nature, fresh air, sunlight, and flowering plants, giving the sick and weary visitors some respite. Other religious charities followed the monastic model, opening their doors to people who were sick, orphaned, disabled, or otherwise disenfranchised from their communities. Like the monasteries, these entities could not provide medical care, and instead they served as charitable hostels providing food, clothing, a place to sleep, and access to gardens or verdant grounds. This may have at least allowed people to reap the restorative benefit of connecting with nature. Although not curative, these opportunities for restful contemplation in nature probably provided a temporary sense of well-being.

Monastic and charity hospitality faded by the fifteenth century. Care of the ill and impoverished fell to civic organizations, poorly equipped to manage the plagues, poverty, and transient populations of the period. Families with the means to do so cared for their ailing loved ones at home, but the disadvantaged suffered with the limited resources available to them (Gerlach-Spriggs et al. 1998). As the Middle Ages gave way to the Renaissance, conditions in health care changed slowly. During this era of innovation in the arts and sciences, approaches to treating illness began to rely on scientific findings.

By the eighteenth century, advocates, including Florence Nightingale, called for improving public health outcomes by promoting a scientific approach to care. Public health reformers promoted the belief that good hygiene, skilled nursing, and differentiating patients according to symptoms would aid in preventing the spread of infection. These practitioners believed that fresh air and sunshine helped prevent infection and were needed for curing disease and healing the patient. With that in mind, the pavilion-style hospital was created and adopted throughout England and North America. The pavilion design, with long, open wards and beds running down each side, provided an orderly space in which nurses could work. Large windows along both sides of the ward allowed fresh, cross-ventilated air to flow across the room, and patients were able to view trees and the sky while convalescing. The addition of restorative gardens and expansive landscapes soon followed. This hospital design was favored for its efficiency and the ability it afforded to maintain a clean, airy atmosphere. Beds often could be rolled outdoors to accessible patios adjoining the building so that patients could receive large doses of fresh air and sunlight (Gerlach-Spriggs et al. 1998).

Patients convalescing in the eighteenth-century pavilion-style hospitals were separated by condition, as was recommended by the public health reformers of the period. Those with infectious disease and those living with mental health conditions were removed from the common wards to be housed in separate quarters. In Europe and England, the specialized public asylums and solaria were designed in the style of great estates of the period, with bucolic, pastoral landscapes. The health care reformers believed that quarantining patients with infectious disease would reduce the spread of disease, thus reducing the number of deaths. The understanding of infectious disease became more sophisticated by the mid-nineteenth and into the twentieth century, through advancements in medicine, such as the discovery of penicillin. At the same time, with advances in the construction industry, including the ability to build taller and bigger buildings, new hospital designs featured the sealed, monolithic buildings, surrounded by parking lots, we are familiar with today (Cooper Marcus and Sachs 2014). The thought that nature played any role in health care became obsolete.

Humane treatment for patients with mental health and behavioral conditions was introduced at the end of the eighteenth and into the nineteenth century as a new approach to the care of psychiatric patients. Socialization and meaningful physical activities became the new normal for psychiatric patients. It was believed that this approach would advance recovery. The theory held that if provided with a safe, socially and physically stable environment, the patient could establish a structured lifestyle that resembled the way that people lived outside the institution. The French physician who first experimented with this approach called it *traitement moral*, which was translated to "moral treatment" when it was brought to the United States (Gerlach-Spriggs et al. 1998).

Benjamin Rush, M.D., a prominent citizen and medical physician, lived and worked in Philadelphia, Pennsylvania, during this time of changing attitudes in psychiatric health care. He had studied medicine in the United Kingdom and traveled to Europe, where he was impressed by the psychiatric hospitals and care provided to those patients.

Returning to Philadelphia, he became a teacher at the Institute of Medical and Clinical Practice, had his own medical practice, and was a prominent civic leader. In fact, Dr. Rush signed the Declaration of Independence.

After joining the staff at Pennsylvania Hospital, Dr. Rush quickly became disheartened by the care of mental health patients there. He convinced the hospital to adopt the moral treatment approach to patient care. He proposed the theory, practiced in some hospitals in Europe, that hands-on, occupational opportunities facilitated the recovery of psychiatric patients. Dr. Rush believed that meaningful physical labor and access to nature were important components of care because they helped create a normal lifestyle for his patients. He wrote a treatise on the treatment of mental health patients in which he wrote that "cutting wood…digging in the dirt…washing and scrubbing floors" often could lead to a cure (Rush 1812, p. 226). He suggested that psychiatric patients be housed in a separate facility from the main hospital, in a farm setting where they could work in the fields, experiencing physical labor outdoors. Years later, Dr. Rush became known as the "Father of American Psychiatry" (Penn Medicine 2021).

Dr. Rush died before he saw the first private psychiatric hospital built in the United States. It was conceptualized by Philadelphia's Quaker community, in 1813, and built under the direction of Thomas Kirkbride, M.D., LL.D., founder of the American Psychiatric Association (Davis 1998). Known now as Friends Hospital, it has continued to serve as a psychiatric hospital for more than 200 years. The design of the building and its grounds took cues from the European and English psychiatric hospitals with their Romantic-style landscapes, complete with long, winding, shaded walkways and wide-open grassy meadows. This gave the patients a chance to engage in a passive form of therapeutic horticulture, enjoying the calming and stress-reducing benefit of being in nature. The active engagement in farming and caring for the grounds was prescribed by doctors following Dr. Rush's treatise. Dr. Kirkbride, having become a strong advocate for the design principles used at Friends Hospital, created a set of guidelines for building asylums in the same manner. By the early twentieth century, 28 states had public asylum campuses built following the Kirkbride Plan (Cooper Marcus and Sachs 2014).

The Menninger Foundation, a psychiatric clinic opened in 1919 in Topeka, Kansas, was known for its innovative approaches to the practice of psychiatry. The positive results of using the landscape for active and passive engagement by patients at Friends Hospital prompted the Menninger Foundation and Kansas State University to collaborate on a

university-level curriculum that incorporated a horticulture component, specifically designed for psychology students. In addition to
coursework in psychology and horticulture, the program required the
completion of a 7-month clinical internship working with patients at the
Menninger Foundation (Shapiro and Kaplan 1998).

The rapid growth of American industrialization in the eighteenth
and nineteenth centuries created dense urban centers where workers'
housing was built in close proximity to the factories where they were
employed. As cities grew, green space and planted ground were replaced by new construction and paved roadways. The result was
cramped living conditions in tenement-style buildings, polluted air,
dirty streets, and long hours on the job in equally confined, noisy, and
unhealthy environments. With these compounding stressors to contend
with on a daily basis and with little means to combat them, working-
class families were becoming disconnected from nature. At the same
time, the wealthy factory owners, businesspeople, and politicians, with
the financial means to escape the urban chaos, built townhouses or elab-
orate apartment buildings on the outskirts of the city and landscaped
vacation retreats miles away in the countryside and in the mountains.
Landscape designers, architects, artists, and writers, who had seen the
magnificent grand estates and landscapes of Europe and England,
brought the Romantic design movement back to the United States and
to these bucolic country estates.

The mid-nineteenth century saw the emergence of an urban social
reform movement. Davis (1998) cited an 1896 book that described the
Children's Aid Society providing horticultural activities to children living in tenement housing. Davis (1998) contended that this was the first
recorded case of engagement in horticultural activities for the purpose
of improving the well-being of disadvantaged youths.

The development of public parks was another aspect of social reform
in cities across the United States. The New York City Parks Commission
believed that, as the city grew, a residential community would grow up
around the 843 undeveloped acres they had purchased and set aside for
parkland, at what was then the northernmost boundary of the city. The
commissioners held a design contest to find a landscape design team
that would be able to manage a project of that scale. The Greensward
Plan, created by landscape architects Frederick Law Olmsted and
Calvert Vaux, was the winning entry (Rogers 1977). It was a bold proposal that incorporated the Romantic landscape design sensibility of
the grand estates in Europe and England.

Along with emphasizing aesthetics and circulation, the Greensward
Plan considered how the park experience would affect people in moral,

social, physical, and emotional ways. Olmsted, the visionary of the team and a believer in the social reform movement, described a verdant landscape with the capacity to provide respite and rejuvenation for working families (Kavanaugh 1994). The park was to be free of noise, pollution, and the hectic pace of the city outside its walls. It was to be accessible to the diverse city population, regardless of financial means or cultural status. To this day, Central Park continues to be referred to as the Lungs of New York City (Rogers 1977).

Until the early 1900s, the use of horticultural activities and time spent engaging in nature had been considered an appropriate treatment modality primarily for patients with psychiatric and behavioral conditions. However, after two world wars, the United States had to tend to a growing number of young men who had lost limbs and sustained severe physical and neurological injuries during their service. Instead of being adequately rehabilitated and sent home, these men were languishing in long-term health care facilities. Fortunately, these facilities provided diversional activities to pass the long days in which limited rehabilitation care was given. One of the leisure activities was engaging in horticultural activity, which was gaining momentum as a practical modality within the emerging practice of occupational therapy (Davis 1998).

A well-respected physician and advocate for an emerging approach to the care of people with physical disabilities was Howard Rusk, M.D. In the early 1940s, Dr. Rusk's professional focus was the practice of physiatry, also known as physical medicine and rehabilitation, a medical specialty involving the prevention, diagnosis, and treatment of disease or injury in the nerves, muscles, bones, and connective tissues (American Academy of Physical Medicine and Rehabilitation 2024). Dr. Rusk opened the Rusk Institute in New York City in 1951. Believing in the treatment of the whole person, Dr. Rusk brought together occupational, physical, and speech therapists to offer prosthetic and vocational training and psychosocial services. While Dr. Rusk was opening his rehabilitation hospital, the occupational therapy training department at Bloomingdale Hospital, in White Plains, New York, was offering training in horticulture skills to its students (Davis 1998). Shortly after opening the hospital, Dr. Rusk had a greenhouse built on the ground floor, known as the Glass Garden. Its first horticulturist was tasked with developing a stand-alone horticultural therapy program separate from the other rehabilitative therapies. Within the walls of the Rusk Institute's Glass Garden, horticultural activities flourished for more than 50 years under the guidance of trained horticultural therapists, many of whom are now leaders and teachers in the field of horticultural therapy (Chambers et al. 2014).

The growing trend to engage people in horticultural activities as part of their treatment plan, whether in rehabilitation, psychiatric, or elder care facilities, piqued the interest of community members passionate about gardening. An influx of garden club volunteers in the 1950s and 1960s created visibility for horticulture and nature engagement in health care settings and assisted the practitioners who were leading the way in creating a new profession (Davis 1998).

Engagement in horticultural activities was being offered as a therapeutic modality in many more settings by the mid-1960s and into the next decade. The 1970s saw a green movement emerge across the United States, with people becoming interested in cleaning up the environment, recycling, and growing and eating organic food (Janick 1992). The first Earth Day events were held in 1970. Enrollment in university horticulture departments increased as interest in agriculture and gardening grew. Organizations and treatment facilities working with patients with physical and psychiatric disabilities, children and older adults, prison populations, and those in schools and in other settings were introducing horticulture as a therapeutic activity in their programming (Haller et al. 2019).

The first national meeting of these practitioners was held in 1973, with the goal of codifying the use of horticulture as a therapeutic tool. The meeting was attended by horticulturists; psychologists; educators; volunteers from garden clubs and expert gardeners; professionals from the fields of occupational, physical, and recreational therapy; those working in correctional facilities; and others. From that meeting, the National Council for Therapy and Rehabilitation Through Horticulture (NCTRH) was formed, with 85 original members. By 1974, NCTRH membership had risen to 335, representing 40 states, England, and Canada (Haller et al. 2019).

The mission of the NCTRH was to formalize the best horticultural therapy practice standards and promote the profession. The organization developed educational publications, created national and international networking opportunities, and held annual conferences. One of the original members of the NCTRH was Richard Mattson, Ph.D., a floriculture professor at Kansas State University. Soon after, Dr. Mattson developed an academic curriculum for horticulture students wanting to explore a profession in horticultural therapy. Several university-level degree programs soon followed the Kansas State University model, offering certificate programs in horticultural therapy (Haller et al. 2019).

All those working in the fields of horticultural therapy, ecopsychology, environmental studies, and similar pursuits understood that people are drawn to nature and gardening and that health benefits are inherent in nature engagement. In order to promote their work, a primary directive from the NCTRH leadership was to publish academic papers in science and medical journals and provide data showing the positive benefits of the practice. Several authors emerged, writing on the subject from a variety of perspectives. The early work, written by horticulturists, psychologists, and environmentalists, continues to be referenced today by researchers, practitioners, and instructors.

THEORETICAL UNDERPINNINGS: THE BUILDING BLOCKS OF SUPPORT FOR THERAPEUTIC HORTICULTURE

The practical theory behind horticultural therapy and therapeutic horticulture is *hortophilia*, a term introduced by neurologist, author, and humanist Oliver Sacks, M.D., who firmly believed in the benefit of the human connection people have with plants. Dr. Sacks pointed to a distinct difference between *biophilia* and *hortophilia*. Whereas *biophilia* (*bio* meaning "life" and *philia* meaning "love of") describes the intrinsic human love of all living things, *hortophilia* (*hortus* meaning "garden" and *philia* meaning "love of") is the deeply embedded human desire to interact with and nurture plants, which calls people of all ages, as seen in Figure 5–3, to engage in horticultural activities such as gardening and maintaining house or office plants (Sacks 2019). This is what makes horticultural therapy distinctive among the many new approaches to nature therapy (Figure 5–4).

One of the earliest and most prolific authors to write about the people-plant relationship was Charles Lewis, horticulturist and director of collections at a prominent arboretum in the suburbs of Chicago, Illinois. Lewis researched human evolution to gain insight into and understanding as to why human beings have a strong connection with plants and a preference for certain types of landscapes. His conclusion was that an evolutionary bond exists that has left a genetic imprint from the time when the species first lived and relied on the land for food, shelter, and safety. Evolutionary scientists identified the region where this took place as the African savanna. Because the population in that region would have been hunter-gatherers, moving from one place to another, their safety depended on being able to quickly assess the land's resources and select the best location for protection and ample food. The savanna landscape included a protected area in which to forage for food and build shelter. In the distance, there would be a wooded area of tall trees with a high canopy and no underbrush. A wide area of open land,

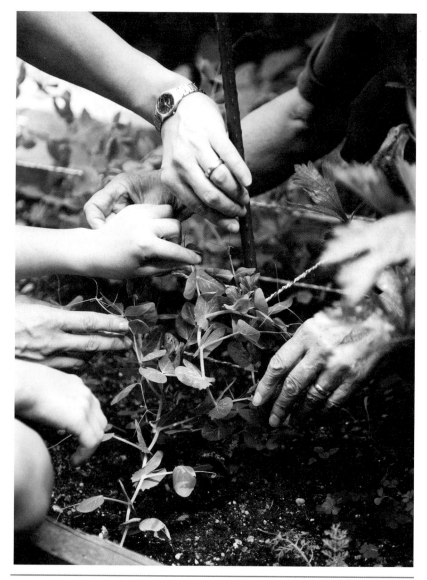

Figure 5–3. Trellising activity promoting cooperation and social support with an intergenerational population.
Source. Photograph courtesy of A. Meore.

between the protected home base and the tall trees, would allow the community to see danger approaching with plenty of time to escape quickly into the protected areas around them.

Researchers have found that when given a choice between the savanna and other types of landscapes, children and many adults will choose the sa-

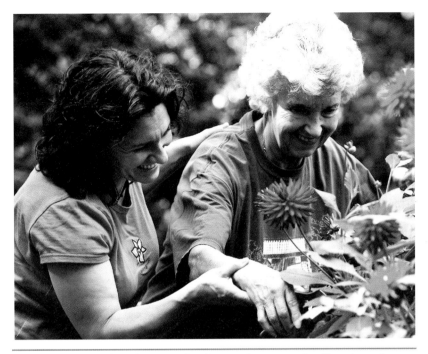

Figure 5-4. Adaptive gardening, using a racheting hand pruner, for older adults in the home garden.
Source. Photograph courtesy of A. Meore.

vanna landscape as a preferred environment. Lewis (1994, 1996) pointed out that many American parks are designed to promote that same sense of safety and refuge that are instilled in us on an evolutionary level.

Stephen Kellert, Ph.D., was one of the first researchers to write and teach extensively on the theory of biophilia. In collaboration with biologist and ecologist E.O. Wilson, Ph.D., he edited *The Biophilia Hypothesis* (Kellert 2018), a text that expanded on the earlier writing of Dr. Wilson, in which he described the innate connection humans have with other living species (Wilson 1984). The collection of essays edited by Drs. Kellert and Wilson were written by scientists examining the theory from diverse areas of expertise, exploring the human connection with all life forms, including plants.

Advances in technology concerned Dr. Kellert. He feared that humanity was losing its connection with the natural world. His continued research led him to examine the built environment. Dr. Kellert (2012) considered ways in which new building designs could contribute positively to people's health and wellness, breaking the trend toward *nature deficit*, a term coined by journalist and author Richard Louv (2008).

Dr. Kellert promoted the idea of building structures with environmentally sensitive materials and designing structures to create an experience with nature when indoors, looking out (Kellert et al. 2008).

Dr. Kellert's most recent book was published posthumously and is a groundbreaking guide to understanding a changing perspective in the way we design and build the environment we live, work, and play in. The essays examine all aspects of the environment, from home and work to community and city, proposing that the future built world should foster the human-nature connection (Kellert 2018).

RELEVANT RESEARCH: QUANTIFYING THE EFFECT OF THERAPEUTIC HORTICULTURE INTERVENTIONS

The seminal 1984 study, "View Through a Window," examining the restorative effect of a view of nature on surgical patients, was conducted by Roger Ulrich, Ph.D., a professor in the Department of Architecture and Centre for Healthcare Architecture, Chalmers University of Technology, in Sweden. At an acute care hospital, Dr. Ulrich reviewed medical records for surgical patients who had gallbladder surgery over the course of a 9-year period. He and his team were able to narrow the field to 46 patients by identifying commonalities in the following characteristics: gender, age, smoker or nonsmoker, obesity or normal weight, and similar traits. In the postsurgical unit, exactly half the beds faced the sky and trees, and the other half faced a brick wall. The study was undertaken to determine whether having a view of nature would have a restorative effect. The researchers identified 23 patients with the natural view and paired them with 23 patients with the wall view. They extracted information from four areas in each medical chart in order to compare outcomes. Following are the findings of the "View Through a Window" study (Ulrich 1984).

- Patients with the view of nature were discharged almost 1 full day sooner than those with the wall view.
- Patients with the view of nature needed a smaller amount and strength of analgesic medication on days 3–5 (on the first 2 days and last 2 days, the difference was insignificant).
- Nursing notes indicated more positive comments from the patients with the natural view and more negative notes from the patients

with the wall view (notes documented mood, level of pain, and need for nursing attention).

- Patients with the view of nature had fewer requests for additional medication for anxiety or other minor postsurgical complications.

Another study by Dr. Ulrich showed that after 5 minutes of viewing a scene with vegetation, stress levels decreased, evidenced by reductions in blood pressure and muscle tension. He encouraged others in the field, including horticulturists and psychologists, to engage in ongoing research by using physiological and health-related measurements to show tangible evidence of the important benefit of plants to improve well-being (Ulrich and Parsons 1992).

Environmental psychologist Rachel Kaplan, Ph.D., and her husband, psychologist Stephen Kaplan, Ph.D., studied the restorative experience of being in nature and the psychological benefit of being "nearby nature" (S. Kaplan 1992). The Kaplans defined "nearby nature" as vegetation that is experienced in a person's ordinary day. It can be indoors or outdoors or viewed through a window. After dozens of studies, they found that having access to nature throughout a person's daily life is an important factor in satisfaction and well-being at work, at home, or at play.

Dr. Stephen Kaplan's work focused on the attention restoration theory, which posits that people experience directed attention fatigue when engaged in prolonged mental effort. Furthermore, connecting with nearby nature restores the ability to direct attention or focus. The Kaplans contended that the availability of nearby nature is not an amenity or decoration but an essential human need because of its ability to reduce attention fatigue. A student studying, an office worker creating documents on a computer, or a patient staying in a hospital will each find relief from attention fatigue if they can look around at images of nature or through a window at a view of nature (R. Kaplan 1992; S. Kaplan 1992, 1995).

In the early twenty-first century, studies supporting the work of earlier theorists and researchers have been published at a furious pace. Researchers from countries and cultures all over the globe are finding evidence of the physiological and psychological benefits of being in nature or nearby nature. For example, a 2011 study published in *Public Health* found decreased levels of cortisol and pulse rates in participants when walking in the forest (Lee et al. 2011). Another study discussed at length later in this chapter found decreased perception of stress, pain, depression, and loneliness (Figure 5–5) among veterans engaging in therapeutic horticulture activities such as the grounding activity shown in Figure 5–6 (Meore et al. 2021).

Therapeutic horticulture: before

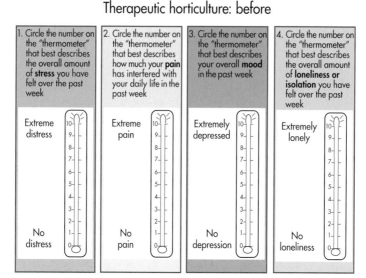

Therapeutic horticulture: after

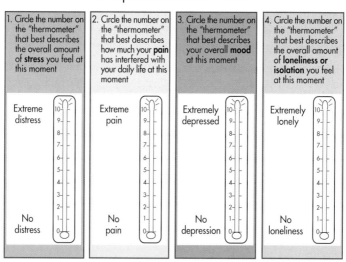

Figure 5–5. Participant-reported outcome thermometers for the four symptom domains (stress, pain, mood, and social isolation) administered before and after each horticultural therapy session.

Source. Reprinted from Meore A, Sun S, Byma L, et al: "Pilot Evaluation of Horticultural Therapy in Improving Overall Wellness in Veterans With History of Suicidality." *Complementary Therapies in Medicine* 59:102728, 2021 33965561. This article is distributed under the terms of the Creative Commons Attribution 4.0 International License (http://creativecommons.org/licenses/by/4.0/).

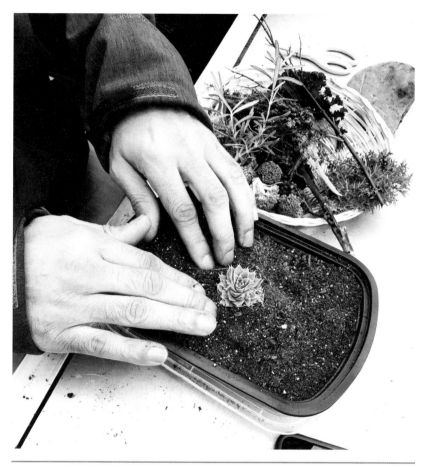

Figure 5–6. **Therapeutic benefits of grounding incorporated into the horticultural therapy process.**
Source. Photograph courtesy of A. Meore.

HORTICULTURAL THERAPY AND THERAPEUTIC HORTICULTURE: COMMONALITIES AND DIFFERENCES

As the profession of horticultural therapy grows, the American Horticultural Therapy Association continues to refine definitions and terminology as it works on developing a credentialing examination. The

American Horticultural Therapy Association has described commonalities and differences between horticultural therapy and therapeutic horticulture, as illustrated in Figure 5–7.

Components of horticultural therapy include the following:

- The participant engages in horticulture-related activities.
- The participant has an identified disability, illness, or life circumstance requiring services.
- The activity is facilitated by an HTR.
- The participation is in the context of an established therapeutic, rehabilitative, or vocational plan, which includes measurable goals and objectives, assessment, and documentation (Haller et al. 2019).

Components of therapeutic horticulture include the following:

- The participant engages in horticulture-related activities.
- The participant has an identified disability, illness, or life circumstance requiring services.
- The activity is facilitated by an HTR or other professional therapist with training in horticulture.
- The participation is in the context of the goals and mission of an organization or the needs of the individual or group and may include health maintenance, well-being, and leisure activity (Haller et al. 2019).

Although there are distinct differences in who is conducting the intervention and for what purpose, there is a strong overlap in the methods and materials used in horticultural therapy and therapeutic horticulture practice. Similar to humanistic psychology, both horticultural therapy and therapeutic horticulture are person-centered practices, and the needs and goals of the individual are the driving force of the intervention. With the patient considered to be at the center of the relationship, the therapist's role in both modalities is to guide and facilitate the engagement with the plant or natural materials, making modifications or adaptations in order to achieve the desired outcome and considering safety in every step of the process.

Both horticultural therapy and therapeutic horticulture can be practiced in diverse and wide-ranging settings, from hospitals and specialized residential communities for people with developmental disabilities, older adults, or others with a specific therapeutic need to correctional facilities, botanical gardens, schools, and community settings (Table 5–1). Programs can be divided into three types: therapeutic, psychosocial, and educational and vocational.

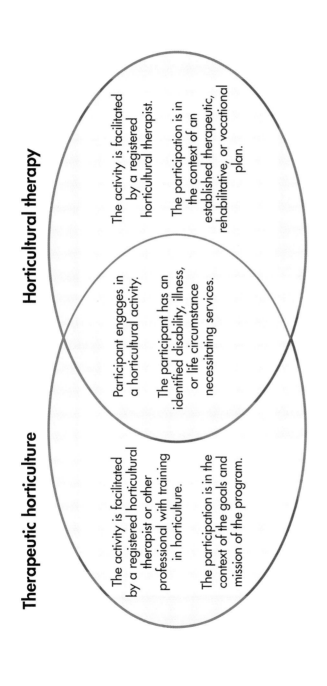

Figure 5-7. Components of therapeutic horticulture and horticultural therapy.

Source. Definitions have been adapted from P. D'Amico, HTM, Program Coordinator, NYBG Horticultural Therapy Certificate Program. American Horticultural Therapy Association: "Definitions and Positions." 2021. Available at: https://www.ahta.org/index.php?option=com_content&view=article&id=86:ahta-definitions-and-positions&catid=20:site-content&Itemid=152.

Table 5–1.   Populations and settings for therapeutic horticulture interventions

Community (social)	Residential (social)	Educational and vocational	Medical
Drug and alcohol rehabilitation support groups	Retirement communities	Vocational school	Acute care hospital
Community gardens	Assisted living facilities	Special needs school	Physical medicine and rehabilitation hospital
Community centers	Skilled nursing facilities	At-risk youth detention center	Pediatric hospital
Religious communities	Halfway houses	Mainstream school (public and private)	Psychiatric hospital
Public parks	Community-based group homes	Incarceration program	Long-term care facility
LGBTQ+ youths	Supported independent living	Religious school	Intermediate care facility
LGBTQ+ families	Developmental disability centers	Garden center vocational program	Cancer care
Farms	Residential schools	Prison vocational training program	Memory care
Food-insecure neighborhoods	Farms	Schools for autistic persons	Hospice care
Refugee communities	Correctional facilities		Practitioner's office
BIPOC communities	Urban neighborhoods		
Day habilitation programs	Patients' homes		
Corporate and other worksites	Homeless shelters		
	Foster homes		
	Domestic violence shelters		

Note. BIPOC=Black, Indigenous, and people of color.

- Therapeutic programs follow a medical model. The focus is on recovery from illness, injury, or life circumstances that negatively affect a person's health.
- Psychosocial programs follow a wellness model. The focus is on introducing a valuable leisure activity that can provide the benefit of overall well-being and improved physical, mental, and spiritual health.
- Educational and vocational programs follow an educational model. The focus is on learning new, meaningful skills in the physical, cog-

nitive, and psychosocial realms that could lead to higher levels of education, job placement, volunteering, or making a meaningful contribution to the community (Haller 1998).

With hortophilia at the core of the therapeutic horticulture practice, horticultural therapists maintain that every patient has the capacity to tap into their innate connection with plants and benefit from the active process of engaging with them, as shown in Figure 5–8. However, people who are so removed from plants and nature as to be described as "nature deficient" (Louv 2008) and averse to nature might need a slow introduction to becoming aware of their connection with the natural world. In such cases, a passive nature experience, such as watching a garden-related video, sampling the scents of the garden, or having a talk session while walking or seated in a garden or park, might be an important first step in providing exposure to nature. With this type of incremental approach, it is likely that plants eventually can be successfully introduced to such a person.

GUIDELINES FOR THE PRACTICAL USE OF THERAPEUTIC HORTICULTURE

The process of engaging in a horticulture-related activity distinguishes therapeutic horticulture from other nature therapies. The practice is flexible and adaptable and is an appropriate resource to address issues in nearly every functional domain (e.g., physical, cognitive, psychological, social, emotional, spiritual, vocational, recreational) (Table 5–2).

Therapeutic horticulture is generally practiced as an active experience, and the patient's relationship with the plant can be multisensory. In the richest sensory environment, this would take place in an outdoor garden bursting with diversity, color, scent, texture, and four-season interest. Other types of outdoor gardens, parks, yards, or even small apartment balconies are adequate spaces in which to engage in a therapeutic treatment session outdoors. An indoor area with plants also may be an appropriate therapeutic setting (e.g., in a greenhouse, atrium, or naturally lit room in an office, school, or residence). The beauty of the people-plant relationship is that even in a room with one plant, a person can have a meaningful, therapeutic experience in relationship with that plant under the guidance of a skilled practitioner. If the care and culture

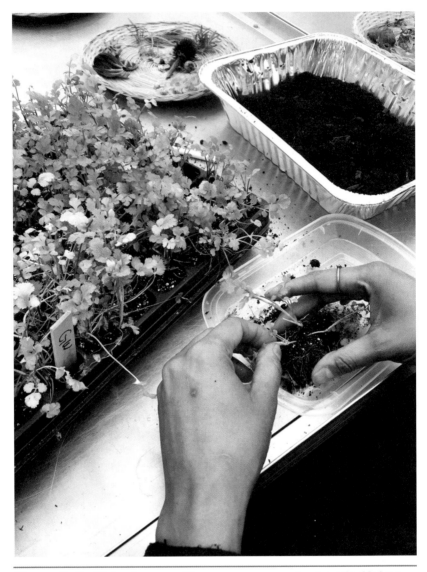

Figure 5–8. Thinning seedlings as an exercise in mindful nature engagement.

Source. Photograph courtesy of A. Meore.

of plants will be a component of the therapeutic practice, it is recommended that the practitioner have at least a rudimentary knowledge of horticulture and be familiar with the activity, tools, plants, and materials that will be used.

Table 5-2. Potential beneficial outcomes of therapeutic horticulture interventions

Cognitive domain	Psychological and emotional domain	Psychosocial domain	Physical domain
Develop new interests	Cultivate well-being	Decrease isolation	Exercise fine motor skills
Learn new skills	Reduce stress and anxiety	Increase socialization	Increase strength and dexterity in hands and fingers
Learn new vocabulary	Reduce restlessness	Promote interaction through a common interest	Increase strength and range of motion at upper extremities
Practice following single-step and multistep instructions	Practice mindfulness	Practice and improve socialization skills	Exercise gross motor skills (e.g., increase strength and range of motion at lower extremities and core and improve coordination, balance, and stability)
Practice sequential tasks	Improve self-confidence and self-esteem	Practice group participation	
Practice goal setting	Improve mood	Practice turn-taking, sharing, and teamwork	
Stimulate curiosity and questioning	Nurture another living thing	Provide opportunities to practice leadership skills	
Exercise short- and long-term memory recall	Explore self-expression through a creative plant-based activity	Provide an opportunity to experience wonder	Provide moderate exercise, helping to increase coordination, strength, stamina, and endurance
Improve sustained focused attention	Develop a sense of responsibility to others and to our environment	Provide an opportunity to observe life cycles	
Improve divided attention	Practice delayed gratification and patience	Provide an opportunity to make metaphoric comparisons to self	
Enhance the understanding of abstract concepts including time, growth, change, and death	Lift spirits for those who have lost a sense of purpose or hope		Provide opportunity for sensory stimulation (vision, hearing, touch, taste, and smell)
Increase awareness of our living environment	Provide a feeling of satisfaction at accomplishing a set goal		Provide outdoor activity and access to fresh air and sunshine
Experience an opportunity to feel a sense of wonder and "being away"	Help to relieve feelings of depression		

Table 5–2. **Potential beneficial outcomes of therapeutic horticulture interventions (continued)**

Cognitive domain	Psychological and emotional domain	Psychosocial domain	Physical domain
		Provide a common language for people to share their cultural traditions Have potential to engage in social or vocational activities such as plant sales, harvest fairs, cooking classes, contests, and social excursions	

PLANNING A THERAPEUTIC HORTICULTURE SESSION

When a therapeutic horticulture session is being planned, several factors must be considered in order to effectively create the opportunity for a positive experience for the participants (Table 5–3). The practitioner first must consider what the therapeutic goals are, what expected outcome is sought, and which type of program will be used. Next, the setting and available resources must be assessed, with a particular focus on potential safety concerns. Finally, the practitioner must consider the activity itself, giving thought to necessary space requirements and possible adaptations, as seen in Figure 5–9, and modifications that would foster patient success. Ideally, a task analysis would be completed before the session to assist the therapist in planning. Task analysis requires therapists to engage in the specific activity they have chosen for the session. Therapists will carefully analyze each step they complete and consider how it will be presented to the participants within the treatment setting. Task analysis examines each step of the process and helps the therapist understand

- Application and benefit
- Complexity
- Most effective mode to present instruction

Table 5–3. **Considerations for planning a therapeutic horticulture session**

Factors to consider	Questions to consider
Goal	What is the desired patient outcome?
	What role does the plant, natural material, or horticultural activity contribute to goal attainment?
Setting and safety	Will the intervention be provided for a group or an individual patient?
	Will the session be conducted indoors or outdoors?
	What resources are available to the therapist (e.g., plants, a garden, water)?
	What safety precautions are needed (e.g., shade for excessive sun if outdoors, potential toxicity of plant material, access to sharp tools)?
Activity	Will this be a passive experience, such as experiencing plants that provide visual, olfactory, tactile, taste, or auditory sensation?
	Will this be an active experience? For example, will the patient engage in caring for the plant, experiencing the reciprocal nurturing and giving aspects of the relationship, in addition to the sensory interactions?
	What materials and tools will be needed?
	What are the step-by-step tasks needed for the activity?
Adaptations and modifications	Will adaptations or modifications be needed to appropriately accommodate the specific needs of the individual or group?

- Practicality of the desired outcome
- Anticipated modifications, adaptations, or necessary safety precautions

Ideally, any treatment setting would have a garden. A simple 3-foot-by-4-foot raised planting bed can provide as much therapeutic value as a horticulturally rich, cultivated garden for growing food or ornamental plants and flowers. Indoor environments appropriate for therapeutic horticulture activities could be a plant-filled greenhouse, atrium, or well-lit room filled with natural light. Plants have the capacity to grow in conditions we would not expect, like an office with incandescent or fluorescent light and no windows. With proper care, some indoor plants will thrive in that challenging environment.

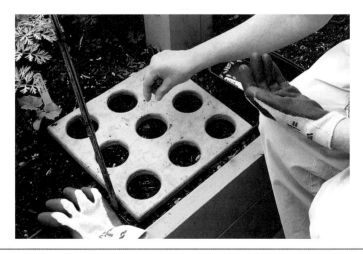

Figure 5–9. Sowing seeds using an adapted tool (seeding frame) to help patients with visual impairment improve fine motor control and engage in activity with peers.
Source.   Photograph courtesy of A. Meore.

Within the wide spectrum of settings in which therapeutic horticulture engagement can occur, it is helpful to consider that horticulture activities can take place in inpatient and outpatient settings (Table 5–1). With the effect of the novel coronavirus disease 2019 (COVID-19) pandemic dictating new ways of delivering health care, many horticultural therapists found success in engaging their patients in horticulture programs virtually. Regardless of the setting, with thoughtful planning and attention to specific individual needs, the adaptability of therapeutic horticulture allows the practitioner to empower the patient to continue engaging with plants beyond the treatment session, such as in the home or community. In this way, the therapeutic benefit carries over to the patient's everyday life, and the patient has an opportunity to reinforce and apply compensatory strategies learned in the therapy session.

PROGRAM EXAMPLE: PSYCHOSOCIAL THERAPEUTIC HORTICULTURE PROGRAM

The Therapeutic Horticulture and Rehabilitative Interventions for Veteran Engagement (THRIVE) Program provides an example of the way an in-person therapeutic horticulture program can be developed to foster continued benefit through at-home nature engagement. The THRIVE Program began in January 2020 as a partnership between a renowned botanical garden and a local urban Department of Veterans Affairs (VA) Medical Center. The purpose of this program is to increase veteran community engagement, promote mentorship and group cohesion, and teach skills rooted in engagement with the natural world that promote a reduction in suicide risk factors.

Once a week, veterans attend a 3.5-hour class with a small cohort of peers at an herb and vegetable garden located within the botanical garden (Figure 5–10). The cohort meets for 4 weeks (Figure 5–11). Each month, a new cohort attends the program. The primary goal of the THRIVE Program is to increase veteran resilience and decrease suicidal ideation through a combination of experiential, didactic, and team-building methods.

Each week's session began with a quiet, contemplative walk around the garden's perimeter, allowing for observation and reflection, culminating in a period of journaling in response to a focus question. After a group sharing of journal responses, participants were introduced to concepts related to the therapeutic nature of the people-plant relationship and engaged in an activity that exemplified the theoretical framework. A second experiential activity followed the lunch break. Lunch was an informal gathering, allowing the veterans to socialize, develop relationships, and deepen cohort bonds. Sessions concluded with group reflections on the day's experience.

The veterans participating in the THRIVE program reported sustained reductions in baseline stress, pain, depression, and loneliness from the first to the fourth week of the program. Additionally, participants reported acute improvement from baseline in symptom domains following the therapeutic horticulture intervention (Figure 5–12).

Clinical Translation: Case Example

Ms. D, a 52-year-old African American woman, has lived her entire life in an urban setting with little access to nature. She is a veteran of Operation Iraqi Freedom and served in the U.S. Air Force. She lives in secure permanent housing with her husband and mother-in-law and has one adult daughter who was recently in an out-of-state inpatient rehabilitation facility for addiction treatment. Her daughter's battle with addiction has been a great source of stress.

Ms. D is a full-time employee of the federal government and worked remotely during the COVID-19 pandemic. She describes this as being a difficult time for her, and eventually she was unable to work because of mental health issues.

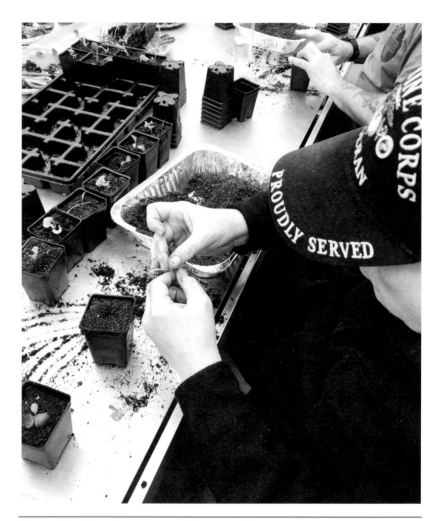

Figure 5-10. Veteran potting seedlings in a therapeutic greenhouse setting.
Source. Photograph courtesy of A. Meore.

Ms. D came to the VA Medical Center in 2009, postdischarge from active service, and was screened by Transitional Care Management. She remained in the Air Force National Guard until 2020. She had been receiving monthly treatment from one psychiatrist at the VA Medical Center since 2009. In addition, she had been seeing a social worker weekly for therapy related to issues of depression and anxiety since 2001.

Ms. D came to the THRIVE Program with diagnoses of chronic PTSD and adjustment disorder with mixed emotional features, a history of sexual trauma, and documented alcohol abuse. She described her alcohol consumption as becoming a problem in 2018, when she began hid-

Week 1

Cohort arrival and orientation	Increase a sense of familiarity and relationship with the garden environment. Introduce focus question for journaling and reflection.
Journaling and reflection	Share reflections and establishing space, place, and belonging. Promote group safety and support.
Theory	Review past concepts. Introduce concepts: attention restoration theory.
Break/lunch	Promote cohort relationships and cohesion.
Garden walk	Increase familiarity and comfort level in garden spaces. Attend to what we pay attention to.
Soil experiential exercises	Create a restorative nature planting. Learn about care and culture of succulent plants.

Orientation

Journaling and reflection

Ice breaker and introductions

Theory

Exercise or activity

Break

Week 2

Cohort arrival and orientation	Orient participants to environment. Introduce focus question for journaling and reflection.
Journaling and reflection	Acknowledge the presence of feelings and emotions as they relate to exposure to nature and the garden. Establish a sense of space and place.
Ice breaker and participant introductions	Multisensory, tabletop plant exploration. Engage participants in learning how to "listen" to emotions as they arise.
Theory	Introduce concepts: Biophilia. Introduction of horticultural therapy as it applies to the VA's Whole Health Model of Care.
Break/lunch	Promote cohort relationships and cohesion.
Greenhouse orientation	Familiarize participants with greenhouse space and plant maintenance tasks.
Soil experiential exercises	Engage in multisensory individual and group experiences utilizing soil and planting mix composition.

Figure 5–11a. **Description of weekly horticultural therapy didactics and activities.**

VA=Department of Veterans Affairs.

Source. Reprinted from Meore A, Sun S, Byma L, et al: "Pilot Evaluation of Horticultural Therapy in Improving Overall Wellness in Veterans With History of Suicidality." *Complementary Therapies in Medicine* 59:102728, 2021 33965561. This article is distributed under the terms of the Creative Commons Attribution 4.0 International License (http://creativecommons.org/licenses/by/4.0/).

ing her drinking from those around her. In one incident, her mother confiscated her car keys to prevent her from driving under the influence. Ms. D did report a reduction in alcohol use prior to beginning the THRIVE Program in 2020. Both her social worker and psychiatrist had referred Ms. D to the THRIVE Program because of her mental health symptoms, which were debilitating at times and prevented her from working. She was prone to panic attacks, exacerbated by her history of asthma. When the COVID-19 pandemic was initially discovered in 2020,

Week 3

Cohort arrival and orientation	Promote memory formation and reflection on garden experience. Introduce focus questions for journaling and reflection.
Journaling and reflection	Share reflections and establishing space, place, and belonging. Promote group safety and support.
Aromatherapy exercise	Engage in multisensory experience using culinary spices. Reinforce the connection between the sense of smell and memory/emotional recall.
Nutrition and cooking	Engage participants in preparing food in groups; educate and provide nutritional information for body and mind.
Break/lunch	Promote cohort relationships and cohesion through the sharing of food and beverages made collaboratively.
Mindful breathing and bulb planting exercise	Reinforce learned horticultural skills and relaxation techniques. Acknowledge and express feelings of gratitude and appreciation.

Orientation

Journaling and reflection

Ice breaker and introductions

Theory

Exercise or activity

Break

Week 4

Cohort arrival and orientation	Increase a sense of familiarity and relationship with the garden environment. Introduce focus question for journaling and reflection.
Journaling and reflection	Share reflections and establishing space, place, and belonging. Promote group safety and support.
Theory	Recap biophilia, attention restoration theory. Introduce mindful nature engagement. Instill an acceptance of personal imperfection and encourage a sense of self-compassion.
Mindful seed harvesting	Foster a sense of purpose and empowerment. Engage in mindful seed harvesting practice.
Break/lunch	Promote cohort relationships and cohesion.
Mindful seed sowing	Allow for the acknowledgment of emotion and permission to release it through mindful seed sowing practice. Bolster a sense of empowerment and skill mastery through seed sowing practice.

Figure 5–11b.   Description of weekly horticultural therapy didactics and activities.
VA=Department of Veterans Affairs.
Source.   Reprinted from Meore A, Sun S, Byma L, et al: "Pilot Evaluation of Horticultural Therapy in Improving Overall Wellness in Veterans With History of Suicidality." *Complementary Therapies in Medicine* 59:102728, 2021 33965561. This article is distributed under the terms of the Creative Commons Attribution 4.0 International License (http://creativecommons.org/licenses/by/4.0/).

stay-at-home mandates were issued throughout the world. Ms. D reported feeling increased anxiety as a result of the high risk of complications she might encounter if she were to contract the virus.

Ms. D also reported difficulties with attention and memory recall that had interfered with her work performance for many years. These difficulties worsened with the increase in psychosocial stressors and exacerbation of depressive symptoms. She was referred for neuropsychological evaluation by her psychiatrist to assess cognitive function and to support differential diagnosis and treatment planning.

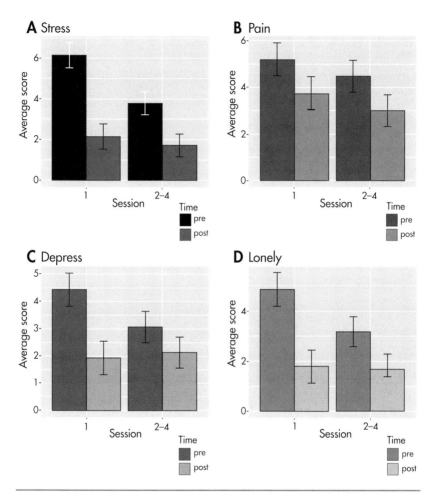

Figure 5–12. **Plots showing data on pre-post patient-reported outcome scores for four symptom domains—(A) stress, (B) pain, (C) mood, and (D) social isolation—at baseline (session 1) and subsequent sessions 2–4 merged, depicted as bar plots for average values from the mixed effect model for each domain with corresponding standard error.**

Source. Reprinted from Meore A, Sun S, Byma L, et al: "Pilot Evaluation of Horticultural Therapy in Improving Overall Wellness in Veterans With History of Suicidality." *Complementary Therapies in Medicine* 59:102728, 2021 33965561. Copyright 2021, Elsevier. This article is distributed under the terms of the Creative Commons Attribution 4.0 International License (http://creativecommons.org/licenses/by/4.0/).

No areas of cognitive impairment were found during the assessment, but Ms. D did show a weakness of memory processes that was attributed to her experiences of severe emotional distress. The neuropsychologist agreed that these memory lapses are often heightened in daily life when one is constantly required to process multiple sources of information at once. Ms. D was strongly encouraged to continue participating actively in her mental health treatment, with a focus on strengthening coping mechanisms for managing psychosocial stressors. It was hoped that therapy would aid in decreasing her experience of cognitive difficulties in daily life. After this appointment, Ms. D was recommended to the THRIVE Program.

Within her mental health treatment plan, Ms. D expressed that she wanted to focus on taking more responsibility for the changes in her life. In addition, she wanted to understand how to use better communication styles and process the deaths of family and friends. During the 3.5 weeks she participated in the THRIVE Program, Ms. D engaged in weekly mindful walks through the garden and wrote her responses to the session's focus question in a journal. All participants' responses were shared within the safety of the group. Each session included an introduction to the theory of the "people-plant relationship" and how it benefits mental health wellness. This was followed by a hands-on, experiential activity, including

- Sensory engagement with plants to identify feeling states
- Activities promoting self-expression and the sharing of "my story" represented in the creation of a tabletop garden
- Mindfulness and grounding practice through a repotting planting exercise
- Creation of an aromatherapy jar using botanicals, which evoked a relaxed and focused response

Ms. D and her fellow veterans were given a lunch break, which allowed the group to socialize, develop relationships, and deepen cohort bonds. Sessions concluded with group reflections on the day's experience.

Each week during the THRIVE Program, Ms. D engaged in verbal interaction and self-expression. She was initially quiet and hesitant to share and speak with other veterans and staff in the program but quickly showed increased interest in the class content, as evidenced by increased eye contact, smiling, verbal contributions, and in-depth writing. She expressed, on several occasions, how the garden made her feel calm and relaxed. During the classes and lunch periods, she engaged socially with the group and openly shared how she felt more socially connected and less lonely being in THRIVE.

During one visit, Ms. D had a few periods when she appeared to have a panic attack. Her breathing quickened, and she had to sit down. She was able to access her inhaler, and the health coach present from the VA Medical Center guided her through a breathing exercise to reduce her anxiety and respiratory discomfort. Ms. D expressed feeling overwhelmed because the garden was a reminder to her of her deceased grandmother, which resurrected a grief reaction related to the more recent deaths of her father, friend, and dog. She expressed that the THRIVE Program assisted her during these feelings and that she was grateful for the supportive presence and experience.

Ms. D attended a discharge education course called Next Steps, which asked her to identify what matters to her and why she wants to remain in good health. During this class, existing VA wellness and support offerings were explained, and she agreed to continue with virtual yoga, exercise, and meditation classes, as well as use VA apps such as PTSD Coach or Mindfulness Coach, in addition to continuing to pursue her new interest in plants and nature.

Per her psychiatrist and social worker, Ms. D has not engaged in any drinking since beginning the program and shared that she greatly benefited from the program. She said that the program introduced her to new things and was "great medicine." She has been able to return to work and expressed that her next plan is to move closer to where her daughter is living so as to have more of an opportunity to repair their relationship and focus on their health and well-being. Ms. D has been attending mental health appointments and weekly wellness classes offered at the VA hospital and continues to show progress in managing her anxiety and depression.

Although Ms. D has a complex medical and personal background, this is not uncommon for the veterans seen in the THRIVE Program. Multiple mental and physical health comorbidities and impaired social relationships are shared by most of the veteran population. Ms. D is one example of how engagement in horticultural therapy can have a profound effect on mental and emotional health and well-being and how these effects can generalize to positively affect other areas of one's life (Byma 2021).

THIS MOMENT: A RESURGENCE OF THE CRITICAL ROLE OF HORTOPHILIA IN DAILY LIFE

Beginning in February 2020, the world experienced a global pandemic, resulting in an abrupt halt to the hectic pace that Western culture has come to know. Quarantine mandates, mask-wearing requirements, social distancing, and thousands of jobs lost forced people to stay at home, away from others. This left many feeling alone and isolated. For those who had the technical knowledge and capacity to do so, computer-based contact was one of the few ways to connect with others. Our homes were transformed into the workplace, the classroom, the gym, and the playroom. All but essential businesses were closed, and hundreds of thousands of our loved ones, friends, and neighbors were losing their jobs or becoming ill and dying. People were frightened, lonely, angry, confused, and bereft of the human relationships that help define us.

In this state of sustained stress, loss, and confusion, people instinctively turned to the outdoors and nature for solace and a sense of normalcy. Most public recreational areas were temporarily closed, resulting in a deep sense of longing. With the extraneous noise of contemporary life silenced, it was the first time that many experienced the draw to the natural world. As restrictions were lifted, people ventured out to parks, public gardens, or their own backyards. Many were inspired to explore gardening for themselves (Figure 5–13). For some, growing food was a way to save money; for others, it was a connection with their childhood or a memory of a parent or grandparent. Still others gardened for exercise or as a way to learn a new hobby or to break up the boredom of long days at home without daily human contact. Unknowingly, these "pandemic gardeners" were practicing hortophilia. The discovery or rediscovery of engaging with plants, for many, is comparable to meeting an old or new friend, offering a sense of connection and control in a time of uncertainty. Although the trauma of living through the COVID-19 pandemic will remain for some time, people across the globe were given the chance to connect with the stability and comfort found in nature and inherent in the people-plant relationship. Therapeutic horticulture provides a universal approach for treating individuals through a wellness model, supporting their physical, cognitive, and behavioral healing.

KEY POINTS

- Horticultural therapy is distinguished from other nature therapies by being an active process involving the physical care of plants or gardens.

- When engaging in the care of a plant, a patient experiences intimacy with nature at the most foundational level, engaging with and nurturing a living thing. This experience lends itself to recognizing metaphors that parallel the human condition and the opportunity to learn from them.

- A registered horticultural therapist (HTR) often practices in clinical settings, collaborating with a treatment team and developing goals, objectives, modifications, adaptations, and safety precautions for an individual or group with specific therapeutic needs.

- Professionals in allied disciplines can use their knowledge of horticulture and understanding of the people-plant relationship to enrich their practice by engaging a patient in therapeutic horticulture.

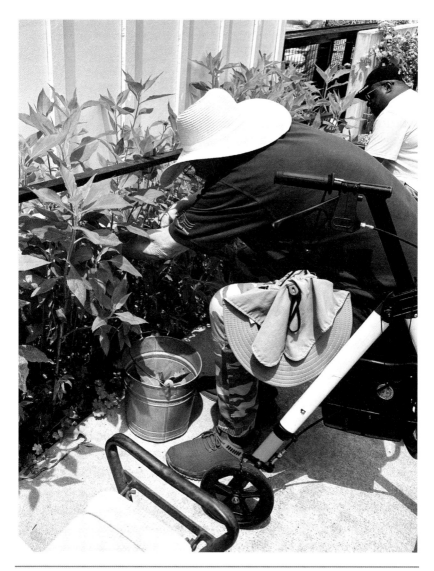

Figure 5-13. Client engaging in focused attention while weeding an overgrown garden border.
The client is using adapted seating because of lower extremity weakness.
Source. Photograph courtesy of A. Meore.

- Engagement in structured horticultural activities may expose a patient to a new activity that they can turn to and use as a tool for health and well-being at any time in their life. Whether it is the care of a few houseplants at home or in the office or the planting and maintenance of a whole garden, patients will understand that a simple, sustainable, and meaningful resource for self-care exists.

QUESTIONS

1. What are the four most important things you must consider when planning a therapeutic horticulture session?

   A. The patient, the plant-based activity, the date, and the availability of water.
   B. The patient's preferences, the setting, the resources needed for a plant-based activity, and the desired outcome.
   C. The setting, the biophilia hypothesis, the plant-based activity, and the patient.
   D. The setting, the patient's preferences, plants, and snacks.
   E. The desired outcome, garden tools, access to water, and seeds.

Correct answer: B. The patient's preferences, the setting, the resources needed for a plant-based activity, and the desired outcome.

> Therapeutic horticulture is a person-centered modality. Therefore, the person and the person's preferences are at the center of the therapeutic relationship. The desired outcome, or goal, is critical because it identifies the purpose of the session. Finally, knowing the setting, materials, tools, and other resources needed allows the therapist to be prepared to introduce the activity, give instructions, and manage the materials and tools while engaging with the participant during the activity.

2. When performed outside the context of a goal-based treatment plan, the use of plants as an intervention for healing is called

   A. Plant science.
   B. Biophilia.
   C. Psychoanalysis.
   D. Therapeutic horticulture.
   E. Ecotherapy.

Correct answer: D. Therapeutic horticulture.

> Therapeutic horticulture is defined as a plant-based activity that differs from horticultural therapy in that an activity session can

be facilitated by an allied professional with training in horticulture. Treatment goals are determined by the mission and desired outcomes of the organization and are generally focused on health maintenance and wellness.

3. Horticultural therapy must include which components?

    A. A plant, a bottle of water, soil, and a pot.
    B. A patient who has gardening experience and a selection of plants.
    C. A patient with a special need, engagement in a horticultural activity, defined treatment goals, and a therapeutic process delivered by a skilled horticultural therapist.
    D. A professional with a degree in horticulture, a patient with an expressed desire to garden, and a greenhouse with classical music playing.
    E. A social worker and a patient who both like working with plants.

Correct answer: C. A patient with a special need, engagement in a horticultural activity, defined treatment goals, and a therapeutic process delivered by a skilled horticultural therapist.

A horticultural therapy session must include a patient with a special need, one or more plants for the patient's engagement in hortophilia, and clearly defined treatment goals and objectives and must be facilitated by a registered horticultural therapist.

REFERENCES

American Academy of Physical Medicine and Rehabilitation: About physical medicine and rehabilitation. Rosemont, IL, American Academy of Physical Medicine and Rehabilitation, 2024. Available at: https://www.aapmr.org/about-physiatry/about-physical-medicine-rehabilitation. Accessed October 1, 2021.

American Horticultural Therapy Association: Definitions and positions, 2020. Available at: https://www.ahta.org/ahta-definitions-and-positions. Accessed September 12, 2021.

Byma L: Case Study—Desiree, Whole Health Program Manager, VISN 2 Whole Health Network Education Coordinator. Bronx, NY, James J. Peters VA Medical Center, 2021

Chambers N, Fried G, Wichrowski M: The Glass Garden. Boston, MA, Arena Books, 2014

Cooper Marcus C, Sachs N: Therapeutic Landscapes: An Evidence-Based Approach to Designing Healing Gardens and Restorative Outdoor Spaces. Hoboken, NJ, Wiley, 2014

Davis S: Development of the profession of horticultural therapy, in Horticulture as Therapy: Principles and Practice. Edited by Simson SP, Straus MC. New York, Food Products, 1998, pp 3–20

Gerlach-Spriggs N, Kaufman RE, Warner SB Jr: Restorative Gardens: The Healing Landscape. New Haven, CT, Yale University Press, 1998

Gesler WM: Healing places, in Therapeutic Landscapes: An Evidence-Based Approach to Designing Healing Gardens and Restorative Outdoor Spaces. Edited by Cooper Marcus C, Sachs N. Hoboken, NJ, Wiley, 2003, p 6

Haller RL: Vocational, social, and therapeutic programs in horticulture, in Horticulture as Therapy: Principles and Practice. Edited by Simson SP, Straus MC. New York, Food Products, 1998, pp 43–68

Haller RL, Kennedy K, Capra CL: The Profession and Practice of Horticultural Therapy. Boca Raton, FL, CRC Press, 2019

Janick J: Horticulture and human culture, in The Role of Horticulture in Human Well-Being and Social Development. Edited by Relf D. Portland, OR, Timber, 1992, pp 19–27

Kaplan R: The psychological benefits of nearby nature, in The Role of Horticulture in Human Well-Being and Social Development. Edited by Relf D. Portland, OR, Timber, 1992, pp 125–133

Kaplan S: The restorative environment: nature and human experience, in Human Well-Being and Social Development. Edited by Relf D. Portland, OR, Timber, 1992, pp 134–142

Kaplan S: The restorative benefits of nature: toward an integrative framework. J Environ Psychol 15:169–182, 1995

Kavanaugh JP: People-plant principles from the past, in People-Plant Relationships: Setting Research Priorities. Edited by Flagler J, Poincelot RP. New York, Food Products, 1994, pp 231–238

Kellert SR: Birthright: People and Nature in the Modern World. New Haven, CT, Yale University Press, 2012

Kellert SR: Nature by Design: The Practice of Biophilic Design. New Haven, CT, Yale University Press, 2018

Kellert SR, Wilson EO (eds): The Biophilia Hypothesis. Washington, DC, Island Press, 1993

Kellert SR, Heerwagen JH, Mador ML (eds): Biophilic Design: The Theory, Science, and Practice of Bringing Buildings to Life. Hoboken, NJ, Wiley, 2008

Lee J, Park BJ, Tsunetsugu Y, et al: Effect of forest bathing on physiological and psychological responses in young Japanese male subjects. Public Health 125(2):93–100, 2011 21288543

Lewis C: The evolution of horticultural therapy in the United States. Paper presented at Fourth Annual Conference of the National Council for Therapy and Rehabilitation Through Horticulture, Philadelphia, PA, September 6, 1976. Available at: https://findingaids.lib.k-state.edu/folder-13-the-evolution-of-horticultural-therapy-in-the-united-states-fourth-annual-conference-of-the-national-council-for-therapy-and-rehabilitation-through-horticulture-philadelphia-pa. Accessed September 2021.

Lewis C: The evolutionary importance of people-plant relationships, in People-Plant Relationships. Setting Research Priorities. Edited by Flagler J, Poincelot RP. New York, Food Products, 1994, pp 239–254

Lewis C: Green Nature, Human Nature: The Meaning of Plants in Our Lives. Champaign, University of Illinois Press, 1996

Louv R: Last Child in the Woods: Saving Our Children From Nature-Deficit Disorder. Chapel Hill, NC, Algonquin, 2008

Meore A, Sun S, Byma L, et al: Pilot evaluation of horticultural therapy in improving overall wellness in veterans with history of suicidality. Complement Ther Med 59:102728, 2021 33965561

Muir J: Mormon Lilies. Liliaceous Wonder-A Mountain Covered With Flowers Gorgeous Lily Gardens-A Sublime Scene-The Queen of All. (Special Correspondence of the Bulletin.) Salt Lake, July, 1877. (1877). *John Muir: A Reading Bibliography by Kimes, 1986 (Muir articles 1866-1986).* 53. Available at: https://scholarlycommons.pacific.edu/jmb/53. Accessed May 30, 2024.

Mulligan WC: The Lattice Gardener. New York, Macmillan, 1995

Penn Medicine: History of Pennsylvania Hospital, stories: Dr. Benjamin Rush. Available at: https://www.uphs.upenn.edu/paharc/features/brush.html. Accessed October 15, 2021.

Rogers EB: The Central Park Book. New York, Central Park Task Force, 1977

Rush B: Medical Inquiries and Observations, Upon the Diseases of the Mind. Carlisle, PA, Dickinson College, 1812

Sacks O: Everything in Its Place, First Loves and Last Tales. New York, Knopf, 2019

Shapiro BA, Kaplan MJ: Mental illness and horticultural therapy practice, in Horticulture as Therapy: Principles and Practice. Edited by Simson SP, Straus MC. New York, Food Products, 1998, pp 157–197

Ulrich RS: View through a window may influence recovery from surgery. Science 224(4647):420–421, 1984 6143402

Ulrich R, Parsons R: Influences of passive experiences with plants on individual well-being and health, in The Role of Horticulture in Human Well-Being and Social Development. Edited by Relf D. Portland, OR, Timber, 1992, pp 93–105

Wilson EO: Biophilia. Cambridge, MA, Harvard University Press, 1984

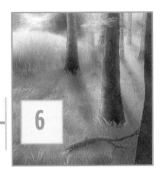

6

Staying Indoors

UTILITY OF BIOPHILIC DESIGN IN MENTAL HEALTH

Kishan Shah, M.D.
Muhammad Aadil, M.D.
Chaden Noureddine, M.D.

I will simply paint my bedroom. This time the colour shall do everything. By means of its simplicity it shall lend things a grand style, and shall suggest absolute peace and slumber to the spectator. In short, the mere sight of the picture should be restful to the spirit, or better still, to the imagination.
—Vincent Van Gogh (1913, p. 31)

Buildings are the de facto human environment of the twenty-first century. Some estimates indicate that most Americans spend 90% of their lives indoors. Although nature's salubrious elements can be easily found outside, constructed environments often exclude them by default (Kellert et al. 2011). Over the years, people have spent less time outdoors. The 2019 Outdoor Foundation survey, which reviewed respondents' outdoor activities over the previous year, marked a nadir in a decade-long downward trend of time spent outdoors. The data showed 1 billion fewer outdoor outings in 2018 than in 2008. Although 35% of Americans reported recreational outdoor outings more than once per week, 32% reported one per month, and 11% went out only one to three times the entire year. Because we spend 90% of our time indoors, we have been connecting less and less with nature both indoors and outdoors (Kellert et al. 2011). The downward trend in recreational outings translates to fewer incidental nature interactions. Sustained nature connectivity then depends on intentionally bringing nature indoors. Luckily, biologists, sociologists, ecologists, and architects have incorporated evidence-based natural elements into architectural and structural designs. In this chapter, we first define the significance of bringing natural elements into indoor environments. Then, we examine the health outcomes of staying indoors and the mental health effects of the coronavirus disease 2019 (COVID-19) stay-at-home orders. Finally, we introduce the innovative ways that we can incorporate nature into indoor environments, through and beyond technological advancements.

BIOPHILIC DESIGN

The *biophilia hypothesis*, coined by biologist Edward O. Wilson (1984), suggests that humans possess an innate tendency to seek connections with nature. In his book *Biophilia*, Wilson (1984) theorized that human beings possess a natural and innate affinity for living systems and seek connections with natural forms of life. The concept of humans being attracted to the living world, or a love for life, has been referenced for centuries, dating back to the writings of the ancient Greeks and Aristotle (Santas 2014). It speaks of a human evolutionary tendency to adapt to the natural world, which is instrumental in promoting physical and mental well-being (Wilson and Kellert 1993).

Biophilic design, in the setting of the biophilia hypothesis, places an emphasis on connecting building occupants and urban environments to the natural world. Because the modern-day natural habitat is an indoor constructed environment surrounded by a vast array of technology, it becomes important to reflect on Wilson's biophilia hypothesis and its application to the current standard living space. The incorporation of biophilic design aims to connect people's affinity toward the natural system to built environments.

Stephen Kellert, a social ecologist who helped pioneer the theory of biophilia, defined *biophilic design* through two different dimensions. The first dimension is "organic and naturalistic," and it is defined by the shapes and forms reflecting biophilia in the built environment. The second dimension is "place based or vernacular," and it is defined by landscapes or buildings and their connection to the ecology or culture of a certain geographic area. The second dimension embodies how an inanimate environment can feel lifelike. These two dimensions of biophilic design can be executed by six different biophilic design elements, which can be further discussed in more than 70 biophilic design attributes. The six biophilic design elements are

1. Environmental features
2. Natural shapes and forms
3. Natural patterns and processes
4. Light and space
5. Place-based relationships
6. Evolved human-nature relationships

Attributes used to study and accomplish these elements include color, water, air, sunlight, plants, animals, biomorphy, geomorphy, bounded and translational spaces, complementary contrast, and light and shadows. Kellert et al. (2011) also emphasized the importance of humans' innate dependence on and propensity toward nature because it plays a crucial role in enhancing emotional, physical, and intellectual well-being and fitness during evolutionary processes.

Biophilic design focuses on creating a habitat for people as biological organisms within a larger ecosystem. The modern ecosystem constitutes a built environment, where the principles of biophilic design seek to foster wellness, health, and fitness. The principles that were discussed by Kellert et al. (2011) frame the foundations of successfully implementing biophilic design within the built environment and include the following:

- Requiring repeated and sustained engagement with nature
- Focusing on human adaptations to the natural world that have advanced people's health, fitness, and well-being

- Encouraging an emotional attachment to particular settings and places
- Promoting positive interactions between people and nature that encourage an expanded sense of relationship and responsibility for the human and natural communities
- Encouraging mutual reinforcing, interconnected, and integrated architectural solutions

Through these principles, biophilic design aims to support the productivity, performance, and resilience of natural systems, especially as building development transforms them. An ecosystem's productivity and resilience are measured by indicators including biological diversity, pollination, biomass, and other ecosystem services. Biophilic design and its principles have both long- and short-term effects on a built environment's conditions and aim to support an overall positive net change to the productivity and resilience of an ecosystem through ecologically sustainable interventions (Kellert and Calabrese 2015).

As discussed by Kellert, biophilic design emphasizes fostering an interconnected and positive relationship with nature in an indoor environment. A biophilic, connective space requires more than simply adding a potted plant or out-of-context picture of nature into the home. Rather, it emphasizes the inclusion of natural light, vegetation, living walls, natural textures and materials, and views of nature. All these elements coexist within a dynamic spatial setting, which is inhabited by one or several social beings. People who have encouraging interactions within this space experience feelings of security and enhanced productivity (Ryan and Browning 2020). Success in biophilic design achieves harmony between various elements of the environment in order to achieve the well-being of its inhabitants (Kellert et al. 2011). The principles of biophilic design are not always followed, because modern-day buildings are not always designed with biophilia in mind (Kellert and Calabrese 2015). In the next section of this chapter, we discuss how an environment devoid of nature may affect the health and well-being of its occupants.

SICK BUILDING SYNDROME

Human intervention and development in natural environments have been motivated by functional needs that tend to stray further away from the inclusion of biophilic elements (Zelnik et al. 2021). This trend has translated to modern architectural designs, and most office buildings, hospitals, schools, shopping centers, and homes tend to be devoid of sensory stimuli and natural forces (Kellert and Calabrese 2015). Buildings that lack biophilic design elements detract from the physical and mental well-being essential for the daily functioning of their inhabitants.

A 2011 study (Elzeyadi 2011) attempted to quantify the hypothesized relationship between sick days taken and employee access to daylight and natural scenery, which are attributes of biophilic design. The study hypothesized that lack of access to dynamic lighting may affect circadian rhythm sensitivity and its manifestation through a set of symptoms, prompting the need for sick days. The three-phase study was conducted inside an office with 120 working spaces, and it assessed both lighting quality and quantity in the working environment and access to scenery through views and windows for 175 employees. It also surveyed employees' health conditions, physical health screenings, and sick days taken through payroll records. The study performed multiple regression and Pearson correlation statistical analyses to examine the relationship between sick leave hours and ratings of lighting quality and views. It found statistical significance for a positive correlation between poor light quality ratings and more sick days taken. Light quality rating and view accessibility variables accounted for 6.5% of the sick leave use variation, which was statistically significant. This study highlighted how being in a building can affect well-being and daily functioning. It also emphasized how, at times, being inside a building devoid of natural elements such as lighting and natural views can manifest into tangible symptoms (Elzeyadi 2011).

Prolonged containment in a deficient indoor environment with poor indoor air quality or contaminants present can result in the manifestation of physical symptoms, which occupants may not be aware of. *Sick building syndrome* (SBS) is a term used to describe a situation in which the inhabitants of a building start to develop acute health- or comfort-related symptoms that are directly linked to the time spent in that building and not caused by another illness. This diagnosis of exclusion requires an important criterion to be met: inhabitants must experience relief of symptoms after leaving the building. SBS can encompass numerous nonspecific symptoms, including headache; dizziness; nausea; eye, nose, or throat irritation; dry cough; dry or itching skin; difficulty concentrating; fatigue; sensitivity to odors; hoarseness of voice; allergies; colds; flulike symptoms; increased incidence of asthma attacks; and personality changes. The manifestation of symptoms can be attributable to various causes, many of which can be reversible. Frequent culprits for SBS are building aerodynamics, including poor ventilation, heating, and air conditioning. Other times, it may include elements such as high levels of dust, tobacco smoke, poor lighting, mold or fungus, volatile chemicals from cleaning products, and high levels of stress. Studies indicate that excessive work-related stress and resulting dissatisfaction can lead to poor interpersonal relationships and correlate to the psychosocial and psychosomatic symptoms of SBS. Common treatment modalities of SBS consist of increasing ventilation rates and subsequent air distribution, as well as removing or modifying the pollutant source. Ways to clean the air in an indoor setting include using frosted glass and skylights for natural light penetration, building a terrace garden, including community spaces, and, most simply, adding indoor plants to the environment (Ghaffarianhoseini et al. 2018).

COVID-19, STAY-AT-HOME ORDERS, AND MENTAL HEALTH

During the COVID-19 pandemic, government measures promoted staying home to reduce the risk of transmitting infection. The social distancing measures and precautions slowed the trajectory of the pandemic, but they also had a direct effect on the social processes that foster mental health. Loneliness and isolation are shown to reduce our psychological well-being and lead to various cardiac, rheumatoid, neurological, and psychiatric disorders including substance use disorders (Mushtaq et al. 2014). Therefore, disruptions in daily interactions, social support availability, and social influences on coping can have significant effects on psychological and emotional well-being. In this section, we review studies that show the effect that stay-at-home orders had on populations' resilience and well-being.

A large-scale online survey approved by an institutional ethics committee investigated 2,392 Chinese people (H.C. Wang et al. 2020). The populations in the study resided in the United Kingdom and China, were staying home, and had no history of mental illness during the initial phase of the pandemic. Participation in the study was voluntary. The study found that participants reported having last left their home 5.47 days ago. During the stay-at-home period, 60.11% experienced depression, 53.09% experienced sleep disturbance, 46.91% reported irritability, and 48.20% reported decreased libido. An astounding 76.12% of participants had developed sleep and circadian disorders. Nearly 80% of the people had indoor activity time of less than 30 minutes per day, and 82.02% did not partake in any outdoor activities. Of the people who were undergoing the stay-at-home mandate, 30% were single, living alone; therefore, they lacked social support. A direct preliminary correlation was found between the frequency and severity of these symptoms and the time spent indoors (H.C. Wang et al. 2020).

A subsequent smaller but similar study (Marroquín et al. 2020) surveyed a nationwide online sample of 435 adults residing in the United States. The study was conducted at the onset of stay-at-home orders, from February 2020 to March 2020. It assessed for correlations of stay-at-home orders and personal distancing with symptoms of depression, generalized anxiety disorder, intrusive thoughts, insomnia, and acute stress. The overarching term *stay-at-home* was considered at both the public policy level, which mandated that travel outside the home be only for acquiring essential goods, and the level of personal distancing, which encouraged personal practices to reduce the spread of the virus. The sample population in this study resided in 46 different states, had a nearly equal gender breakdown, had an average age of 39.2 years, and had a median household income of $40,000–$59,000. Clinical cutoffs were juxtaposed with multiple regression analyses to ascertain the following clinically relevant symptoms: 38.4% of the sample reported symptoms of mild depression (with 27.4% in clinical range), 22.8% of the sample reported symptoms of mild anxiety (with 15.6% showing moderate symptoms), and 38.6% of the sample reported symptoms of insomnia within the clinical range. The development of mental health problems has myriad implications for physical health, such as increased risk of metabolic diseases (Penninx and Lange 2018). This risk cannot be overstated, because the ensuing reduced immunity increases the risk for COVID-19 infection (Marroquín et al. 2020).

The two studies highlighted and quantified how staying home can affect well-being. Although the studies did not specifically evaluate the role that biophilia may have had on the degree of effect, they showed a clear and significant relationship between time spent indoors and the severity of symptoms.

A 2021 Turkish study (Afacan 2021) evaluated the relationship between biophilic design and mood transcendence and gerotranscendence during the COVID-19 pandemic. *Gerotranscendence* is defined as a "shift in meta-perspective from a materialistic and rational view to a more cosmic and transcendent one, normally followed by an increase in life satisfaction" (Tornstam 1989, p. 55). The study included 450 Turkish older adults (65–95 years). Participants were stratified based on their living spaces' biophilic profiles, which were categorized as either indoor biophilic, outdoor biophilic, or nonbiophilic. Each participant completed two sets of questionnaires, once before the COVID-19 pandemic, in 2018, and once during the COVID-19 pandemic, from June

2020 to October 2020. The two questionnaires were the 37-item short-ened version of the Profile of Mood States and the 10-item Gerotrans-cendence Scale. The highest positive correlation was found between fatigue and depression mood states and residence in a nonbiophilic environment. The home environment's biophilic profile also had a dynamic correlation with both the aging experience of participants and their mood state, because outdoor biophilic features of the home were correlated with the highest rate of recovery from mood effects of the pandemic, compared with the indoor biophilic and nonbiophilic groups, whereas indoor biophilic features were correlated with the most improved recovery from feelings of depression and anger (Afacan 2021).

Although the study was conducted exclusively on an older adult patient population, it is important to note that this exact population was considered at elevated mortality risk from COVID-19 (Yanez et al. 2020). Despite its generalization limitations, the study showed that biophilic design could have affected adult health during the COVID-19 pandemic, which forced people to stay indoors in unprecedented ways. The study also showed that the incorporation of biophilic elements indoors can increase psychological well-being.

BENEFITS OF NATURE INDOORS

The National Aeronautics and Space Administration (NASA) Clean Air Study, led by Bill Wolverton, Ph.D., aimed to optimize the air quality of poorly ventilated spaces such as the closed systems used in space travel. New construction during the latter half of the twentieth century also had poor ventilation because of a design ethos that heavily insulated buildings to maximize energy efficiency. The construction materials for both sealed space habitats and modern buildings release volatile irritants that concentrate in unventilated indoor spaces, a phenomenon known as *off-gassing*. Wolverton theorized that houseplants could act as low-cost air purifiers by passively absorbing harmful toxins and organic chemicals. The initial study showed that houseplants dramatically decreased concentrations of benzene, trichloroethylene, and formaldehyde in a closed experimental chamber (Wolverton et al. 1989). When researchers attempted to scale the experiment to real-world conditions, passive absorption by plants did not consistently outperform natural air exchange in removing indoor air pollutants (Budaniya and Rai 2022).

One literature review estimated that a 1,500-square-foot house would need 680 houseplants to reach the same chemical removal rate as indoor-outdoor air exchange. Even though plants are impractical indoor air purifiers by passive absorption, they may show promise as part of active filtration systems. Biowalls are one such system, in which a wall of vegetation is arranged over a series of fans that continuously draw air through the roots and soil. Regardless of whether plants purify air, research has shown psychological benefit to having plants indoors (Cummings and Waring 2020).

A study conducted by Oh et al. (2019) explored the potential effect of plant visualization and imagery on attention. It focused on the visual effect of real plants in comparison to artificial plants, a plant photograph, and the absence of plants. The study included 23 elementary school students, 11–13 years old, to ascertain whether viewing green plants led to physiological benefits. These students were evaluated via electroencephalography (EEG) during exposure to each 3-minute visual stimulus. Results found that viewing real plants significantly decreased theta waves of the frontal lobe, which is associated with increased concentration and attention. Additionally, viewing real plants had a significant association with comfort and other positive mood states (Oh et al. 2019).

A similar study considered the physiological and psychological effects of viewing bamboo plant scenery, which is a popular Chinese landscape design. Videos of bamboo scenery, differing in length, were shown to 180 Chinese university students. Each study group watched a video of distinct urban bamboo scenery collected from separate urban bamboo forests. The study monitored psychological indicators through the Profile of Mood States questionnaires while monitoring various physiological indicators through EEG, skin conductance, blood pressure, and pulse. On average, EEG activity quickly dropped, within a minute of watching the videos. Blood pressure values significantly decreased within 3 minutes of watching the video, which was hypothesized to be due to decreased sympathetic nervous activation. All study groups except one showed decreased sweat production, which was hypothesized to be related to decreased feelings of anxiety. Finally, results showed different physiological responses after watching distinct urban bamboo scenery videos collected from different areas (Y. Wang et al. 2020).

A study by Song et al. (2017) investigated the heart rates and physiological changes in the right and left prefrontal cortex activity of 15 female university students while they were exposed to visual stimulation with roses. In the experiment, 25 fresh, unscented red roses were trimmed to a length of 40 cm and arranged in a glass vase on a desk. Each participant was asked to sit and stare at the roses for 3 minutes and then to stare at an empty desk. Their physiological responses were measured for both experimental conditions. The results showed that while they viewed fresh roses, oxyhemoglobin concentration in the right prefrontal cortex decreased within minutes, which verified the hypothesis that visual stimulation with roses relieved prefrontal activity (Jo et al. 2019).

A study by Zhang et al. (2017) investigated physiological responses to wooden and nonwooden indoor environments. The researchers prepared rooms with different wood coloring as follows: 1) 100% dark brown wood, 2) 50% light brown wood and 50% painted white, 3) 100% light brown wood, and 4) a nonwooden room (painted white) as a control. The study used the autonomic nervous system, respiratory system, and visual system as the physiological indicators. Twenty healthy adults participated in the experiment and were asked to complete work tasks in one of the rooms, and exposure time for each room was set to 90 minutes. Their systolic blood pressure and heart rate were found to be lower in the wooden rooms than in the nonwooden room, and the oxyhemoglobin saturation levels were higher in the wooden rooms than in the nonwooden room. These physiological findings showed the visual relaxation effect of the wooden environments (Jo et al. 2019).

Comprehensive literature validates that in most studies that used display stimuli, such as photographs, three-dimensional images, virtual reality, and videos of natural landscapes, viewing natural scenery led to more relaxed body responses compared with viewing control displays of stimuli (Jo et al. 2019).

Exposure to real, natural stimuli, such as green plants, flowers, and wooden materials, had more positive effects on the prefrontal cortex and autonomic nervous activities compared with the control. These findings reinforce the increasing evidence on the health and physiological benefits of bringing nature indoors.

The benefits of introducing and modifying biophilic design elements extend beyond laboratory settings. A study conducted in suburban Pennsylvania examined the records of patients after cholecystectomy. The study assessed the records of 46 surgical patients, half of whom had access to natural scenery through window views and half of whom had a brick wall view. The study found that the patients whose room looked out on natural scenery took fewer moderate and strong analgesic doses and had shorter postoperative hospital stays (Ulrich 1984). The use of windows is only one example of the therapeutic use of natural and biophilic elements in the health care setting. The literature suggests that design elements including functional ventilation systems, adequate acoustic environments, effective lighting, and nature distraction show evidence-based improvement in hospital outcomes (Ulrich et al. 2008).

As the built environment, including the home and the healing space, becomes more technologically connected, the possibilities of bringing natural elements indoors become increasingly attainable.

MENTAL HEALTH THROUGH TECHNOLOGY

Technological innovation is playing a significant role in creating indoor environments that are beneficial for mental health. A smart home automation system automates electrical, electronic, and technological-based tasks by using various hardware and software technologies (Techopedia 2018). The entire system is completely customizable and can be easily managed with a smartphone or web-enabled device. A smart home provides multiple possibilities for controlling devices in the living space, which can include a thermostat, lighting, security alarms, heating units, and other appliances. The incorporation of biophilic philosophy into the smart home system can be very beneficial to mental health, especially for those who spend extended time indoors. For example, applications can be used to set the brightness of the light at home depending on the time of day or season. For people with seasonal affective disorder or depression, light therapy (exposure to artificial light) has been studied and found to be beneficial (Kurlansik and Ibay 2012). Having a home automation device can also help with mindfulness practices by regularly reminding individuals to take mindful breaths or by playing calming music or sounds that assist with anxiety and poor focus. In people with a history of trauma or PTSD, having such technology at hand can decrease the intensity of flashback episodes and can remind people to use positive coping skills (Leighanne et al. 2020). One can set security alarms and video cameras at home, monitor outdoor activities, or even view a live stream of a pet camera to reduce anxiety and increase the sense of security (Nelson and Allen 2018). Another important use of indoor technology is for older adults and people with disabilities, who can access many options for indoor entertainment, relaxation, exercise, and safety. It provides a sense of security and removes the stress and anxiety that may arise if someone is living alone. Smartwatches can even alert emergency services or family members if they detect a fall or an abnormal electrocardiogram finding (Liu et al. 2016).

A recent study (Yin et al. 2020) aimed to assess the effects of bringing biophilic elements indoors via virtual reality. Participants were exposed to stressor tasks and then assigned to one of four virtual offices: one nonbiophilic base office and three offices enhanced with various biophilic design elements. Physiological recovery was tracked by using biomonitoring sensors measuring indicators such as heart rate variability, blood pressure, and skin conductance. Anxiety was measured via the short version of the State-Trait Anxiety Inventory. The groups exposed to biophilic environments had significantly better physiological and psychological recovery than their counterparts (Yin et al. 2020).

As technological advancements develop more sophisticated tools for smart homes, people will have more options to customize their living spaces. Future research will determine the optimal applications of these technologies to promote well-being.

BRINGING THE OUTSIDE IN

Incorporation of biophilic design into one's home can increase psychological and physical well-being and can be accomplished in multiple ways, most of which are affordable and readily available for patients and providers alike. In the home setting, patients can be advised to use lights and shadows to create an environment more akin to the natural world (Kellert and Calabrese 2015). Keeping windows unobstructed during the day allows the natural light cycle to enter the home. Continuous exposure to natural lighting is associated with improved sleep and increased daytime activity (Boubekri et al. 2014). Daylight can aid in circadian rhythm regulation, as the suprachiasmatic nuclei synchronize the biological rhythm in response to input from the environment's ambient light (Blume et al. 2019). Natural sounds and sights can provoke positive psychological states, with the potential to increase well-being and aid stress recovery (Franco et al. 2017). Patients may be able to acquire plants, indoor green walls, water fountains, and natural materials such as wood or stone, which offer textural sensory pattern variations experienced in nature. A study aiming to compare responses after interactions with indoor plants compared with computer tasks showed a significant reduction in psychological and physiological stress when participants interacted with plant-related tasks (Lee et al. 2015). Patients may interact with plants through gardening because it offers visual, tactile, and olfactory contacts with natural elements. Patients can introduce art within their home. In the fast-paced lifestyle most people live, in conjunction with an ever-changing global landscape that deviates further from connectedness to nature, it becomes imperative to take the simple, small steps to maintain a steady presence of nature in the indoor environment for the well-being of all those who occupy it (Ryan and Browning 2020).

Through more creative measures, patients can be encouraged to emulate the shapes, order, and complexity found in nature by replacing the straight lines and rectangles found in their homes with more complex shapes and geometric patterns. Shapes and color are both attributes of biophilic design (Kellert and Calabrese 2015). Additionally, with the development of technology, patients can engage with nature through video games and virtual reality, which, as discussed earlier, can be effective and innovative ways to add biophilic elements into the indoors.

These environmental modifications should not be limited to the home environment, because biophilic design principles and attributes can be applied to the health care setting, such as a hospital or clinic. A provider can modify the auditory environment of the healing space by introducing music and artificial nature sounds. Acoustic modification can also be attained by reducing noise levels, which can act as a stressor. This can be achieved by the use of acoustic panels and noise-source control of some loud equipment, such as alarms, pagers, and monitors. Additionally, one can use natural lighting as a positive distraction, because it can offer stimulation, which reroutes attention from stressors including pain and negative feelings. Daylight in the health care setting has been shown to be beneficial in a multitude of ways, because it decreases stress, the use of pain medication, depression, and length of stay. It also has been linked to increased job satisfaction and productivity. Another way to visually modify the space in accordance with biophilic design elements is to introduce natural imagery in the healing space. This can be achieved through windows overlooking a park or garden if they are available. An alternative way to achieve natural imagery is to add indoor plants and artwork of natural scenery (Ulrich et al. 2010).

In his book *Biophilia*, Wilson (1984, pp. 11–12) stated, "The natural world is the refuge of the spirit, remote, static, richer even than human imagination." This refuge does not have to be limited to the outdoors. The principles of biophilia and biophilic design allow simple modifications of the built environment, which can transform the home and the healing space into a space that is reminiscent of the natural world.

Clinical Translation: Case Example

Mr. A, an older man, is admitted to the hospital for treatment of Lyme disease after a syncopal episode. Psychiatry is consulted to assess for depression. Since admission, Mr. A has been consistently pessimistic, expressed suicidal thoughts, complained of poor sleep, and appeared generally suspicious and oppositional toward the treatment team. Although he has not refused any treatment, he tells the primary team that he would rather go home and die than spend another day in the hospital. On psychiatric evaluation, he is alert, oriented, and able to describe his diagnosis and the treatment offered. Cognitive examination shows deficits in concentration and short-term recall.

Mr. A is initially guarded and skeptical of the consult team, remarking in dismay, "So they think I'm crazy? I don't need the looney doctor." His family reports that before his illness, he was a cheerful, gregarious, and optimistic person.

In the assessment for factors contributing to his hopeless outlook, Mr. A particularly notes outdoor activities as a passion of his and admits feeling worried that he will never return to them. He has a fantasy of living out his last days at a lake house and dying while out fishing on a boat. He firmly believes that the doctors will never let him leave the hospital, and he will never be able to experience his cherished lake house again.

Although Mr. A rejects any challenges to his pessimistic attitude, his affect brightens when he is discussing what he loves about the outdoors, and his conversation is readily redirected toward that topic. The consult team instructs nursing to keep the window blinds open during the day to expose Mr. A to the view and allow sunshine to reinforce a regular circadian rhythm. They recommend that family bring mementos of Mr. A's outdoor hobbies and interests, including pictures of loved ones and pictures of the lake house and surrounding nature.

The family, primary care team, and nurses are counseled to ally with Mr. A on his goal to return to the outdoors by communicating the treatments and interventions offered as steps to get him back to his lake house.

Over the next 2 weeks, reports from family and nursing indicate that Mr. A has been less ornery, better rested, and more cooperative. Although he continues to have bouts of low mood and hopelessness, he is more trusting of the treatment team and feels more at ease in his hospital room. He no longer wants to die outside but rather to take his grandchildren fishing. The pictures of nature added a soothing element to the unfamiliar hospital environment. Encouraging Mr. A to reflect on his experiences in nature disrupted his depressive ruminations and informally led to self-directed guided imagery.

KEY POINTS

- Wilson's biophilia hypothesis suggests that the human psyche is adapted to find comfort in sensory stimuli found in nature. In contrast, the built environment can induce stress because of separation from those natural stimuli.

- The built environment consists of spaces where human activity has significantly altered the topography, material composition, or biodiversity of the landscape.

- Built environments can be hazardous to human health if designed without consideration of ecological needs. Examples on a smaller scale include constructions with poor airflow, low-light conditions, or materials that release volatile compounds. Large cities that concentrate many buildings, factories, and automobiles expose residents to air, noise, and light pollution.

- Biophilic design incorporates natural elements into the built environment to promote physical and mental well-being and minimize hazards associated with classic architectural practices.

- Biophilic design principles can improve health care outcomes when applied to clinical settings; for example, Ulrich et al. found that patients coalescing from surgery in a room with a window had a shorter length of stay.

QUESTIONS

1. What is one way in which home automation can facilitate biophilic design indoors?

    A. Adjusting home brightness in accordance with the time of day or season.
    B. Setting security cameras in your home.
    C. Having a voice-activated doorbell.
    D. Using a smartwatch to monitor your heart rate.
    E. Having an electric car charging station.

Correct answer: A. Adjusting home brightness in accordance with the time of day or season.

    Biomimicry is an approach to innovation that includes adjusting home brightness to emulate nature's patterns and strategies. One can facilitate biophilic design by adjusting light levels and even color temperature through home automation to attain a dynamic range of natural daylight re-created in an interior setting.

2. In the absence of a pollutant, what is the best remedy for sick building syndrome?

    A. Including artwork centered on nature.
    B. Raising the dose of an albuterol inhaler.
    C. Increasing ventilation.
    D. Purchasing a cactus plant.
    E. Increasing fluid intake.

Correct answer: C. Increasing ventilation.

In the absence of chemical contaminants, sick building syndrome is most commonly caused by poor ventilation. People subjected to poor indoor air quality report symptoms that include headache, dizziness, nausea, skin irritation, and mental fatigue, which mimic other conditions that first must be ruled out. If the symptoms tend to recur while in a particular building, the cause is probably sick building syndrome. To create a healthier indoor space, it is recommended to add natural ventilation to the space or even mechanical ventilation.

3. Incorporation of nature indoors has the most benefit for which body system?

    A. Digestive system.
    B. Autonomic nervous system.
    C. Musculoskeletal system.
    D. Endocrine system.
    E. Reproductive system.

Correct answer: B. Autonomic nervous system.

The autonomic nervous system is part of the peripheral nervous system and helps regulate circulation, respiration, digestion, metabolism, secretions, and body temperatures. Various studies have shown that simply viewing natural scenery through display stimuli, such as photographs, three-dimensional images, virtual reality, and videos of natural landscapes, can lead to more relaxed body responses.

REFERENCES

Afacan Y: Impacts of biophilic design on the development of gerotranscendence and the Profile of Mood States during the COVID-19 pandemic. Aging Soc 43(11):1–25, 2021

Blume C, Garbazza C, Spitschan M: Effects of light on human circadian rhythms, sleep and mood. Somnologie (Berl) 23(3):147–156, 2019 31534436

Boubekri M, Cheung IN, Reid KJ, et al: Impact of windows and daylight exposure on overall health and sleep quality of office workers: a case-control pilot study. J Clin Sleep Med 10(6):603–611, 2014 24932139

Budaniya M, Rai AC: Effectiveness of plants for passive removal of particulate matter is low in the indoor environment. Build Environ 222:109384, 2022. Available at: https://doi.org/10.1016/j.buildenv.2022.109384. Accessed April 28, 2024.

Cummings BE, Waring MS: Potted plants do not improve indoor air quality: a review and analysis of reported VOC removal efficiencies. J Expo Sci Environ Epidemiol 30(2):253–261, 2020 31695112

Elzeyadi I: Daylighting-bias and biophilia: quantifying the impacts of daylighting and views on occupants health. Paper presented at Thought and Leadership in Green Buildings Research, Greenbuild 2011, Washington, DC, U.S. Green Building Council, 2011

Franco LS, Shanahan DF, Fuller RA: A review of the benefits of nature experiences: more than meets the eye. Int J Environ Res Public Health 14(8):864, 2017 28763021

Ghaffarianhoseini A, Alwaer H, Omrany H, et al: Sick building syndrome: are we doing enough? Archit Sci Rev 61(3):99–121, 2018

Gogh VV: The Letters of a Post-Impressionist Being the Familiar Correspondence of Vincent van Gogh. Translated by Ludovici A. New York, Houghton Mifflin, 1913. Available at: https://archive.org/details/lettersofpostimp00goghuoft/page/10/mode/2up. Accessed July 24, 2023.

Jo H, Song C, Miyazaki Y: Physiological benefits of viewing nature: a systematic review of indoor experiments. Int J Environ Res Public Health 16(23):4739, 2019 31783531

Kellert S, Calabrese E: The Practice of Biophilic Design. London, Terrapin Bright, 2015

Kellert SR, Heerwagen J, Mador M: Biophilic Design: The Theory, Science and Practice of Bringing Buildings to Life. Hoboken, NJ, Wiley, 2011

Kurlansik SL, Ibay AD: Seasonal affective disorder. Am Fam Physician 86(11):1037–1041, 2012 23198671

Lee MS, Lee J, Park BJ, et al: Interaction with indoor plants may reduce psychological and physiological stress by suppressing autonomic nervous system activity in young adults: a randomized crossover study. J Physiol Anthropol 34(1):21, 2015 25928639

Leighanne J, Wallace T, Morris J, et al: Smart home stress assist: a real-time intervention for PTSD. J Technol Pers Disabil 8:40–52, 2020

Liu L, Stroulia E, Nikolaidis I, et al: Smart homes and home health monitoring technologies for older adults: a systematic review. Int J Med Inform 91:44–59, 2016 27185508

Marroquín B, Vine V, Morgan R: Mental health during the COVID-19 pandemic: effects of stay-at-home policies, social distancing behavior, and social resources. Psychiatry Res 293:113419, 2020 32861098

Mushtaq R, Shoib S, Shah T, et al: Relationship between loneliness, psychiatric disorders and physical health? A review on the psychological aspects of loneliness. J Clin Diagn Res 8(9):WE01–WE04, 2014 25386507

Nelson BW, Allen NB: Extending the passive-sensing toolbox: using smart-home technology in psychological science. Perspect Psychol Sci 13(6):718–733, 2018 30217132

Oh YA, Kim SO, Park SA: Real foliage plants as visual stimuli to improve concentration and attention in elementary students. Int J Environ Res Public Health 16(5):796, 2019 30841505

Outdoor Foundation: 2019 Outdoor participation report. 2019. Available at: https://oia.outdoorindustry.org/2019-Participation-Report. Accessed December 29, 2020.

Penninx BWJH, Lange SMM: Metabolic syndrome in psychiatric patients: overview, mechanisms, and implications. Dialogues Clin Neurosci 20(1):63–73, 2018 29946213

Ryan CO, Browning WD: Biophilic design, in Sustainable Built Environments. Encyclopedia of Sustainability Science and Technology Series. Edited by Loftness V. New York, Springer, 2020, pp 43–85

Santas A: Aristotelian ethics and biophilia. Ethics Environ 19(1):95–121, 2014

Song C, Igarashi M, Ikei H, et al: Physiological effects of viewing fresh red roses. Complement Ther Med 35:78–84, 2017

Techopedia: What is a home automation system? June 12, 2018. Available at: https://www.techopedia.com/definition/29999/home-automation-system. Accessed June 24, 2022.

Tornstam L: Gero-transcendence: a reformulation of the disengagement theory. Aging (Milano) 1(1):55–63, 1989 2488301

Ulrich RS: View through a window may influence recovery from surgery. Science 224(4647):420–421, 1984 6143402

Ulrich RS, Zimring C, Zhu X, et al: A review of the research literature on evidence-based healthcare design. HERD 1(3):61–125, 2008 21161908

Ulrich RS, Berry LL, Quan X, et al: A conceptual framework for the domain of evidence-based design. HERD 4(1):95–114, 2010 21162431

Wang HC, Ting W, Li Z, et al: Mental health problems of individuals under the stay-home policy. Psychiatry Investig 17(7):712–713, 2020 32654439

Wang Y, Jiang M, Huang Y, et al: Physiological and psychological effects of watching videos of different durations showing urban bamboo forests with varied structures. Int J Environ Res Public Health 17(10):3434, 2020 32423106

Wilson EO: Biophilia. Cambridge, MA, Harvard University Press, 1984

Wilson EO, Kellert SR: The Biophilia Hypothesis. Washington, DC, Island Press, 1993

Wolverton BC, Douglas WL, Bounds K: A Study of Interior Landscape Plants for Indoor Air Pollution Abatement (No REPT-6). Washington, DC, NASA, 1989

Yanez ND, Weiss NS, Romand JA, et al: COVID-19 mortality risk for older men and women. BMC Public Health 20(1):1742, 2020 33213391

Yin J, Yuan J, Arfaei N, et al: Effects of biophilic indoor environment on stress and anxiety recovery: a between-subjects experiment in virtual reality. Environ Int 136:105427, 2020 31881421

Zelnik YR, Mau Y, Shachak M, et al: High-integrity human intervention in ecosystems: tracking self-organization modes. PLoS Comput Biol 17(9):e1009427, 2021 34587157

Zhang X, Lian Z, Wu Y: Human physiological responses to wooden indoor environment. Physiol Behav 174:27–34, 2017

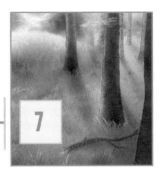

7

The Wild Outdoors

WILDERNESS THERAPY

Alexis Bocian-Reperowitz, M.D.
Stephanie Ruthberg, M.D., M.S.
Diego Garces Grosse, M.D.

> *But there are no words that can tell*
> *the hidden spirit of the wilderness,*
> *that can reveal its mystery, its melancholy, and its charm.*
> —President Theodore Roosevelt (1910, p. xi)

HISTORY OF WILDERNESS THERAPY

The idea of young or immature members of society returning to nature to gain purpose, confidence, and maturity has been practiced by societies across the globe for millennia. The quintessential example is the vision quest, practiced by native tribes and Indigenous cultures across the world for more than 8,000 years (Fernee et al. 2017). During vision quests, adolescent members of society travel alone into nature. This solitary experience represents a point of transition from childhood to adulthood during which participants become more connected to the natural world and gain independence and self-sufficiency. Although vision quests are not common practice in industrialized America, our society has continued to idealize outdoorspersons throughout history. The archetype of an outdoorsperson is one who is rugged, confident, capable, and steadfast. Rooted in patriarchal values, these people traditionally have been male, such as Davy Crockett, Henry David Thoreau, Meriwether Lewis and William Clark, Bear Grylls, and Steve Irwin. But consider Sacagawea's role in Lewis and Clark's expedition and Harriet Tubman's refuge in nature to free slaves. Undoubtedly, their competencies in wilderness play into this mental image of an outdoorsperson. How did their time in the wilderness help these men and women build their qualities, and how can we use the natural world to help young members of society find these qualities within themselves?

In the early 1960s, this idea that time in nature can help young people develop more competencies and confidence became the foundation of Outward Bound, the first widely acknowledged organization for wilderness therapy in modern America. Outward Bound was founded by Kurt Hahn in the 1940s to help Welsh sailors survive World War II (Freeman 2010). It was based on the principle that "training *through* rather than *for*" hardships builds practical skills (Freeman 2010). Since its inception, Outward Bound has branched beyond teaching skills to military recruits and built a business in America around the promise that time in the wilderness can teach the sought-after qualities of the idealized outdoorsperson to young people. Outward Bound programs focus on remote wilderness experiences with novel challenge group tasks for young men and women in addition to time alone in the wilderness to help them develop core character components and confidence (Freeman 2010). Since this modern inception of wilderness therapy, the field has continued to evolve based on research, feedback from patients and families, and patient needs.

In the 1960s through the early 1990s, the field was growing rapidly, with more than 500 unique wilderness therapy programs opening across the United States by 1996 (Russell 2001). During this time, there was no clear definition of wilderness therapy or governing body holding these programs to a set of standards. Many terms even began to be used interchangeably with *wilderness therapy*, including *adventure-based therapy*, *challenge courses*, and *wilderness experience programs* (Powch 1994). Although no clear definition or execution of wilderness therapy existed during this period, the one thing that was clear was that young members of society were craving wilderness experiences to help improve their mental health and self-esteem.

In the mid-1990s, the journey to establish a more standardized definition and process of wilderness therapy began. Other terms such as *adventure-based therapy* and *wilderness experience programs* that previously had been used interchangeably with *wilderness therapy* were determined to be distinct components of, but not interchangeable with, wilderness therapy (Powch 1994). Additionally, in the 1990s, governing bodies were created to help monitor the quality and standardize the experience of wilderness therapy (Russell 2001). Since this time, a standardized definition and procedure for wilderness therapy have been established, edited, and reestablished innumerable times. It has been more challenging for researchers and clinicians to standardize and define wilderness therapy compared with other forms of therapy because of the unique setting. Unlike other forms of therapy that can be extremely standardized and replicated, novel wilderness experiences and challenges cannot be. One of the most comprehensive definitions of wilderness therapy to date states that "treatment takes place in a semi-unpredictable wilderness environment. The programs are commonly run by a multidisciplinary therapist team….The intervention is multi-faceted, consisting of primitive outdoor life, various sequenced tasks and challenges, and structured individual and group-based therapeutic work," and these components interact nonlinearly to produce context-dependent outcomes (Fernee et al. 2017, p. 115). This definition encompasses the major components of therapy while leaving enough ambiguity for the variability that results from the uncontrollable nature of wilderness experiences.

As a definition and standardization for wilderness therapy began to be explored, so did the patient population it was effective for. In the mid-1990s, clinicians indicated that potential candidates for wilderness therapy should go through a clinical assessment, and an individualized treatment plan should be established (Davis-Berman and Berman 1994). The population most targeted for wilderness therapy since its inception has been adolescents. Over time, wilderness therapy has been found to provide the most benefits as a second-line treatment for adolescents who have had unsuccessful experiences with traditional counseling or mental health treatment (Fernee et al. 2017). Many of the adolescent patients referred to wilderness therapy have experienced administrative trouble in school, conflicts at home, trouble with the law, or defiance of authority (Cook 2008). Patients referred to wilderness therapy also have low self-esteem and poor communication skills. Therefore, the most common diagnoses associated with wilderness therapy are oppositional defiant disorder, conduct disorder, ADHD, and substance abuse. Patients with other diagnoses including severe emotional disorders, depression, and depression with suicidal ideation also may be referred to wilderness therapy. Although this is the major group of patients targeted for wilderness therapy, it has shown to be effective in other populations as well. Wilderness therapy can be used for male and female patients and is effective for family therapy and veterans or survivors of sexual assault with PTSD (Joye and Dietrich 2016; Powch 1994). Recently, Johnson et al. (2020) found support for trauma-informed wilderness therapy as a meaningful intervention for adolescents. For all populations, the unique structure and process of wilderness therapy make it effective for patients who did not respond to first-line treatments.

PROCESS AND STRUCTURE OF WILDERNESS THERAPY

The process of wilderness therapy is inextricably intertwined with the natural environment. Because the natural environment cannot be precisely replicated and controlled, wilderness therapy cannot be precisely defined and proceduralized in the same way as other forms of mental health therapy. Wilderness therapy relies on the interaction between environments that are unfamiliar to patients, the patients themselves, the group, and the leaders. It uses these variables while applying traditional methods of group system model, interpersonal behavior, group psychotherapy, family systems, and cognitive-behavioral therapy to help patients develop positive coping skills and meet their individual treatment goals (Russell 2001). What truly separates wilderness therapy from other forms of therapy is the environment in which it occurs.

In other, more traditional forms of therapy, the central focus of the therapy is the relationship between the patient and the clinician or between the patient and the other members of their therapeutic group. In wilderness therapy, the relationship between the patient and the therapeutic environment is the central relationship. As previously described, the patient populations are teenagers or young adults with a background of conflict between themselves and authority figures. These patients often view traditional therapists as authority figures and transfer their distrust of authority figures onto them, which hinders their experience in traditional therapy. In wilderness therapy, the "natural consequences experienced in wilderness living allow staff to step back from traditional positions of authority to which the client is accustomed" (Russell 2001, p. 74). Instead of patients being expected to follow the rules of authority figures, their self-care and personal responsibility are facilitated by natural consequences in the wilderness. This allows authority figures to no longer be seen as oppositional to the patients' goals but as teammates to reach common goals and overcome natural obstacles. Additionally, these patients who have had multiple experiences with mental health care often perceive a societal stigma toward mental health treatment. This stigma is avoided by moving treatment to a wilderness setting (Russell and Phillips-Miller 2002). The most current definitions require that wilderness therapy be performed in an unfamiliar wilderness environment. This is not limited to the woods and can include desert, mountain, and ocean landscapes that are remote and foreign to the patients (Fernee et al. 2017). The most important aspect of the location in which wilderness therapy is practiced is that it is novel to the patient, so it presents a new set of challenges and experiences.

Although the exact procedure is flexible, most wilderness therapy programs have a similar flow and process rooted in evidence to help patients. The first phase of wilderness therapy occurs while the patient adapts to a novel environment. As treatment progresses and the patients have adjusted, they work with peers and counselors to undergo a series of challenges presented by the natural world. Finally, the patients work with the counselors and peers to gain perspective on the experience and plan for reentry into their previous lives and environments.

At the start of wilderness therapy, the relationship between the patient and the natural environment is central to the therapeutic experience. This is often considered the "cleansing phase" of wilderness therapy (Russell 2001, p. 75). Wilderness can be considered a "restorative environment for at-risk youth who have high levels of anxiety and are stressed from mental fatigue caused by too much direct attention" (Russell and Farnum 2004, p. 41). The removal from society and placement in a new and isolated environment of wilderness have benefits for patients with a wide variety of presenting conditions. For patients with substance abuse diagnoses, wilderness therapy removes them from the environments that perpetuate the patterns that led to their addictions. It also removes access to said substances (Russell 2001). During this initial cleansing phase, patients eat a healthy diet, exercise as a consequence of living in the wilderness, and learn basic survival and self-care skills. This can allow patients to develop a sense of confidence in themselves, and the healthier lifestyle can make them feel physically more confident.

Often, patients are overwhelmed in their home environments by attention, responsibilities, and social pressures from in-person interactions, technological communication, and social media (Gabrielsen and Harper 2018). The initial natural environment–focused phase of wilderness therapy also gives patients time and inner quiet to reflect on life, their choices, and their sense of self (Fernee et al. 2017). This can be particularly helpful for patients with anxiety, depression, and other diagnoses related to interpersonal interactions by allowing a quieting of the mind to develop increased awareness and personal insight. Patients usually describe this as a positive and transformative experience during which they have time and mental space to gain perspective, mentally confront past challenges, and increase their appreciation for their positive life experiences (Russell and Phillips-Miller 2002). Once the cleansing phase is completed, patients move on to the next stages of wilderness therapy with a clear mind.

After the initial phase of therapy in which the relationship between the patient and the wilderness is central, the focus of the therapeutic experience slowly shifts to the relationship between the patient and their self-image, as well as the relationship between the patient and the other members of their therapeutic group. This phase of wilderness therapy is usually achieved through group challenge activities, most commonly hiking and camping (Fernee et al. 2017). Although the activities may vary, it is important that they provide a simple and continuous movement that is new to the patient and that they can improve over time. This shift was explored in an in-depth analysis of a wilderness therapy centered on backpacking over 6–8 weeks in a group (Caulkins et al. 2006). Hiking is an uninterrupted, simple movement that allows patients' minds to wander, reflect on their choices, reevaluate what they had placed importance on in the past, and decide what they planned to do differently moving forward. It is also important that the physical demands of the experience are new to the patients (Fernee et al. 2017). Novel and repetitive physical activities allow patients to build a skill over time and gain physical strength. Patients report feeling that as the act of hiking each day becomes easier, they feel a sense of accomplishment and self-efficacy that will allow them to stay calm and persevere

(Fernee et al. 2017). This leads the patients to develop mental resilience that they can apply to their everyday lives outside wilderness therapy.

As patients work to accomplish novel and challenging wilderness tasks and build their sense of self, they work alongside staff and peers. Wilderness therapy is generally done in small groups with an approximate 2:1 patient-to-counselor ratio specifically to allow for the social self to develop (Russell 2001). Patients who benefit from wilderness therapy typically have had previous high-conflict relationships with caregivers, authority figures, and peers. The teamwork needed to conquer the environmental challenges in wilderness therapy while living alongside the peers and counselors helps the patients overcome this lack of trust and connection in interpersonal relationships. Working for a common goal and living alongside counselors and peers in nature help patients see others as team members who go through challenges with them (Russell 2005). This allows patients to build trust in counselors so that they can develop the social skills to share their feelings and hardships.

Because of their high-conflict relationships before therapy, many patients have limited social support. The new and rugged environment requires communication and cooperation for safety and comfort (Russell 2001). The therapeutic group working toward a common goal through cooperative acts helps them build prosocial skills. After expeditions, patients report feeling "cared about" and having a group of people they can trust and share with (Cook 2008). Once the patients start to trust their counselors and peers, they can build on that trust by developing communication skills and cooperation that will help them navigate their strained interpersonal relationships in everyday life. The trusted counselors help by teaching the patients prosocial ways to "manage anger, share emotions, and process interpersonal issues within the group" in an environment in which the patients feel emotionally safe and supported (Russell 2001, p. 75). They then encourage the patients to use these skills and build relationships with their families and caregivers outside therapy through facilitated contact.

Once the patients complete the first phases of wilderness therapy, they spend the final weeks preparing to transition back to their real-world environments. This is accomplished through one-on-one counseling with the now trusted counselors, as well as group therapy (Russell 2001). The patients and therapists work together to create a plan to accomplish their specific goals once they return to their home environments (Russell 2001). The staff also facilitates patients' transition into outpatient therapy when they return home. This allows patients to transfer their trust in their wilderness therapy counselors to their outpatient mental health providers in their communities.

Each patient works with the therapeutic team to set their own goals, so one standard outcome cannot be used as a measure of success or failure of a wilderness program. Unlike many other forms of therapy that work toward a cure, when patients leave wilderness therapy, they are not considered "cured" or "fixed" (Russell 2005). Instead, wilderness therapy creates a foundation of communication skills, self-efficacy, and personal responsibility that patients can use when tackling future challenges (Davis-Berman and Berman 2012). The initial cleansing experience and the relationship the patient develops with the natural world provide time for the patient to think and reflect. Many patients look back on this stage of therapy as the time when they realized that their past behavior was a symptom of other issues in their lives, and they understand that they want to make a change (Russell 2001). As the patients gain physical strength and competencies through living in and interacting with the natural environment, they develop increased self-esteem and self-concept, which helps them resist previous choices and negative influences when they return to life outside the wilderness setting (Russell 2001). As patients move through therapy, they develop communication skills and prosocial behavior that help them build a more consistent and strong support group in their everyday lives. Once patients feel that they are in a supportive environment, they can address mental health challenges with staff, which provides positive therapeutic experiences that encourage patients to continue traditional therapy when they return to their community. The gains that patients experience in wilderness therapy hold true over time. Two years after the completion of wilderness therapy, 87% of the patients who completed wilderness therapy said that they were still doing well and consistently working toward the goals outlined in their wilderness therapy treatment plan (Russell 2005). As patients gain distance from the wilderness therapy experience, they continue to reflect and make discoveries about themselves and their strengths. Even patients who stated that they did not enjoy wilderness therapy while participating reported social and emotional gains 2 years after completion.

CONTROVERSIES

Although research largely favors the positive experience and long-term gains of participants, wilderness therapy is not without controversy. One major cause of controversy is the ambiguity in definition, procedure, and goals of wilderness therapy. This ambiguity provides patients who need nontraditional therapy with a more flexible therapeutic environment, but it can leave room for misconceptions of what true wilderness therapy is. It also allows the media to portray wilderness therapy as a sort of bootcamp where patients are physically and emotionally broken down with cruelty (August 2003). This view of wilderness therapy gained more media traction in the 1990s, when five teenage patients enrolled in various wilderness therapy programs died. Four of them died as a result of complications of dehydration or heatstroke, and one patient died after losing footing on a dangerous hike (August 2003). These tragedies were inexcusable and led to various changes in oversight and the advancement of healthy wilderness therapy environments. First, the Outdoor Behavioral Healthcare Research Cooperative was founded in 1999 at the University of Idaho (Russell 2001). Their goal is to fund research into wilderness therapy programs to set safe standards and give accreditation to programs that meet these standards. Also, many wilderness programs now work with insurance companies and the states in which they operate to meet standards and become accredited as adolescent residential treatment programs. Some of these standards include required calories per day, medical and professional clinical staff supervision and check-ins, and individualized treatment plans (Russell 2001). As wilderness therapy has progressed since its inception in the 1960s, it has begun to strike a balance as a second-line treatment that is not only flexible enough to meet the unique needs of patients but also standardized enough to show positive and measurable outcomes.

APPLICATIONS FOR THE PHYSICIAN

Traditional wilderness therapy requires dedicated time and resources that may not be easily accessible, especially in urban centers. Cox et al. (2017) found that the frequency of exposure to nature is a stronger predictor than duration for a variety of health outcomes. Thus, it is useful to consider quotidian interventions that physicians can incorporate into their outpatient practices. For example, providers can conduct walking sessions outdoors or give instructions to patients on exercises that they can do outside, such as outdoor meditation and prescribed walks and hikes. Making small changes to models of therapy and treatment to incorporate more frequent exposure to the natural world are no substitute for an intensive multiday outdoor excursion but may approximate the benefits of wilderness therapy to a broader population.

Clinical Translation: Case Example

Laura, a 15-year-old girl with a history of unspecified anxiety disorder and oppositional defiant disorder, has been at four different schools in the past 5 years because of behavioral conduct issues and has tried various medications and therapies with limited success. At this time, wilderness therapy would be an appropriate intervention. She would benefit from the small group dynamic with like-minded peers and the establishment of a new role model in one of the counselors. The novel physical terrain may allow her to shed her maladaptive defense mechanisms and replace them with new coping strategies that she can continue to build on after wilderness therapy is completed.

KEY POINTS

- Wilderness therapy is not a new idea. Young people have been turning to nature to gain purpose and personal growth for millennia.

- The patient population traditionally consists of adolescents with a background of conflict between themselves and authority figures.

- Wilderness therapy must be performed in an unfamiliar wilderness environment and is often done in groups. Trust in counselors or leaders is used to model better behaviors for the patients and generalize to their home environments.

- Benefits of wilderness therapy extend far beyond the experience itself.

- Misconceptions and previously unregulated safety in these programs have limited the reach of wilderness therapy in the past.

QUESTIONS

1. Which of the following patients best exemplifies the population in which wilderness therapy is most effective?

    A. A 12-year-old with active suicidal ideation and new-onset self-harm behavior.

    B. A 32-year-old with long-standing bipolar disorder well controlled by lithium.

C. A 16-year-old who fights with their parents, frequently skips school, and was not compliant with traditional talk therapy.
D. A 20-year-old who dropped out of college, has started using cocaine, and has had no previous mental health treatment.
E. A 72-year-old army veteran with early-stage dementia.

Correct answer: C. A 16-year-old who fights with their parents, frequently skips school, and was not compliant with traditional talk therapy.

Wilderness therapy programs are tailored to address externalizing behavioral disorders such as conduct disorder by facilitating personal growth removed from the systems in which problematic behaviors were learned. Patients with acutely elevated suicide risk (A) should be stabilized before considering a wilderness program. A patient with a well-controlled mood disorder (B) would not benefit from the intensive residential structure of a wilderness program and may risk disrupting access to their medications. Wilderness therapy is not the first-line treatment for a new-onset substance use disorder (D). The wilderness setting poses physically and mentally demanding challenges and is not equipped with the mobility and safety considerations necessary for treatment of cognitive decline in an older patient (E).

2. A patient in wilderness therapy is reflecting on their experience while hiking a 100-mile trail during a group discussion with other patients and a counselor in the wilderness environment. This is most consistent with what phase of wilderness therapy?

A. The initial, cleansing phase of wilderness therapy.
B. The second stage of wilderness therapy, in which self-image and interpersonal relationships are the therapeutic focus.
C. The third stage of wilderness therapy, in which patients prepare to transition back to their home environment.
D. The fourth stage of wilderness therapy, in which patients maintain the interpersonal skills they gained during their wilderness experience.

Correct answer: B. The second stage of wilderness therapy, in which self-image and interpersonal relationships are the therapeutic focus.

The initial, cleansing phase (A) focuses on concrete tasks of doing physical exercise, eating a nutritious diet, and learning survivalist hiking skills. Introspection and self-reflection begin during the second stage of therapy while still in the wilderness. Answer choices C and D describe maintenance of treatment at the conclusion of the wilderness excursion.

3. Which of the following standards is most likely to help a wilderness therapy program receive accreditation as an adolescent residential treatment center?

    A. Required calories burned per day.
    B. Staff are certified wilderness experts.
    C. Wheelchair-accessible hiking trails.
    D. Weekly visits with parents.
    E. Individualized treatment plans.

Correct answer: E. Individualized treatment plans.

Wilderness programs must meet clinical standards to be accredited as adolescent residential treatment centers. These standards include developing individualized treatment plans for each client so that their progress can be measured against concrete treatment goals. Other standards include minimum caloric intake per day, not expenditure (A), and regular check-ins with medical professionals, not family members (D). Although having certified wilderness experts on staff may lend credibility and improve safety of the program, this is not a feature associated with accreditation as an adolescent residential treatment center (B). Wilderness programs often include rugged terrain that may not be wheelchair accessible. Accessible trails are not a requirement for residential treatment program accreditation (C).

REFERENCES

August I: Utah wilderness therapy deaths. Salt Lake Tribune, July 13, 2003. Available at: https://archive.sltrib.com/story.php?ref=/news/ci_7139316#:~:text=Since%201990%2C%20five%20teens%20have,given%2090%2Dday%20conditional%20licenses. Accessed March 7, 2022.

Caulkins MC, White DD, Russell KC: The role of physical exercise in wilderness therapy for troubled adolescent women. Journal of Experiential Education 29(1):18–37, 2006

Cook EC: Residential wilderness programs: the role of social support in influencing self-evaluations of male adolescents. Adolescence 43(172):751–774, 2008 19149144

Cox DTC, Shanahan DF, Hudson HL, et al: Doses of nearby nature simultaneously associated with multiple health benefits. Int J Environ Res Public Health 14(2):1–13, 2017 28208789

Davis-Berman J, Berman DS: Research update: two-year follow-up report for the wilderness therapy program. Journal of Experiential Education 17(1):48–50, 1994

Davis-Berman J, Berman DS: Reflections on a trip: two decades later. Journal of Experiential Education 35(2):326–340, 2012

Fernee CR, Gabrielsen LE, Andersen AJ, et al: Unpacking the black box of wilderness therapy: a realist synthesis. Qual Health Res 27(1):114–129, 2017 27354386

Freeman M: From "character-training" to "personal growth": the early history of Outward Bound 1941–1965. Hist Educ 40(1):21–43, 2010

Gabrielsen LE, Harper NJ: The role of wilderness therapy for adolescents in the face of global trends of urbanization and technification. Int J Adolesc Youth 23(4):409–421, 2018

Johnson EG, Davis EB, Johnson J, et al: The effectiveness of trauma-informed wilderness therapy with adolescents: a pilot study. Psychol Trauma 12(8):878–887, 2020 32496098

Joye S, Dietrich Z: Promoting resilience among veterans using wilderness therapy. Wilderness Environ Med 27(3):427, 2016

Powch IG: Wilderness therapy. Women Ther 15(3–4):11–27, 1994

Roosevelt T: African Game Trails. New York, Syndicate Publishing, 1910

Russell KC: What is wilderness therapy? Journal of Experiential Education 24(2):70–79, 2001

Russell KC: Two years later: a qualitative assessment of youth well-being and the role of aftercare in outdoor behavioral healthcare treatment. Child Youth Care Forum 34:209–239, 2005

Russell KC, Farnum J: A concurrent model of the wilderness therapy process. Journal of Adventure Education and Outdoor Learning 4(1):39–55, 2004

Russell KC, Phillips-Miller D: Perspectives on the wilderness therapy process and its relation to outcome. Child Youth Care Forum 31:415–437, 2002

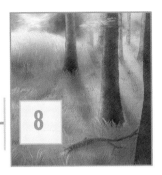

8

The Wet Outdoors

HARNESSING THE POWER OF
OUR AQUEOUS SURROUNDINGS

Mary-Anne E. Hennen, M.D.
Ryan Behmer Hansen, M.D.
Elizabeth Fam Filtes, M.D.
Celena Q. Ma, M.D.

*The water you touch in a river is the last of that which has
passed, and the first of that which is coming.
Thus it is with time present.*
—Leonardo da Vinci (1888)

The intimate history between humanity and water is extensive. Marine biologist and author Wallace J. Nichols stated, "There's something about water that draws and fascinates us" (Nichols and Cousteau 2014, p. 8). But why are we so hydrocentric? It might be unsurprising that many of us are drawn to and find solace in water, given that the human body is nearly 70% water (National Oceanic and Atmospheric Administration 2021; Nichols and Cousteau 2014; Water Science School 2019). Water is the most abundant substance on Earth. Water covers more than 70% of Earth's surface, and more than 80% of our oceans remain largely unexplored (National Oceanic and Atmospheric Administration 2021; Nichols and Cousteau 2014; Water Science School 2019). Water has remained shrouded in a clandestine, even sacred status since early human history and has often held a restorative role in various cultures, belief systems, and societies. Water also has been misused, with harmful results. In this chapter, we take a deep dive into the complex relationship between water and humankind, including the cultural, historical, and spiritual identity of water; its physiological effects; the dark historical role of water in psychiatric treatment; and how it has been adapted to take on its contemporary role in mental health.

WATER AND HUMANITY THROUGHOUT HISTORY

Many early civilizations were built near bodies of water: Jericho, West Bank, around springs of water; ancient India near the Ganges River; and, perhaps most prominently, the ancient Egyptians, whose entire society revolved around the comings and goings of the Nile River. This was no coincidence. Living near water gave inhabitants access to drinking water, water for agriculture, and a place to bathe. It also contributed to the culture and development of these early societies. It led to the birth of various trades and innovations, including fishing, shipbuilding, and irrigation. Water connected civilizations through trade between Asia, Africa, and the Middle East and led to the age of exploration. Voyagers came back home with stories from abroad; listeners became intrigued by the possibilities that travel through water brought.

Beyond the practical and anthropological necessity of water, many religions attached spiritual meaning to water, and it was highly regarded in many belief systems. In Greek mythology, Poseidon, the god of the sea, is one of the most powerful gods (Columbia University Press 2015). In animism, water is considered an entity that connects people through relationships (Schweitzer 2015; Zip Water 2017). For the three

Abrahamic religions, water was not only sacred but also precious because of its scarcity in the Middle Eastern deserts where Semitic, semi-nomadic clans developed the monotheistic traditions as the Fertile Crescent started to dry up. In Judaism, water represents purity and life (Kabbalah Center 2022). In Christianity, baptism through water signifies a declaration of faith and rebirth (Rouwhorst et al. 2009). In Islam, water signifies wisdom and is referred to as an integral part of one's self (Jah 2020; Zip Water 2017). In Hinduism, water is sacred and has purifying and cleansing powers (Sharma and Tiffin 2007). Buddhism emphasizes the calmness and serenity of water, with water offerings as common practice in their shrines (Unno 1998).

Perhaps the predecessor to many modern practices, Greco-Roman bathhouses were a central feature throughout the Roman Empire. What began with the ancient Greeks' conviction that hygiene and cleanliness were essential in maintaining good health was further transformed into the magnificent baths made famous by the Romans (Cartwright 2013). Water continued to shape the development of civilization in the 1700s and 1800s, as "spa towns" emerged throughout Europe. Bathing practices, which were believed to have healing properties and previously had been reserved for more wealthy citizens, began to become more common among less-well-to-do members of society (Wallaya 2020). Water's composition varied geographically. The granite-filtered water that ran through Malvern, United Kingdom, was reputed to be miraculously pure, containing "nothing at all." A medicinal quality was ascribed to "liquid gold," a term reverently applied to the sulfurous waters that ran into the baths near Vienna, Austria (Wallaya 2020). People traveled to these spa towns for the physical rewards they promised.

Over the last 200 years, humans have found various ways to leverage the power of water to improve physical and mental health, as we describe later in this chapter. Yet there has always been a duality to water. It was established early on that water could also spread disease (e.g., cholera, typhoid) and cause death (World Health Organization 2002). The connection between water quality and health was first noted by Alcmaeon of Croton in 470 B.C. (Codellas 1932). Access to healthy water continues to be an essential public health concern today.

THE DARK AND STORMY HISTORY OF WATER IN PSYCHIATRY

In 1951, the development of the first antipsychotic medication, chlorpromazine, revolutionized the way we think about the treatment of mental illnesses. It opened a world of possibilities in using targeted pharmacotherapy (Ban 2007). In the era before this shift, psychiatric treatment revolved around nonpharmacological therapies, such as rest cures, phototherapies, electrotherapy, hypnosis, diet cures, and hydrotherapies (Harmon 2009; McGuire 1997). In light of new understandings of mental illness and its treatment, these therapies have since been discontinued or revised, but their history remains relevant because they inform modern techniques. For the purposes of this section, we focus more closely on those that are water related. As mentioned earlier, the way that water has been used by psychiatrists and other practitioners to treat psychiatric illness is complex, and a lot of troubled history is found behind many of these "therapies." In this section, we explore how water in the hands of doctors has shown potential for both significant therapeutic benefit and substantial harm.

One way that water was used historically to benefit psychiatric patients was by reducing the use of more abrasive treatments. As early as the 1890s, Emil Kraepelin and Alois Alzheimer were proponents of warm water "duration baths" (Clarfield 2005). These baths were intended to be maintained at a fairly constant temperature, about 93°F, according to Kraepelin's recommendation. Alzheimer noted that the use of these baths would lessen the need for restraint and isolation in psychotic patients, thereby resulting in more humane care (Clarfield 2005).

Many contemporaries of Kraepelin and Alzheimer rejected the duration baths, however. Especially in the United States, cold water wraps and other less comfortable therapies were used more often (Clarfield 2005). Common therapies included sponging, hot and cold packs, enteroclysis (the practice of injecting water or other liquids into the intestine), hypodermoclysis (the practice of injecting water subcutaneously), cabinet sweats, tubs (the practice of submerging in a bathtub for a limited amount of time), and swimming pools (Jackson 1915; see descriptions of these therapies later in this section). The spectrum of indications for these therapies was broad. According to a 1915 article published in the *Journal of the American Medical Association*, the indications for hydrotherapy treatment included "depression, excitement, elimination, autointoxication and when a relaxation is desired or mental diversion and exercise" (Jackson 1915, p. 1651). The importance placed on hydrotherapy in this same article is striking. J. Allen Jackson (1915, p. 1651), at the time serving as chief resident physician for the Philadelphia Hospital for the Insane, wrote, "'Lunatic asylum' is the proper nomenclature for an institution which has no hydrotherapy outfit; to call such an institution a hospital would be a misnomer and, to say the least, exceedingly out of place." Although these modalities were considered essential therapeutic mental health treatments in their day, many are now considered problematic, radical, and inhumane.

There was a logic to the use of water as a therapeutic technique to treat mental illness. It was believed that exposing the body to different temperatures would produce different reactions throughout the body and alleviate psychotic and affective symptoms (Harmon 2009; Jackson 1915). Water temperatures during these treatments ranged from 40°F to 100°F, depending on the indication. Cold temperatures were believed to be useful in treating mania, hysteria, agitation, and psychosis because they slowed blood flow to the brain and slowed mental activity. Hotter temperatures were indicated for depression, anxiety, insomnia, and autointoxication because they were thought to be cleansing and stimulating of blood flow to the brain, which would promote motivation and clarity of mind. Some of these early aqueous treatments were simple, such as sponging and hot and cold packs that would be wrapped on a patient's body for hours at a time. These strategies have even been adapted for use today in settings such as spas and bathhouses. Other, more invasive treatments such as enteroclysis and hypodermoclysis were considered therapeutic in that they would maintain adequate hydration and could remedy autointoxication.

Other treatments were more demoralizing, often used punitively, and left a much darker mark on the history of psychiatric treatment. For example, the infamous "sprays" were often compared with showers, but they were actually a degrading, traumatizing experience for patients, who stood naked in a showerlike stall while a nurse used a powerful hose to blast the patient with water at a specific temperature for several minutes at a time (Cox et al. 2019; Jackson 1915; Nelson and Erickson 1949). "Shock baths" were essentially ice-cold dunk tanks into which mentally ill patients would be dropped unexpectedly and without warning in the hopes of shocking the mental ailment out of them (Cox et al. 2019). "Continuous baths" consisted of suspending a patient in a hammocklike apparatus inside a bathtub for hours to even days at a time, with water temperatures maintained continuously between 95°F and 100°F (Allen 1937; Harmon 2009). "Cabinet sweats" were conducted in locked boxes or cabinets, also known as "fever cabinets," that were heated with high-wattage light bulbs on the inside that increased the internal temperature to 105°F; patients would be placed inside with only their head sticking out of a hole in the top for about 10 minutes at a time, then quickly moved to showers (Jackson 1915).

Given the severity and duration of these intensive treatments, it is not difficult to imagine how any negligence or bias on the part of the treating party could result in patient abuse and mistreatment. Although these treatments may seem barbaric and undignified now, they were respected and trusted methods in their time and were considered an indispensable tool in the arsenal of treatments for mental illness (Jackson 1915). As we will see, several of these treatments have been abandoned to the dark past, but others have been adapted and have paved the way for contemporary therapies. Examples include the "shock baths" and "continuous baths," which could be seen as crude, poorly devised predecessors of the mammalian diving reflex and flotation restricted environmental stimulation technique (REST) therapies, respectively.

CURRENT THERAPIES AND PRACTICAL GUIDELINES

We now focus more closely on the evidence for water therapies to improve health. When one considers water-based therapeutic modalities, two major terms may come to mind: *hydrotherapy* and *balneotherapy*. Although these terms are often used interchangeably, they are actually two subtly distinct concepts. Hydrotherapy is a therapeutic strategy that uses simply water in its various forms—liquid, ice, and vapor—in different applications for the promotion of health and treatment of diseases (Mooventhan and Nivethitha 2014). Balneotherapy, on the other hand, is a distinct traditional medicinal practice that specifically entails using certain natural thermal mineral waters and clays for therapeutic effects (Yang et al. 2018). In the next section, we first delve deeper into the physiological effects of water on different body systems. Then, we look more carefully at the differences between water-based treatment modalities, their benefits, and the different aspects of these therapies summarized in Table 8–1.

Physiological Effects of Water on Various Body Systems

Although those who administered water therapy in historic times did not fully understand its underlying therapeutic mechanisms, modern observational tools and research instruments have allowed us to better appreciate how hydrotherapy can have beneficial effects. In this section, we share these findings, organized by body system.

Cardiovascular System

The physiology of the cardiovascular system is intimately connected with water. For example, in order to maintain constant deep tissue temperature, exposure of small surface areas to cold produces a vasodilatory effect in the underlying vasculature, resulting in increased blood flow to the tissues beneath the site of exposure (Weston et al. 1994).

Table 8–1. Comparison of modern water-based therapeutic modalities

	Flotation restricted environmental stimulation technique	Cold water exposure or immersion	Aquarium therapy	Water-based exercises	Balneotherapy
Method	Patient floats supine in a magnesium sulfate-saturated pool held at about 93°F–95°F. Other stimuli (e.g., light, sound, and pressure on spinal cord) are minimized.	Patient submerges in cold water for a prolonged time or is exposed to cold water in the form of liquid or solid (ice).	Patient observes a "blue space" (i.e., water, fish, vegetation) (Cracknell et al. 2018).	Patient swims or participates in large muscle activities, usually led by a trained instructor or therapist, in a pool or other body of water (Silva et al. 2019).	Patients bathe in warm (≥68°F) mineral springs. Ambience, water pH, temperature, and mineral composition naturally vary (Clark-Kennedy et al. 2021).

Table 8–1. Comparison of modern water-based therapeutic modalities (*continued*)

	Flotation restricted environmental stimulation technique	Cold water exposure or immersion	Aquarium therapy	Water-based exercises	Balneotherapy
Equipment and materials needed	Tank (typically 270 cm×150 cm×130 cm) or body of saturated saltwater Control over temperature, sound, light Earplugs (Jonsson and Kjellgren 2016)	Cold water or ice in bucket or container (McKee et al. 2015) Open bodies of water such as the sea (Kelly and Bird 2021) Ice pack (Kyriakoulis et al. 2021; Linehan 2015); ideal water temperature thought to be ~50°F–59°F (Kyriakoulis et al. 2021; Linehan 2015)	Aquarium (small or large, in home, or dedicated facility open to the public) Aquarium maintenance	Pool or other body of water with sufficient depth Trained instructor or supervisor present	Hot mineral spring or spa

Table 8–1.	Comparison of modern water-based therapeutic modalities *(continued)*				
	Flotation restricted environmental stimulation technique	Cold water exposure or immersion	Aquarium therapy	Water-based exercises	Balneotherapy
Origination	John C. Lilly created the first saltwater isolation tanks in 1954, aiming to study human consciousness in the absence of external stimuli.	Unknown	The first public aquarium was opened in 1853 as part of the London Zoo (Karydis 2011).	Unknown	Unknown; used for centuries in ancient Greece, Rome (Gianfaldoni et al. 2017), China, and Japan

Table 8–1. Comparison of modern water-based therapeutic modalities (*continued*)

	Flotation restricted environmental stimulation technique	Cold water exposure or immersion	Aquarium therapy	Water-based exercises	Balneotherapy
Possible indications	Generalized anxiety disorder Major depressive disorder PTSD Panic disorder Social anxiety disorder Chronic pain conditions Insomnia (Jonsson and Kjellgren 2016)	Borderline personality disorder Other emotional dysregulation–related disorders Anxiety-related disorders, panic disorder (Kyriakoulis et al. 2021)	Overall not well studied in clinical psychiatric populations (Clements et al. 2019)	Major depressive disorder (Silva et al. 2019) Overall not well studied in clinical psychiatric populations (Jackson et al. 2022)	Chronic pain conditions Rheumatic disorders Dermatological problems Fibromyalgia, chronic pain (Clark-Kennedy et al. 2021) Generalized anxiety disorder (Dubois et al. 2010)

Table 8–1.	Comparison of modern water-based therapeutic modalities *(continued)*				
	Flotation restricted environmental stimulation technique	Cold water exposure or immersion	Aquarium therapy	Water-based exercises	Balneotherapy
Proposed therapeutic mechanism	Reduces physiological stress by attenuating environmental stimuli. Attention and thoughts are guided toward a here-and-now state, promoting relaxation (Kjellgren et al. 2008). Whole-body heating and patient expectations also may contribute to short-term therapeutic effects (Loose et al. 2021).	Mammalian diving reflex: in response to breath-holding with full submersion in water (Panneton 2013) or in response to isolated facial exposure to cold stimuli (McKee et al. 2015), a series of reflexes occurs, including bradycardia, increased parasympathetic tone, and decreased arterial blood pressure, followed by peripheral vasoconstriction (Panneton 2013).	Various theories may explain its restorative properties, including the following: • Attention restoration theory • Stress recovery theory • Biophilia hypothesis (Cracknell et al. 2018) • Attachment theory (applied to the human–marine animal relationship) (Clements et al. 2019) • Simple distraction (Clements et al. 2019)	Promotes social interaction, decreases oxidative stress (Silva et al. 2019) Buoyancy and hydrostatic pressure may permit patients with pain or orthopedic or neurological problems to engage in otherwise more difficult physical activity.	Absorption of bioactive organic molecules may contribute to various physiological or healing mechanisms (Cheleschi et al. 2020). Natural spring microbiome may be beneficial (Cheleschi et al. 2020).

Table 8–1. Comparison of modern water-based therapeutic modalities (*continued*)

	Flotation restricted environmental stimulation technique	Cold water exposure or immersion	Aquarium therapy	Water-based exercises	Balneotherapy
Proposed therapeutic mechanism (*continued*)	Decreased functional connectivity between somatomotor and default mode networks (Al Zoubi et al. 2021)	Cold shock may improve mood through activation of the hypothalamic-pituitary-adrenal axis (Kelly and Bird 2021).		Decreased inflammation and pain may contribute to general well-being.	Decreased inflammation and pain may contribute to general well-being. Whole-body heating and patient expectations may also contribute to short-term therapeutic effects. Natural environment may confer restorative benefits, as in aquarium therapy.

Table 8–1. Comparison of modern water-based therapeutic modalities (*continued*)

	Flotation restricted environmental stimulation technique	Cold water exposure or immersion	Aquarium therapy	Water-based exercises	Balneotherapy
Frequency and duration	12 sessions (45 min twice a week) have been proposed (Bood et al. 2007). Duration of ~7 weeks is common (Kjellgren et al. 2020).	Ideal frequency and duration are unknown. Acute improvement in mood is seen after ≤20 min of immersion in cold seawater (Kelly and Bird 2021). For reduction of extreme emotions, can be done as needed for 15–30 s (Linehan 2015).	Ideal frequency and duration are unknown.	Varies 2–3 weekly sessions of 40–60 min for 8–14 weeks have been used (Jackson et al. 2022; Silva et al. 2019).	Varies In published research, several protocols use 20- to 30-min sessions for ~15–20 sessions over 3–4 weeks (Bender et al. 2014).

Table 8–1.   Comparison of modern water-based therapeutic modalities (*continued*)

	Flotation restricted environmental stimulation technique	Cold water exposure or immersion	Aquarium therapy	Water-based exercises	Balneotherapy
Barriers and contraindications	Active suicidality with plan or intent History of neurological condition that may interfere with protocol Skin condition or open wound that causes pain with exposure Discomfort or fear of water Acute intoxication	Caution use for those with • Hypertension • Previous cerebrovascular disease (McKee et al. 2015) • Anorexia or heart disease (Kelly and Bird 2021) • Concurrent use of β-blockers or other heart-slowing medications • Cold urticaria	Barriers include monetary costs (e.g., price of admission for public aquarium or cost to purchase, install, and maintain a home aquarium).	Severe cardiac disease Active suicidality with plan or intent Severe epilepsy Skin condition or open wound that causes pain with exposure Discomfort or fear of water Acute intoxication Allergy to pool additive Cold urticaria	Allergy to minerals or water content Impaired thermal regulation Intoxication Water phobia

Table 8–1. Comparison of modern water-based therapeutic modalities (*continued*)

	Flotation restricted environmental stimulation technique	Cold water exposure or immersion	Aquarium therapy	Water-based exercises	Balneotherapy
Possible beneficial effects	Stress reduction Alleviation of chronic pain Anxiolysis (Jonsson and Kjellgren 2017) Improved mood and subjective well-being (Kjellgren et al. 2020) Improved sleep (Kjellgren et al. 2020)	Bradycardia Anxiolysis Decrease in panic symptoms (Kyriakoulis et al. 2021) Acute mood improvement (Kelly and Bird 2021) Reduced extreme emotions (Linehan 2015)	Positive emotions Connectedness to natural environments and other beings (Cracknell et al. 2018) Relaxation, stress reduction (Clements et al. 2019) Anxiolysis (Barker et al. 2003; Clements et al. 2019)	Anxiolysis Improved mood Higher self-esteem Higher sense of well-being (Jackson et al. 2022) Decrease in physical pain	Improved sleep Reduced stress Anxiolysis Improved mood (Clark-Kennedy et al. 2021) Reduced chronic pain symptoms General sense of well-being (Bender et al. 2014; Cheleschi et al. 2020)

Table 8–1. Comparison of modern water-based therapeutic modalities (continued)

	Flotation restricted environmental stimulation technique	Cold water exposure or immersion	Aquarium therapy	Water-based exercises	Balneotherapy
Possible adverse effects	Currently being assessed in clinical trials (NCT03899090) "Intensification phase," in which chronic pain symptoms or psychological problems, in the absence of usual stimuli, become more apparent; may occur early in treatment (Jonsson and Kjellgren 2017).	Hypertensive crisis, stroke (McKee et al. 2015) Arrhythmias and myocardial infarction (Kelly and Bird 2021) Hypothermia (with colder water or more prolonged exposures)	Small risk of aquarium-associated bacterial infection (may be minimized with hygienic practices) (Clements et al. 2019) Small risk of injury while installing or maintaining aquarium (if patient is responsible for this)	Rarely, short-term fatigue after treatment; potential for increased pain (Reger et al. 2022) Allergic reaction to pool additives Risk of drowning or falls (minimized with nonslip mats, supervision)	Rarely, mild and transient skin irritation or exacerbation of psoriasis (Clark-Kennedy et al. 2021) Risk of drowning or falls (minimized with nonslip mats, supervision)

Table 8–1.	Comparison of modern water-based therapeutic modalities *(continued)*				
	Flotation restricted environmental stimulation technique	**Cold water exposure or immersion**	**Aquarium therapy**	**Water-based exercises**	**Balneotherapy**
Advantages	Effects of treatment may be realized with minimal effort or specific instructions.	Minimal equipment needed, quick technique	Few contraindications or adverse effects May be available to clients for long periods of time and at their convenience	Physical activity confers other (nonpsychiatric) health benefits.	Effects of treatment may be realized with minimal effort or specific instructions.

In patients with congestive heart failure, warm water baths and low-temperature sauna bathing at 140°F for 15 minutes was found to improve cardiac function, increase 6-minute walking distance, and reduce plasma levels of brain natriuretic peptide (Iiyama et al. 2008; Mooventhan and Nivethitha 2014).

Cold water immersion has been shown to increase heart rate, blood pressure, metabolism, and peripheral catecholamine concentration and to decrease cerebral blood flow (Bleakley and Davison 2010; Mooventhan and Nivethitha 2014). Acute immersion in warm water similarly increases blood pressure but generally reduces heart rate (Mooventhan and Nivethitha 2014).

Nervous System

The human nervous system is also sensitive to water in its various forms. Applying water in cold modalities, such as ice massage, ice packs, or cold water immersion, on the calf for 10 minutes reduces the skin's temperature, thus reducing the amplitude of action potentials and in turn increasing their latency and duration. Cold water immersion is the most effective way to produce therapeutic effects associated with reducing motor nerve conduction (Herrera et al. 2010; Mooventhan and Nivethitha 2014).

Adjusting the water temperature in hydrotherapy is theorized to modulate pain. Temperature and pain are peripherally sensed through thermal receptors and nociceptors, respectively. The sensory signals are transmitted to the brain via the lateral spinothalamic tract. Stimulating the thermal receptors through immersion in a temperature extreme competes with the pain signal traveling along the same spinal tract, thus reducing the experienced pain.

Hydrotherapy also relieves mechanical stress on muscles and joints because of water's buoyancy. In patients with multiple sclerosis, 40 sessions of an aquatic exercise program were found to improve fatigue, spasms, pain, depression, disability, and overall functional autonomy (Bender et al. 2005; Castro-Sánchez et al. 2012).

Adapted cold showers send an overwhelming amount of electrical impulses from the peripheral nerve endings of the dense cold receptors in the skin to the brain, effectively working as a mild electroshock therapy, and may result in antidepressive or antipsychotic effects, as well as analgesic effects by suppressing neurotransmission in the mesolimbic system (Shevchuk 2008).

Cold immersion can also activate parts of the reticular activating system, which is the system responsible for regulating sleep-wake transitions and arousal, thereby promoting wakefulness, mobility, and energy.

Respiratory System

Water-based therapies can exert substantial and quantifiable changes in pulmonary functioning as a result of both temperature- and pressure-mediated effects. When water temperature is greater than body temperature, oxygen transport is improved through a concordant increase in cardiac output. Conversely, when water temperature is less than body temperature, oxygen transport is interrupted (Mooventhan and Nivethitha 2014). Water temperatures also affect breathing parameters. For example, vital capacity (the volume of air exhaled after a maximal inhalation) decreases as temperature decreases. Tidal volume (the volume of air moved into or out of the lungs during quiet breathing) has a parabolic relationship with temperature, such that tidal volume increases at temperatures above and below neutral temperature (Choukroun et al. 1989; Mooventhan and Nivethitha 2014).

Cold water immersion has been found to increase the respiratory minute volume and decrease end-tidal carbon dioxide partial pressure, which are indicative of a more efficient respiratory effort (Bleakley and Davison 2010). Repeated stimulation with cold water has been shown to reduce infections, increase peak expiratory flow, and improve quality of life in patients with chronic obstructive pulmonary disease (Goedsche et al. 2007; Mooventhan and Nivethitha 2014).

Musculoskeletal System

Application of cold water can cause physiological reactions such as a decrease in local metabolic function, local edema, nerve conduction velocity, and muscle spasms and an increase in local anesthetic effects. Immersion in water colder than 59°F has been shown to significantly delay the onset of muscle soreness after exercise (Bleakley and Davison 2010; Bleakley et al. 2012). Studies have found that immersing one's legs into warm water maintained at approximately 111°F for 45 minutes before repetitive flexion-extension exercise significantly reduced markers of muscle damage attributable to exercise, including creatine kinase levels in the blood, muscle soreness, jump height, and maximum voluntary contraction force (Mooventhan and Nivethitha 2014; Skurvydas et al. 2008).

Aquatic exercise is a practical alternative for people with obesity who have high risk of falling or have joint pain, because the buoyancy of the water reduces the overall weight put on bones, joints, and muscles. The warmth and the pressure of the water also may reduce swelling, leading to overall muscle relaxation (Mooventhan and Nivethitha 2014).

Gastrointestinal System

Water has been shown to have a significant effect on the human gastrointestinal system. After hot water compress treatment, bowel sounds increased by 1.7 times, suggesting that this treatment can help those with constipation by promoting gas release or defecation (Mooventhan and Nivethitha 2014). Drinking warm water is also effective for the treatment of colonic spasms and has no side effects (Church 2002).

Patients with hemorrhoids or anal fissures found a significant decrease in anal burning and pain after using sitz baths with warm water between 59°F and 86°F (Mooventhan and Nivethitha 2014). In those with anorectal disorders, pain relief was more significant and longer lasting when sitz baths were done at higher temperatures (104°F, 113°F, or 122°F) for 10 minutes at a time. This effect may be a result of anal sphincter relaxation with increased bath temperature due to the thermosphincteric reflex, a reaction in which thermal signals decrease internal sphincter electromyographic activity (Shafik 1993).

In summary, water affects physiology in many ways. Therefore, various mechanisms likely underlie each of the modern water therapies, which are described in the next section.

Hydrotherapy

Flotation Therapy

Flotation REST is one type of hydrotherapy. During flotation REST, participants float inside a dark, quiet tank filled with water saturated with magnesium sulfate (Epsom salts). The water is usually heated to skin temperature, about 93°F–95°F. Sensory signals from visual, auditory, olfactory, gustatory, thermal, tactile, vestibular, gravitational, and proprioceptive channels are minimized. Theoretically, this reduction in physiological stress guides participants' thoughts to the here and now, promoting a state of relaxation (Kjellgren et al. 2008). Contrarily, this reduction in physiological stress may bring about a resurgence of chronic pain or psychological issues, making it harder for some patients to relax, especially early in treatment (Jonsson and Kjellgren 2017). Default mode networks (DMNs) are parts of the brain that are activated while a person is awake but not engaged in any specific task and is focused on internal mental state processes, such as self-referential processing; DMNs are often related to difficulty in disengaging from self-centered thoughts. Altered DMN activity has been implicated in depression and anxiety (Coutinho et al. 2016). Decreased functional connectivity between somatomotor networks and DMNs brought about by flotation

REST (Al Zoubi et al. 2021) also may reduce anxiety. A typical flotation REST regimen may include twelve 45-minute sessions over the course of 6–7 weeks (Bood et al. 2007; Kjellgren et al. 2020).

Flotation REST may reduce stress and sleep difficulties, muscle tension, and pain, as well as anxiety and depression (Al Zoubi et al. 2021; Jonsson and Kjellgren 2017). Related sleep improvements in patients with insomnia may persist even 4–6 months after treatment cessation (Kjellgren et al. 2020). Its use may result in mood improvements characterized by increases in relaxation, happiness, and well-being. Effects tend to be more significant in participants who are most severely anxious. Therefore, indications for which flotation REST is being investigated include generalized anxiety disorder (GAD), major depressive disorder (MDD), PTSD, panic disorder, chronic pain conditions, and insomnia. It may be used as an adjunct treatment along with pharmacotherapy or psychotherapy. Possible adverse effects of flotation REST are being investigated in clinical trials.

Cold Water Exposure or Immersion

Cold water immersion or exposure is another type of hydrotherapy. It can be done in various ways, including immersion in large ice or water buckets, seas, ponds, oceans, or lakes in winter, or the application of ice packs or wraps to the skin. Either partial-body (such as hands or face) or whole-body exposure can be performed. Multiple theories have been proposed for the positive effects of this hydrotherapy. The shocking cold effect has been theorized to lead to positive changes in mood through activation of the hypothalamic-pituitary-adrenal axis (Kelly and Bird 2021). A mammalian diving reflex also may be activated with either cold water exposure (especially on the face) or water immersion (and related breath-holding) (McKee et al. 2015). The diving reflex actually consists of a predictable series of physiological reflexes, leading to bradycardia, an increase in parasympathetic tone, a decline in arterial blood pressure, and peripheral vasoconstriction (Panneton 2013). It promotes the survival of all mammals in an oxygen-deprived state by preferentially circulating blood to the brain and heart. In humans, it can also be used as a means of emotional regulation, as part of dialectical behavior therapy (DBT; Linehan 2015). The diving reflex can be used as a means of managing extreme emotions in stressful situations, particularly for patients with borderline personality disorder. One technique involves self-submersion of the face in icy, cold water for 30 seconds while holding a deep breath (Linehan 2015). This technique theoretically allows its user to have immediate relief from overwhelming feelings and be in a calmer state of mind. Another technique involves holding an ice cube in the hand until it melts. This can be used as an intense and uncomfortable stimulus to break dissociative episodes because it helps patients connect to their present and physical reality. Presumably, techniques that activate the mammalian diving reflex or aim to break dissociative episodes would be best used on an as-needed basis.

Immersion in cold seawater for up to 20 minutes has been shown to induce acute improvements in mood (Kelly and Bird 2021). Other potential benefits of cold water application include slowing of heart rate, anxiolysis, decrease in self-reported panic (Kyriakoulis et al. 2021), and reduction of extreme emotions (Linehan 2015). Thus, cold water immersion or application could be useful for patients with borderline personality disorder or an emotional dysregulation–related disorder. It also may have some utility for anxiety-related symptoms or for panic disorders (Kyriakoulis et al. 2021).

Cold water exposure is not without risks, and caution should be exercised in the use of this technique for patients with heart-slowing medications, cold urticaria, heart disease, hypertension, or a history of cerebrovascular disease. The ideal frequency and duration of cold water immersion are unknown; however, prolonged exposure to excessively cold water may be harmful and should be avoided. Depending on the temperature of and exposure time to the water, patients may be at risk for hypothermia. Possible adverse effects include hypertensive crisis, stroke (McKee et al. 2015), arrhythmias, and cold shock–associated myocardial infarction (Kelly and Bird 2021).

Aquarium Therapy

Aquarium therapy is another type of hydrotherapy. Its participants observe a "blue space" containing water, aquatic creatures, or vegetation. The aquarium itself may be small or large and in home or public. Aquarium therapy promotes improvements in both physical and mental health, specifically in providing relief from stress, insomnia, pain, and anxiety (Cracknell et al. 2016). More specifically, it draws on the *biophilia hypothesis*, a term coined by Edward O. Wilson in 1984 to describe his theory that human beings have an innate tendency to seek out and establish connections with other forms of life (Grinde and Patil 2009; Logan and Selhub 2012). It can then be surmised that a significant aspect of what is believed to make aquarium therapy effective is the actual marine life with which one interacts. Although research supports the role of biodiversity and species richness in promoting superior well-being outcomes, "a growing literature on psychological benefits of blue/aquatic environments, mostly derived from testing landscape scenery (via photographs or in situ)" suggests that there may be inherent psychological benefits of aquatic, blue environments even before marine life is added (Cracknell et al. 2016, p. 1247).

It is no coincidence that doctors' offices, hospitals, clinics, workspaces, and various environments traditionally perceived as stressful often feature fish tanks and aquariums; studies on aquarium therapy have found that patients who are exposed to waiting rooms that have aquariums tend to experience less pain and stress during their visits (Cracknell et al. 2016). A recent zoological study found that visitors to a touch tank aquarium had psychological benefits backed by physiological changes suggesting increased energy, increased happiness, and decreased stress (Coolman et al. 2020). Another theory that may explain why aquariums are found to be therapeutic is attention restoration theory (ART). ART implies that "prolonged or intense periods of directed attention, the type of forced concentration that leads to mental fatigue, distraction, and irritability, can be alleviated by experiencing a restorative setting" (Cracknell et al. 2016, p. 1245). For environments to be considered restorative settings, according to Kaplan (1995), they must have four key factors: 1) fascination (ability to effortlessly hold one's attention), 2) being away (removed physically or mentally from one's daily routine), 3) extent (meaningfully and richly connected to a landscape), and 4) compatibility (harmoniousness with one's beliefs or inclinations). Aquarium therapy, which takes the viewer away to a soothing, exquisitely related aquatic world of myriad creatures of different colors, shapes, and sizes, satisfies all four of these criteria and is capable of offering broad therapeutic benefits.

Aquariums also have been found to be calming for patients with behavioral and stimulation disturbances, such as those with ADHD or autism and older patients with agitation. The variety of species, brightly colored fish, and induction of natural fascination make aquariums an effortless focal point for patients and minimize disruptive behaviors by decreasing psychomotor agitation, hyperactivity, and aggression (Cocker 2012). In a study of patients with Alzheimer's disease, various beneficial changes were observed after a fish tank was introduced into the activity room; patients who were prone to lethargy were more alert, and those who tended to be restless and pacing spent more time sitting and watching the fish (Edwards and Beck 2002). Although the emotion-enhancing, relaxation-inducing, and anxiolytic effects of aquarium therapy are promising, a recent systematic review (Clements et al. 2019) suggested that such effects are not very well studied in clinical psychiatric populations. Thus, their therapeutic utility for the treatment of MDD, GAD, PTSD, bipolar disorder, and panic disorder may be a fruitful area for further research.

In an ideal world, everyone would have equal access to live aquariums, by visiting large public aquariums or keeping smaller aquariums in their homes, but many populations are unable to access these resources. When considering alternative applications of this type of aquarium therapy for patients who do not live near any aquariums or bodies of water, virtual hydrotherapy delivered as technologically simulated aquariums may be a viable alternative. Several popular computer screensavers that were popular in the 1990s and 2000s featured aquatic creatures and fish simply moving about in front of a serene, underwater background. These screensavers were well liked for their soothing, whimsical nature and are still common today. Whether aquarium therapy is provided in real life or a virtual format, it is a safe form of hydrotherapy, with fewer risks and contraindications than cold water immersion, flotation REST, water-based exercises, and balneotherapy.

Water-Based Exercise and Pain

Water-based exercise has proven to be effective in promoting physical and mental health. One study showed that moderate-intensity, water-based exercise improved the physical and psychological domains of quality of life, depressive symptoms, aerobic capacity, and muscular strength of women (Takeshima et al. 2002). Swimming training also has been shown to improve mental health parameters, cognition, and motor coordination in children with ADHD (Huang et al. 2017). Water-based exercise also has been helpful for relieving pain in patients with various musculoskeletal diseases (Cochrane et al. 2005). For example, hydrotherapy was superior to land-based exercise for relieving the pain of osteoarthritis (Carbonell-Baeza et al. 2012). Eight months of physical training in warm water was shown to improve physical and mental health in women with fibromyalgia. Improvement in physical pain often can translate into mitigation of emotional distress, including anxiety and depressive disorders that are often comorbid in patients with severe pain (Sheng et al. 2017; Von Korff and Simon 1996).

Balneotherapy

Although there are many similarities between balneotherapy and hydrotherapy, they are recognized as distinctive therapies. Balneotherapy is a traditional medicinal practice that specifically entails bathing or submerging a patient into thermal mineral waters and clays in order to achieve therapeutic effects (Yang et al. 2018). One might imagine locations such as hot springs, ice baths, spas, beaches, pools, lakes, and rivers for this type of therapy. It is a respected part of many cultural practices, traditionally associated with hot springs, ice baths, and cold water springs. In modern Western society, one might visualize a spa when thinking about balneotherapy. Peloidal clays associated with balneotherapy can be likened to the contemporary practice of applying facial masks. One might expect that these things are colloquially associated with relaxation, stress relief, wellness, mindfulness, and general mental well-being, and several studies have been done to support this connection (Clark-Kennedy et al. 2021; Rapolienė et al. 2016; Yang et al. 2018).

Known benefits of balneotherapy include physiological changes in blood pressure and heart rate and alleviation of chronic pain and musculoskeletal conditions. In addition, it has been found to be beneficial in the treatment of depression, stress, fatigue, insomnia, and other mental health conditions (Clark-Kennedy et al. 2021; Yang et al. 2018). According to Rapolienė et al. (2016, p. 1), balneotherapeutic approaches result in a "reduction in the number and intensity of stress-related symptoms, a reduction in pain and general, physical, and mental fatigue, and an improvement in stress-related symptoms management, mood, activation, motivation, and cognitive functions."

Of course, although possible contraindications are few, clinicians must consider them before recommending balneotherapy for their patients. Those who have a history of skin hypersensitivities should be cautious when considering balneotherapy. Moreover, patients with acute dermatological conditions such as infections, blistering, ulcers, or open wounds should avoid initiating balneotherapy until they are adequately treated because engaging in this therapy too early may worsen their dermatological conditions.

SPECIAL CONSIDERATIONS AND LIMITATIONS

Throughout this chapter, we have described the potential benefits and applications of specific water-based therapies. Not only the risks and benefits of these therapies but also the practical limitations and barriers to their use must be considered. Carbonell et al. (2020) proposed several categorical challenges in mental health care systems that affect patient participation. Among these are structural barriers, health culture, and the biomedical model. Water-based therapies, as potential treatments in mental health care, are no exception to these limitations. Each of these barriers, as they pertain to water therapy, is discussed briefly below. Nonetheless, although water therapies are subject to certain limitations, they are also useful for circumventing some of the limitations of other psychiatric therapies. When relevant, we discuss these advantages as well.

Structural Barriers

Structural barriers include financial cost and accessibility. For most of the water therapies described, treatment costs could be prohibitive, or access may be limited. Patients who want to engage in aquatic exercises may not have access to a safe pool or body of water. For example, an estimated 11% of households in a small Bolivian town in 2019 obtained their water from a river that is used to wash clothes and bodies, to wash cars, and to function as an informal latrine (Cairns 2018). Its use increases exposure to pathogens, a risk that may outweigh any psychiatric benefits to be gained from aquatic exercises. Other water therapies are more resource intensive than aquatic exercises, requiring not just clean water but also particular equipment. Home aquarium therapy is limited by the high cost for installation and labor-intensive upkeep. Public aquariums may be equally inaccessible if none are nearby or if the price of admission is too high. Those who want to benefit from flotation REST may not have access to the highly controlled stimulus-reducing environment in which it is performed.

Water is a scarce resource in many communities across the globe because of problems of infrastructure, allocation, and prioritization (Wutich 2020). The laws we enact, policies we create, and institutions we support influence the availability of water. Funding and reimbursements are products of our laws, policies, and institutions, and these processes also have a bearing on accessibility. Low payment and funding support for mental health services contribute generally to structural barriers (Carbonell et al. 2020). We could not find reimbursement or referral data for water therapies such as balneotherapy, flotation REST, or water-guided psychotherapy. Reimbursement for music therapy, another possible adjunctive treatment for depressive or anxious disorders, has been shown to vary significantly by state (Sena Moore and Peebles 2020). It is quite possible that water therapy reimbursement rates also vary geographically, contributing to limited access to therapeutic modalities for some patients.

Other structural barriers may exist for those with musculoskeletal impairments, phobias, or allergies. Any of these problems, if severe enough, may cause disability, thereby limiting the accessibility of certain water therapies. Patients with allergies to certain pool additives may not be able to do water-based exercises in these pools. Likewise, patients with cold urticaria should not engage in cold water immersion. Some patients with severe water phobias may not be well suited for any of the water therapies discussed in this chapter. Other patients with severe water phobias might actually benefit from carefully guided exposure to some of the water therapies as part of a process of systematic desensitization. For these patients, aquarium-related therapy, which involves only minimal direct contact with water, might be a good place for the therapist to start. Patients with certain musculoskeletal impairments may need additional accommodations in order to maneuver into the flotation REST pool. We list these barriers, and others, in Table 8–1.

One of the advantages of most water therapies is that they may be done without a mental health clinician physically present. There is a significant shortage of mental health clinicians and a growing demand for their services. Therefore, water therapies may be more readily available than many other psychiatric interventions. Some water therapies can be self-administered (such as cold water immersion, as described in the DBT workbook by Linehan [2015], or balneotherapy), or they may be performed with the help of prerecorded video instructions (such as water-based exercises). For patients who live near public-access bodies of water or swimming pools, certain water-based therapies may even be free of cost. Certain water therapies, for some patients, might be among the most accessible psychiatric interventions.

INFLUENCE OF THE BIOMEDICAL MODEL

The predominance of the biomedical model may either encourage or discourage the use of water therapies. The biomedical approach tends to ignore sociocultural and psychological factors associated with health. Thus, flotation REST, water-guided psychotherapy, or aquarium therapy—therapies that may be known best for their psychological benefits—may be discounted by some clinicians and patients.

Simultaneously, awareness of how water therapies affect various physiological systems (as we outlined in this chapter) is growing, and the link between physiological systems and psychiatric realms such as mood, anxiety, and sense of well-being is becoming more evident. The use of water therapies fits into the biomedical model seamlessly. Both physicians and their patients may increasingly recognize their benefits.

Most patients use biomedical models of treatment (Carbonell et al. 2020). For patients who prefer not to, or who are open to alternative methods of treatment, and for those who consider water therapies as outside traditional biomedical practice, the water therapies may be particularly valued.

HEALTH CULTURE

Mental illness is stigmatized worldwide. This may present another important barrier to the uptake of water therapies. The use of cold water immersion for the stated purpose of regaining emotional control, or to break a dissociative spell, requires an implicit acceptance by patients that they have a psychiatric problem. Patients may fear that participation in some of the water-based therapies signals to important figures in the patients' life that they are "mentally ill." Many may want to avoid this label and similar ones. Attendance at flotation REST sessions may be difficult to hide. Flotation REST also may be difficult for patients to explain to others if they are reluctant to discuss their psychiatric issues with family or friends.

Engagement in other water-based therapies could be done without raising any eyebrows. In fact, some water therapies are widely practiced, so they may be more easily accepted and could even be explained as being used for nonpsychiatric benefits. Water-based exercises, for example, are not necessarily associated with mental illness and are practiced by many people without mental illness for cardiovascular benefits.

Framing these treatments through a patient-centered approach, rather than an illness-focused one, may reduce the stigma associated with treating mental health symptoms.

Clinical Translation: Case Example

A 59-year-old woman with a history of MDD, borderline personality disorder, and chronic pain from severe osteoarthritis presents to her psychiatrist's office, reporting ongoing symptoms despite medication compliance. She has been followed up consistently at the clinic for 6 years, with limited response to multiple antidepressant and mood stabilizer medication trials. She asks her provider whether any other treatment options are available besides medications and psychotherapy. Her provider recently read some studies about the potential benefits of certain water-based therapies, such as flotation REST and water-based exercise for depression and chronic pain conditions and cold water immersion and balneotherapy for borderline personality disorder. She counsels her patient about these modalities, informing her of possible benefits, adverse effects, and contraindications, as well as reinforcing DBT techniques and mindfulness practices. The patient requests further information and referrals for flotation REST and balneotherapy, which her physician provides. At her 1- and 2-month follow-up appointments, she reported some improvement in her depressive symptoms, lability, impulsiveness, and relationship stability.

KEY POINTS

- The history of hydrotherapy in psychiatry was dark, but many modern therapeutic treatments are used today.

- Flotation restricted environmental stimulation technique, cold water immersion or exposure, aquarium therapy, water-based exercises, virtual water therapy, and balneotherapy are all examples of modern hydrotherapy techniques.

- Hydrotherapies have shown promise for improving psychiatric-related symptoms including depression, anxiety, sleep, self-esteem, and overall sense of well-being.

- Some hydrotherapies are helpful in alleviating pain in patients with comorbid, chronic medical conditions.

- Water therapies, like all other pharmacological and nonpharmacological therapies, are subject to certain practical limitations.

QUESTIONS

1. According to Kaplan's criteria for attention restoration theory (ART), an environment must have four key factors to be considered restorative. Which of the following is not one of these key factors?

    A. Extent of connection.
    B. Compatibility.
    C. Being removed.
    D. Proximity.
    E. Fascination.

Correct answer: D. Proximity.

According to Kaplan's criteria for ART, an environment can be considered a restorative setting if it has the following key factors:

fascination (E), being removed (C), extent of connection (A), and compatibility (B) (Kaplan 1995). Of the answer choices listed, only proximity (D) is not an essential factor for an environment to be restorative.

2. Flotation restricted environmental stimulation technique (REST) therapy is being studied for applications in all of the following except:

    A. Insomnia.
    B. Specific phobias.
    C. PTSD.
    D. Generalized anxiety disorder.
    E. Major depressive disorder.

Correct answer: B. Specific phobias.

Some studies have suggested that flotation REST therapy may be helpful in many different conditions, including generalized anxiety disorder (D), major depressive disorder (E), PTSD (C), panic disorder, social anxiety disorder, chronic pain conditions, and insomnia (A) (Jonsson and Kjellgren 2016). It has not been suggested in the treatment or adjunctive treatment of specific phobias (B).

3. Cold water exposure or immersion therapy may be helpful in treating some anxiety-related or panic disorders, as well as emotional dysregulation disorders. However, potential adverse effects are associated with this treatment. Which of the following is a possible adverse effect?

    A. Arrhythmia and myocardial infarction.
    B. Fatigue.
    C. Bacterial infection.
    D. Hyperthermia.
    E. Skin irritation or allergic reaction.

Correct answer: A. Arrhythmia and myocardial infarction.

Known possible adverse effects in cold water immersion or exposure therapy include arrhythmia and myocardial infarction (Kelly and Bird 2021) (A), hypertensive crisis, stroke (McKee et al. 2015), and risk of hypothermia with colder and more prolonged exposures. Hyperthermia would not be an expected adverse effect in this case (D). Skin irritation or allergic reaction is more likely to be associated with water-based exercises and balneotherapy (E). Of the remaining answer choices, fatigue is more commonly associated with water-based exercises (B), and bacterial infection is more commonly associated with aquarium therapy (C).

REFERENCES

Al Zoubi O, Misaki M, Bodurka J, et al: Taking the body off the mind: decreased functional connectivity between somatomotor and default-mode networks following floatation-REST. Hum Brain Mapp 42(10):3216–3227, 2021 33835628

Allen CN: Psychological factors in continuous bath hydrotherapy for psychotic patients. J Abnorm Soc Psychol 31(4):418–422, 1937

Ban TA: Fifty years chlorpromazine: a historical perspective. Neuropsychiatr Dis Treat 3(4):495–500, 2007 19300578

Barker SB, Rasmussen KG, Best AM: Effect of aquariums on electroconvulsive therapy patients. Anthrozoos 16(3):229–240, 2003

Bender T, Karagülle Z, Bálint GP, et al: Hydrotherapy, balneotherapy, and spa treatment in pain management. Rheumatol Int 25(3):220–224, 2005 15257412

Bender T, Bálint G, Prohászka Z, et al: Evidence-based hydro- and balneotherapy in Hungary—a systematic review and meta-analysis. Int J Biometeorol 58(3):311–323, 2014 23677421

Bleakley CM, Davison GW: What is the biochemical and physiological rationale for using cold-water immersion in sports recovery? A systematic review. Br J Sports Med 44(3):179–187, 2010 19945970

Bleakley C, McDonough S, Gardner E, et al: Cold-water immersion (cryotherapy) for preventing and treating muscle soreness after exercise. Cochrane Database Syst Rev 2012(2):CD008262, 2012 22336838

Bood SÅ, Sundequist U, Kjellgren A, et al: Effects of flotation REST (restricted environmental stimulation technique) on stress related muscle pain: are 33 flotation sessions more effective than 12 sessions? Soc Behav Pers 35(2):143–156, 2007

Cairns MR: Metering water: analyzing the concurrent pressures of conservation, sustainability, health impact, and equity in use. World Dev 110:411–421, 2018

Carbonell Á, Navarro-Pérez JJ, Mestre MV: Challenges and barriers in mental healthcare systems and their impact on the family: a systematic integrative review. Health Soc Care Community 28(5):1366–1379, 2020 32115797

Carbonell-Baeza A, Ruiz JR, Aparicio VA, et al: Land- and water-based exercise intervention in women with fibromyalgia: the al-Andalus physical activity randomised controlled trial. BMC Musculoskelet Disord 13(1):18, 2012 22336292

Cartwright M: Roman baths. World History Encyclopedia, 2013. Available at: https://www.worldhistory.org/Roman_Baths. Accessed May 11, 2024.

Castro-Sánchez AM, Matarán-Peñarrocha GA, Lara-Palomo I, et al: Hydrotherapy for the treatment of pain in people with multiple sclerosis: a randomized controlled trial. Evid Based Complement Alternat Med 2012:473963, 2012 21785645

Cheleschi S, Gallo I, Tenti S: A comprehensive analysis to understand the mechanism of action of balneotherapy: why, how, and where they can be used? Evidence from in vitro studies performed on human and animal samples. Int J Biometeorol 64(7):1247–1261, 2020 32200439

Choukroun ML, Kays C, Varène P: Effects of water temperature on pulmonary volumes in immersed human subjects. Respir Physiol 75(3):255–265, 1989 2717815

Church JM: Warm water irrigation for dealing with spasm during colonoscopy: simple, inexpensive, and effective. Gastrointest Endosc 56(5):672–674, 2002 12397274

Clarfield AM: A warm bath. J Am Geriatr Soc 53(6):1075–1076, 2005 15935042

Clark-Kennedy J, Kennedy G, Cohen M, et al: Mental health outcomes of balneotherapy: a systematic review. International Journal of Spa and Wellness 4(1):69–92, 2021

Clements H, Valentin S, Jenkins N, et al: The effects of interacting with fish in aquariums on human health and well-being: a systematic review. PLoS One 14(7):e0220524, 2019 31356652

Cochrane T, Davey RC, Matthes Edwards SM: Randomised controlled trial of the cost-effectiveness of water-based therapy for lower limb osteoarthritis. Health Technol Assess 9(31):1–114, 2005

Cocker H: The positive effects of aquarium visits on children's behaviour: a behavioural observation. Plymouth Student Scientist 5(2):165–181, 2012

Codellas PS: Alcmaeon of Croton: his life, work, and fragments. Proc R Soc Med 25(7):1041–1046, 1932 19988748

Columbia University Press: Columbia Electronic Encyclopedia, 6th Edition, Vol 1. New York, Columbia University Press, 2015

Coolman AA, Niedbalski A, Powell DM, et al: Changes in human health parameters associated with an immersive exhibit experience at a zoological institution. PLoS One 15(4):e0231383, 2020 32302324

Coutinho JF, Fernandesl SV, Soares JM, et al: Default mode network dissociation in depressive and anxiety states. Brain Imaging Behav 10(1):147–157, 2016 25804311

Cox SC, Hocking C, Payne D: Showers: from a violent treatment to an agent of cleansing. Hist Psychiatry 30(1):58–76, 2019 30247072

Cracknell D, White MP, Pahl S, et al: Marine biota and psychological well-being: a preliminary examination of dose-response effects in an aquarium setting. Environ Behav 48(10):1242–1269, 2016 27818525

Cracknell DL, Pahl S, White MP, et al: Reviewing the role of aquaria as restorative settings: how subaquatic diversity in public aquaria can influence preferences, and human health and well-being. Human Dimensions of Wildlife 23(5):446–460, 2018

da Vinci L: The Notebooks of Leonardo Da Vinci—Complete, Vol 1. Translated by Richter JP. Project Gutenberg, 1888. Available at: https://www.gutenberg.org/ebooks/5000. Accessed January 1, 2004.

Dubois O, Salamon R, Germain C, et al: Balneotherapy versus paroxetine in the treatment of generalized anxiety disorder. Complement Ther Med 18(1):1–7, 2010 20178872

Edwards NE, Beck AM: Animal-assisted therapy and nutrition in Alzheimer's disease. West J Nurs Res 24(6):697–712, 2002 12365769

Gianfaldoni S, Tchernev G, Wollina U, et al: History of the baths and thermal medicine. Open Access Maced J Med Sci 5(4):566–568, 2017

Goedsche K, Förster M, Kroegel C, et al: Repeated cold water stimulations (hydrotherapy according to Kneipp) in patients with COPD. Forsch Komplement Med 14(3):158–166, 2007 17596696

Grinde B, Patil GG: Biophilia: does visual contact with nature impact on health and well-being? Int J Environ Res Public Health 6(9):2332–2343, 2009 19826546

Harmon RB: Hydrotherapy in state mental hospitals in the mid-twentieth century. Issues Ment Health Nurs 30(8):491–494, 2009 19591022

Herrera E, Sandoval MC, Camargo DM, et al: Motor and sensory nerve conduction are affected differently by ice pack, ice massage, and cold water immersion. Phys Ther 90(4):581–591, 2010 20185615

Huang CJ, Huang CW, Tsai YJ, et al: A preliminary examination of aerobic exercise effects on resting EEG in children with ADHD. J Atten Disord 21(11):898–903, 2017 25359761

Iiyama J, Matsushita K, Tanaka N, et al: Effects of single low-temperature sauna bathing in patients with severe motor and intellectual disabilities. Int J Biometeorol 52(6):431–437, 2008 18196282

Jackson JA: Hydrotherapy in the treatment of mental diseases: its forms, indications, contraindications and untoward effects. J Am Med Assoc 64(20):1650–1651, 1915

Jackson M, Kang M, Furness J, et al: Aquatic exercise and mental health: a scoping review. Complement Ther Med 66:102820, 2022 35218906

Jah CA: Water in Islamic culture. Riyadh, Saudi Arabia, EcoMENA, 2020. Available at: https://www.ecomena.org/water-islam. Accessed May 11, 2024.

Jonsson K, Kjellgren A: Promising effects of treatment with flotation-REST (restricted environmental stimulation technique) as an intervention for generalized anxiety disorder (GAD): a randomized controlled pilot trial. BMC Complement Altern Med 16:108, 2016 27016217

Jonsson K, Kjellgren A: Characterizing the experiences of flotation-REST (Restricted Environmental Stimulation Technique) treatment for generalized anxiety disorder (GAD): a phenomenological study. Eur J Integr Med 12:53–59, 2017

Kabbalah Center: What does water symbolize in Judaism? June 12, 2020. Available at: https://kabbalahcenter.net/kabbalah-water. Accessed June 27, 2022.

Kaplan S: The restorative benefits of nature: toward an integrative framework. J Environ Psychol 15(3):169–182, 1995

Karydis M: Organizing a public aquarium: objectives, design, operation and missions. A review. Global NEST Journal 13(4):369–384, 2011

Kelly JS, Bird E: Improved mood following a single immersion in cold water. Lifestyle Med 3(1):e53, 2021

Kjellgren A, Lyden FJ, Norlander T: Sensory isolation in flotation tanks: altered states of consciousness and effects on well-being. Qual Rep 13:636–656, 2008

Kjellgren A, Norell-Clarke A, Jonsson K, et al: Does flotation-rest (restricted environmental stimulation technique) have an effect on sleep? Eur J Integr Med 33:101047, 2020

Kyriakoulis P, Kyrios M, Nardi AE, et al: The implications of the diving response in reducing panic symptoms. Front Psychiatry 12:784884, 2021 34912254

Linehan MM: DBT® Skills Training Handouts and Worksheets, 2nd Edition. New York, Guilford, 2015

Logan AC, Selhub EM: Vis Medicatrix naturae: does nature "minister to the mind"? Biopsychosoc Med 6(1):11, 2012 22472137

Loose LF, Manuel J, Karst M, et al: Flotation restricted environmental stimulation therapy for chronic pain: a randomized clinical trial. JAMA Netw Open 4(5):e219627, 2021 33988708

McGuire MT: A history of psychiatry: from the era of the asylum to the age of Prozac. JAMA 278(11):949–950, 1997

McKee K, Nelson S, Batra A, et al: Diving into the Ice Bucket Challenge: intraparenchymal hemorrhage and the mammalian diving reflex. Neurohospitalist 5(3):182–184, 2015 26288676

Mooventhan A, Nivethitha L: Scientific evidence-based effects of hydrotherapy on various systems of the body. N Am J Med Sci 6(5):199–209, 2014 24926444

National Oceanic and Atmospheric Administration: How Much of the Ocean Have We Explored? Silver Spring, MD, National Oceanic and Atmospheric Administration, 2021. Available at: https://oceanservice.noaa.gov/facts/exploration.html#:~:text=More%20than%20eighty%20percent%20of,the%20mysteries%20of%20the%20deep. Accessed May 11, 2024.

Nelson PA, Erickson DJ: Hydrotherapy for psychiatric patients. Med Clin North Am 33:1121–1130, 1949 18145654

Nichols WJ, Cousteau C: Blue Mind: The Surprising Science That Shows How Being Near, in, on, or Under Water Can Make You Happier, Healthier, More Connected, and Better at What You Do. Boston, MA, Little, Brown, 2014

Panneton WM: The mammalian diving response: an enigmatic reflex to preserve life? Physiology (Bethesda) 28(5):284–297, 2013 23997188

Rapolienė L, Razbadauskas A, Sąlyga J, et al: Stress and fatigue management using balneotherapy in a short-time randomized controlled trial. Evid Based Complement Alternat Med 2016:9631684, 2016 27051455

Reger M, Kutschan S, Freuding M, et al: Water therapies (hydrotherapy, balneotherapy or aqua therapy) for patients with cancer: a systematic review. J Cancer Res Clin Oncol 148(6):1277–1297, 2022 35171330

Rouwhorst G, Poorthuis M, Schwartz JJ, et al: A remarkable case of religious interaction: water baptisms in Judaism and Christianity, in Interaction Between Judaism and Christianity in History, Religion, Art and Literature. Edited by Poorthuis M, Schwartz JJ, Turner J. Leiden, The Netherlands, Brill, 2009, pp 103–126

Schweitzer PP: Arctic: sociocultural aspects, in International Encyclopedia of the Social and Behavioral Sciences, 2nd Edition. Edited by Wright JD. New York, Elsevier, 2015, pp 927–932

Sena Moore K, Peebles L: A preliminary overview of music therapy reimbursement practice in the United States. Music Ther Perspect 39(1):69–77, 2020

Shafik A: Role of warm-water bath in anorectal conditions: the "thermosphincteric reflex." J Clin Gastroenterol 16(4):304–308, 1993 8331263

Sharma M, Tiffin H: Polluted river or goddess and saviour? The Ganga in the discourses of modernity and Hinduism, in Five Emus to the King of Siam: Environment and Empire. Edited by Tiffin H. Leiden, The Netherlands, Brill, 2007, pp 31–50

Sheng J, Liu S, Wang Y, et al: The link between depression and chronic pain: neural mechanisms in the brain. Neural Plast 2017:9724371, 2017 28706741

Shevchuk NA: Hydrotherapy as a possible neuroleptic and sedative treatment. Med Hypotheses 70(2):230–238, 2008 17640827

Silva LAD, Tortelli L, Motta J, et al: Effects of aquatic exercise on mental health, functional autonomy and oxidative stress in depressed elderly individuals: a randomized clinical trial. Clinics (São Paulo) 74:e322, 2019 31271585

Skurvydas A, Kamandulis S, Stanislovaitis A, et al: Leg immersion in warm water, stretch-shortening exercise, and exercise-induced muscle damage. J Athl Train 43(6):592–599, 2008 19030137

Takeshima N, Rogers ME, Watanabe E, et al: Water-based exercise improves health-related aspects of fitness in older women. Med Sci Sports Exerc 34(3):544–551, 2002 11880822

Unno T: River of Fire, River of Water: An Introduction to the Pure Land Tradition of Shin Buddhism. New York, Doubleday, 1998

Von Korff M, Simon G: The relationship between pain and depression. Br J Psychiatry Suppl 168(30):101–108, 1996 8864155

Wallaya N: Explore history and healing in some of Europe's oldest spa towns. National Geographic, July 26, 2020. Available at: https://www.national-geographic.co.uk/travel/2019/12/five-historic-european-spa-towns-to-visit. Accessed April 24, 2022.

Water Science School: The Water in You: Water and the Human Body. Boulder, CO, U.S. Geological Survey, 2019. Available at: https://www.usgs.gov/special-topics/water-science-school/science/water-you-water-and-human-body#science. Accessed May 11, 2024.

Weston M, Taber C, Casagranda L, et al: Changes in local blood volume during cold gel pack application to traumatized ankles. J Orthop Sports Phys Ther 19(4):197–199, 1994 8173566

World Health Organization: Emerging Issues in Water and Infectious Disease. Geneva, Switzerland, World Health Organization, 2002

Wutich A: Water insecurity: an agenda for research and call to action for human biology. Am J Hum Biol 32(1):e23345, 2020 31697009

Yang B, Qin QZ, Han LL, et al: Spa therapy (balneotherapy) relieves mental stress, sleep disorder, and general health problems in sub-healthy people. Int J Biometeorol 62(2):261–272, 2018 28936572

Zip Water: The importance of water in different cultures. Zip Water, February 10, 2017. Available at: https://www.zipwater.com/zip-effect/the-importance-of-water-in-different-cultures. Accessed May 10, 2024.

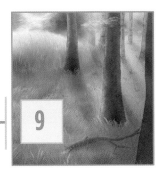

9

The Friendly Outdoors

ANIMAL-ASSISTED THERAPY

Rafael Coira, M.D., J.D.
Diego L. Coira, M.D.

> *There's something about the outside of a horse*
> *that's good for the inside of a human.*
> —A human

> *When I'm with a horse, they don't care if I'm awkward or if*
> *I have scars. They don't care about my achievements or if I*
> *fit in at school. I can leave my social anxiety at the stable door*
> *because I don't have to prove anything to a horse.*
> —A human

CULTURE, PSYCHOLOGY, AND CONTEXT

Darwin

For better and worse, the Darwin family left an indelible effect on the field of psychiatry. Erasmus Darwin, physician and grandfather of the famous Charles, is perhaps best known for his treatise *Zoonomia; or The Laws of Organic Life*, a book that reads like a textbook of neuropsychiatry and, in broad strokes, managed to lay out Charles's later theory of natural selection (Darwin 1794). Erasmus is also remembered for proposing the later barbarically used rotation therapy for mental illness, and Charles's half-cousin Francis Galton coined the term *nature versus nurture* and twisted Charles's famous work (Darwin and Kebler 1859) into a justification for eugenics.

In his own work, Charles Darwin emphasized the similarities of intelligence and temperament between humans of different races. He was passionately against slavery and lamented the atrocities committed by his fellow Europeans on the basis of race (Schwartz 2009). In the book most relevant to the subject at hand, *The Expression of the Emotions in Man and Animals*, he examined the similarities of emotional expression between humans and animals (Darwin 1897). In so doing, he managed to lay out the theoretical bedrock of several fields of psychiatry. He laid the basis for psychoanalysis, casually inspired the theory of attachment, firmly explained social psychology, and in the same sentence emphasized the cruciality of interspecies communication. Let us examine a case study from this text to illustrate the roots of animal-assisted therapy (AAT).

Charles Darwin described the dog in Figure 9–1 this way:

> He walks upright and very stiffly; his head is slightly raised, or not much lowered; the tail is held erect and quite rigid; the hairs bristle, especially along the neck and back; the pricked ears are directed forwards, and the eyes have a fixed stare. Let us now suppose that the dog suddenly discovers that the man he is approaching is not a stranger, but his master; and let it be observed how completely and instantaneously his whole bearing is reversed. Instead of walking upright, the body sinks downwards or even crouches, and is thrown into flexuous movements; his tail, instead of being held stiff and upright, is lowered and wagged from side to side; his hair instantly becomes smooth; his ears are depressed and drawn backwards, but not closely to the head; and his lips hang loosely. From the drawing back of the ears, the eyelids become

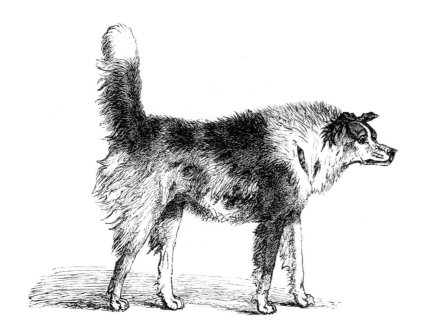

Figure 9–1. Half-bred Shepherd dog approaching another dog with hostile intentions.

Artist: Mr. A. May.

Source. Reprinted from Darwin C: The Principle of antithesis, the second of the three principles of expression, in *The Expression of the Emotions in Man and Animals: With Photographic and Other Illustrations.* New York, D. Appleton, 1897, p. 54. Image provided by Wellcome Library, London. Available at: https://wellcomecollection.org/works/f83m56bw. Copyrighted work available under Creative Commons Attribution only license CC BY 4.0 (http://creativecommons.org/licenses/by/4.0/).

elongated, and the eyes no longer appear round and staring. (Darwin 1897, pp. 50–51; see Figure 9–2)

Further along, he writes, "We will now consider how the principle of antithesis in expression has arisen. With social animals, the power of intercommunication between the members of the same community— *and with other species*, between the opposite sexes, as well as between the young and the old—is of the highest importance to them" (Darwin 1897, p. 60, emphasis added). The implication is that these means of interspecies communication are genetically inherited because they have proven useful for survival.

In these passages, Charles Darwin described two of the key theoretical underpinnings of AAT: the biophilia hypothesis and social signaling between species. Let us look at each in turn.

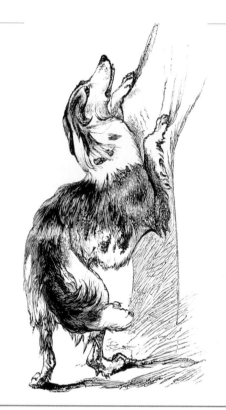

Figure 9–2. The same half-bred Shepherd Dog as in Figure 9–1 caressing his master.
Artist: Mr. A. May.
Source. Reprinted from Darwin C: *The Expression of the Emotions in Man and Animals: With Photographic and Other Illustrations.* New York, D. Appleton, 1897, p. 55. Image provided by Flickr Commons. Available at: https://commons.wikimedia.org/wiki/File:The_expression_of_the_emotions_in_man_and_animals_(1872)_(14598419260).jpg. No known copyright restrictions exist.

Biophilia

Biophilia has been mentioned elsewhere in this book. It is most associated with Edward Wilson and his book of the same title. One definition is a theoretical tendency for humans to affiliate with living things. A more functional understanding would perhaps deemphasize the concept of drive and focus more on emotional salience. It can be argued that on the species level, over tens of thousands of years, there has been evolutionary pressure for humans to unconsciously and consciously assign emotional salience to certain aspects of nature that have a large impact on survival. One such category would be living things (setting aside the complexity of defining life). More crudely put, we are probably evolutionarily wired to notice things that can eat us and things that can help us escape being eaten.

Social Signaling

The concept of social signaling has perhaps been best elucidated by Thomas Lynch, the creator of radically open dialectical behavior therapy. He defined social signaling as any action or behavior that is carried out in the presence of another person, and he believed that it was so central to emotional well-being that he declared it the primary mechanism of change in his form of therapy (Lynch 2018). One of the many keys in the approach is that people who alter their social signaling can activate their own social safety system, which is characterized by high parasympathetic activation in a low sympathetic tone. Perhaps more crucial is that these social signals will then be picked up (often unconsciously) by the people around the individual, engaging their own social safety system and creating a positive feedback loop wherein they are likely to be more expressive, engaged, and, consequently, socially connected. That improved social connectedness, Lynch theorized, is the path to wellness for many people. All of this is rooted in evolutionary psychology.

As noted earlier, more than a century prior, Charles Darwin was not only beating the same drum but also explicitly emphasizing the cruciality of interspecies communication for survival. These tendencies for sending immediately identifiable clear social signals to other individuals of the same species and individuals of other species are genetically inherited because they have proven effective for survival. The snarling teeth and guttural growl of a rabid dog will activate a human's fight, flight, or freeze response before they have even processed the threat. Conversely, when DreamWorks Animation needs to melt the hearts of audiences, they need only trot out Puss in Boots' trademark pleading, nondominant posture and sad eyes. It is undeniable that the social signals of other species can dramatically change humans' neural activation and, with it, their mood and emotions. Evolution provides the framework, but we now examine some of the details.

NEUROBIOLOGY

Mirror Neurons

We have probably all observed in ourselves the near-instantaneous transfer of emotional arousal between species, as described earlier. But how does it happen? Mirror neurons are one of the possible linchpins.

Mirror neurons are neurons that fire both when an individual is performing an action and when the individual is observing another person perform a similar action. They were first identified in the premotor region of the macaque monkey, and many functional MRI studies have strongly supported the existence of mirror neurons in similar regions in humans (Kilner et al. 2014) and other species. Further studies have expanded the concept to a flexible mirror network involving multiple brain regions and functional domains (Bonini et al. 2022). One fascinating finding in the field is that the deactivation of mirror neurons in the observer can actually downregulate an emotional response in the observed animal, that is, the animal receiving the initial stimulus (Carrillo et al. 2019). Carrillo et al. (2019) showed that a rat receiving a fearful and painful shock has reduced freezing behavior if the emotional mirror neurons in the anterior cingulate cortex of an observer rat are deactivated. This remarkable finding indicates that the social transmission of information and emotions is bidirectional. It is highly likely that the flow of emotions between species involves these mirror networks.

Physiology

The physiological effects of human interaction with animals are well established and can be examined across several measures. For example, interaction with animals can modulate blood pressure (Friedmann et al. 1983); furthermore, pet ownership can blunt the hypertensive effect of stress, whereas angiotensin converting enzyme inhibitors may not (Allen et al. 2001). Similarly, interaction with dogs can decrease heart rate (Handlin et al. 2011). Of course, it is no surprise that interaction with dogs can also increase heart rate (Kaminski et al. 2002; Somerville et al. 2008). Pet visitation on a pediatric cardiology unit has been shown to decrease respiratory rate as well (Wu et al. 2002), and in the oncological setting, animal interaction has been shown to increase the oxygen saturation of patients receiving chemotherapy.

The ability of animal interaction to modulate vital signs and, by proxy, sympathetic tone is sufficient for any psychiatrist to leverage to the benefit of their patients' health. However, it is important to measure more general outcomes. To that end, it is useful to mention a pair of studies that have shown a mortality benefit to humans. Impressively, the first showed that pet ownership is associated with higher 1-year survival rates after discharge from a coronary care unit (Friedmann et al. 1980). In a more preventive vein, pet ownership also has been shown to decrease the risk of dying from cardiovascular disease in healthy adults (Ogechi et al. 2016).

Neurotransmitters and Hormones

Several studies have focused on the effect of animals on human cortisol in a variety of treatment populations. The presence of a dog has been shown to decrease cortisol levels in humans, even when a human friend has not (Polheber and Matchock 2014). Service dogs have been shown to decrease cortisol levels in autistic children (Viau et al. 2010) and veterans with PTSD (O'Haire and Rodriguez 2018).

Oxytocin, which is associated with affiliative behavior, is another frequent outcome measure in AAT research and has been shown to be increased in a variety of human-animal interactions (Odendaal 2000). Quite interestingly, the same author showed an increase in oxytocin, β-endorphin, prolactin, phenylacetic acid, and dopamine levels, not just in humans but also in the dogs involved (Odendaal and Meintjes 2003).

CLINICAL PRACTICE

Defining Terms and Legal Framework

Animal-assisted activities are a field that is plagued with a patchwork of terms of art and overlapping legal frameworks. Intermittent media reports and patients' own varying levels of knowledge can confuse the treating psychiatrist. The following is an attempt to clarify some of the most relevant terms.

Animal-assisted therapy is itself a term of art. It can be considered a narrower term within the broader field of animal-assisted interventions or animal-assisted activities. The inclusion of *therapy* in the term denotes several key features. *Therapy* implies that a trained professional is delivering a treatment to a patient. Several notable activities fall outside the definition of AAT. For example, animal visitation in hospital wards is typically delivered by a handler and is made available to many patients without a specific targeted treatment goal. This does not mean that this intervention is not beneficial or informative. A similar potentially beneficial activity that most people are familiar with to some degree is animal-assisted education.

Those that do fall squarely within the narrow umbrella of AAT are animal-assisted physical therapy, animal-assisted occupational therapy, and animal-assisted psychotherapy. The latter, which is most relevant in this chapter, necessarily implies that the treatment is being delivered by someone who is already trained in psychotherapy and has some level of education, experience, or training in incorporating animals into the well-established practice of psychotherapy.

Another term worth mentioning is *pet therapy*. This term is often used interchangeably with AAT or sometimes as an overarching term that loosely encompasses all animal-assisted interventions. The term *pet therapy* has lost favor in the literature and is inherently confusing in the context of attempts to accurately delineate practices. The word *pet* connotes a nonclinical relationship between animal and human, whereas *therapy* is used to specify a clinical intervention.

Another way to divide the field is to examine which category of animal is used. Common terms include *service animal, emotional support animal (ESA)*, and *therapy animal*. Unlike the former two, *therapy animal* is not a legal term. A therapy animal is the type of animal used in AAT. A therapy animal is not necessarily specially trained for AAT but often can be. It is not restricted by species. The most common therapy animals are dogs and horses.

A service animal has a specific legal and clinical definition. For the purposes of the Americans With Disabilities Act (ADA), a service animal is a dog that is individually trained to do work or perform a task for a person with a disability. A miniature horse can also be a service animal under the ADA, with stricter provisions. By definition, a service animal is trained for a specific task and is legally covered only for a person who has a disability. The ADA requires that governments, businesses, and nonprofit organizations that serve the public allow service animals to accompany the person in all public areas. In a hospital, for example, this includes examination rooms, patient rooms, and the cafeteria but not an operating room or a unit where the animal could compromise a sterile environment. Many more details and nuances are included in the statutory and case law surrounding service animals, including overlapping state laws that could broaden the definition of service animal. The Air Carrier Access Act has some more stringent rules about service animals aboard airplanes.

An ESA is generally defined as an untrained animal that supports a person who is disabled by an emotional or mental disorder. An ESA is not recognized as a service dog under the ADA, and therefore the ADA does not require facilities to allow ESAs, although some institutions do choose to allow them. An ESA has protection under several federal laws including Section 504 of the Rehabilitation Act, the Fair Housing Act, and the Individuals With Disabilities Education Act.

A physician is most likely to encounter an ESA in clinical practice in the context of a patient seeking an "ESA letter" for a "no pets waiver." Under both the Fair Housing Act and Section 504, a landlord with a no pets policy is generally required to waive that policy for a person who has an ESA for a mental or emotional disability. A physician or other mental health professional may be called on to provide what is known as an "ESA letter." This letter would generally assert that the person has a mental or emotional disability and that the presence of the animal is needed to lessen the burden of that disability. Sample letters often can be obtained from federal government websites including that of the U.S. Department of Housing and Urban Development (www.hud.gov). The term *disability* in the context of an ESA is less strict than in other areas of the law a physician may encounter, such as in the context of seeking Social Security benefits. For an ESA, a physician's assertion in an ESA letter generally suffices. Of course, a physician should examine the patient and execute sound clinical judgment in asserting a nexus between the patient's disability or limitations and the benefit the animal provides. An ESA also may be allowed in the school setting if it were determined to be part of the student's Individualized Education Program.

The clinician should be broadly aware of the above terms and refresh their recollection when they arise in clinical practice. As noted earlier, by far the most common animals used in AAT are dogs and horses, and thus they merit special attention here.

Levinson: "The Dog as a 'Co-Therapist'"

Much credit for popularizing and legitimizing AAT is given to psychologist Boris Levinson. In his 1962 article "The Dog as a 'Co-Therapist,'" Levinson (1962) described his inadvertent discovery of his dog's clinical prowess. A child had become progressively withdrawn to the point that hospitalization was being considered when his parents brought him to Levinson for an interview. On his arrival, Levinson's dog leaped to the child and began licking his face. Rather than shy away, this previously withdrawn child began to engage with the dog. The child would return to the office to see the dog, at first apparently oblivious to Levinson, but gradually Levinson was included in the play.

Levinson's dog was able to establish an instant alliance with a child who may have been very difficult to reach, and that alliance was then transferred onto Levinson, who could then use his skill to help the child. This description is consistent with the concept of the animal serving as a "social lubricant" or icebreaker. Levinson further defined the ways in which dogs help children develop. At various times, he said, a dog can serve as a companion, friend, servant, admirer, confidant, toy, teammate, slave, scapegoat, mirror, trustee, or defender for the child. Furthermore,

> Even though the dog urinates, defecates, masturbates, and has public and almost indiscriminate sex relations, he is loved and accepted. In identify-

ing with the loved dog, the child is bound to make comparisons and ask why he who has not transgressed as much cannot be accepted? If the dog does not feel guilty, why should the child? (Levinson 1962, p. 61)

Equine-Assisted Therapy

Equine-assisted therapy (EAT) can be delivered in a variety of ways. Methods include groundwork, herd observation, and riding. Groundwork includes activities such as grooming, feeding, and lunging. There is no limit on the psychotherapeutic schools that can be integrated with equine-assisted psychotherapy.

Therapeutic horseback riding can improve balance and motor functioning (Stergiou et al. 2017). In autistic children, EAT has resulted in improvement in socialization, engagement, maladaptive behaviors, and problem-solving (Trzmiel et al. 2019). Many studies have focused on the military veteran population and have found efficacy for EAT in psychosocial outcomes (Kinney et al. 2019). Some evidence indicates that EAT is beneficial in children with ADHD (Helmer et al. 2021), but heterogeneity in outcome variables and methodological quality limits the conclusion (Pérez-Gómez et al. 2021).

SPECIAL CONSIDERATIONS

Before engaging in AAT, it is important for clinicians to consider liability. They may be surprised to find that their malpractice insurance carrier already covers them for AAT, but the clinician should explicitly have this conversation with their insurance carrier and memorialize AAT in their policy. Other liability insurance coverage concerns may be relevant, such as coverage for the facilities used, and the nature of the activities should be made clear.

Insurance billing for AAT remains somewhat of a gray area in that no specific reimbursable billing codes are available for AAT. However, AAT is commonly reimbursed by health insurance carriers through standard billing codes, whether it is performed by physical therapists, occupational therapists, or psychotherapists. Therefore, clinicians must ensure that they are providing and documenting the treatment required for those billing codes. This may in effect shortchange the providers, particularly in EAT, where the costs of maintaining equestrian facilities can be high, yet no additional compensation is provided for what the growing body of literature suggests is an added benefit. The quality and specificity of research must improve if AAT is to be reimbursed in its own right, as electroconvulsive therapy is, for example.

Clinical Translation: Case Example

A 20-year-old woman attending a local private university who has generalized anxiety disorder and social anxiety disorder is receiving escitalopram, 20 mg/day, and individual psychotherapy with moderate response. She agreed to participate in a 12-week program of equine-assisted psychotherapy. The treatment was provided by a board-certified psychiatrist with significant experience in working with horses and with postgraduate training in equine-assisted mental health. The patient was seen weekly for a 1-hour session at an equestrian facility. She had no experience with horses. In the first session, she was introduced to horses and the horse environment. Sessions 2–6 consisted of mindfulness-based cognitive-behavioral therapy facilitated by working with horses doing groundwork (i.e., grooming and leading a horse in the arena). In sessions 7–9, role-play and an obstacle course were used to work on interpersonal communication and problem-solving. Sessions 10 and 11 included mounted work. Session 12 was designed as a herd observation to view and interpret the dynamics of the horses' behavior as it pertained to her own relationships. At the end of the 12-week program, the patient had experienced significant improvement in both generalized and social anxiety disorder symptoms, greater satisfaction with treatment, and a closer alliance with her psychiatrist.

KEY POINTS

- Social signals are passed between humans and animals, often at an unconscious level, and have a powerful ability to affect physiology.

- Strong evidence indicates that human interaction with animals can powerfully affect measures of health such as modulating blood pressure, decreasing heart rate, and increasing oxygen saturation.

- Animal interactions can modulate hormones and neurotransmitters in humans, for example, increasing oxytocin, prolactin, β-endorphin, and dopamine levels and decreasing cortisol levels.

- Having a pet has been shown to have a mortality benefit in the context of cardiac rehabilitation.

- Animal-assisted psychotherapy should be delivered by a person skilled in psychotherapy, with additional training or experience in the use of animals in the delivery of psychotherapy.

QUESTIONS

1. Which type of psychotherapy can be delivered through equine-assisted psychotherapy?

    A. Psychodynamic psychotherapy.
    B. Mindfulness-based cognitive-behavioral therapy.
    C. Dialectical behavior therapy.
    D. Motivational interviewing.
    E. All of the above.

Correct answer: E. All of the above.

Any school of psychotherapy can potentially be enhanced by delivery through equine-assisted psychotherapy. For example, herd observation can facilitate projection and the uncovering of unconscious beliefs about relationships (A). Many people experience a greater capacity for mindful awareness (B) in the horse environment, which is filled with sights, sounds, smells, and motion that draw the senses to the present moment and the reflection of social signals between the horse and the human that can draw awareness of physiological states. Dialectical behavior therapy (C) is a skill-based treatment approach that emphasizes mindfulness and translates research from many areas of psychiatry into skills. Motivational interviewing (D) is a psychotherapeutic technique for treatment of addiction that relies on a nonjudgmental stance. Equine assistance provides an additional neutral body incapable of judgment that reinforces the supportive tone of the therapy session. There are nearly limitless ways in which equine-assisted psychotherapy could be conceptualized as applying to dialectical behavior therapy skills, such as building mastery in the equine environment as a means to reduce vulnerability to the emotional mind.

2. A patient is admitted to the hospital with his service dog. In what area of the hospital is the dog *not* permitted to be present?

    A. The patient's room.
    B. The operating room.
    C. The cafeteria.
    D. The waiting room.
    E. All of the above.

Correct answer: B. The operating room.

The Americans With Disabilities Act (ADA) requires a hospital to permit the presence of a service dog in any area of the hospital that is open to the public. This would include the patient's room (A), the cafeteria (C), and the waiting room (D) but not an operating room (B). Allowing the dog in the operating room probably would not follow other requirements of the ADA, such as the dog not interfering with the operation of the facility and being in direct control of the patient, who may be incapacitated during the procedure. A family member or friend of the patient could care for the dog during the procedure, but the hospital would not be required to allow that person or the dog in the operating room. An interesting question arises if a patient with a service dog is admitted to an inpatient psychiatric unit. The dog likely would be excluded from the unit, but it would be wise to take a nuanced approach rather than set a strict policy (Muramatsu et al. 2015).

3. Which of the following are requirements for a psychiatrist to deliver animal-assisted psychotherapy?

    A. Training in psychotherapy.
    B. A specially trained animal.
    C. Training or experience in animal-assisted therapy.
    D. A and C.
    E. All of the above.

Correct answer: D. A and C.

In order to effectively and safely deliver animal-assisted psychotherapy, a clinician must be skilled in the delivery of psychotherapy (A) and have the necessary training or experience to integrate the animal into the treatment (C). Training organizations provide high-quality training for people seeking to specialize in animal-assisted therapy; however, no specific training is currently required, and as in other forms of psychotherapy, the skills can be attained through tutelage and supervision by an experienced practitioner. Although the animal may have specialized training (B), it is not always necessary. For example, a person skilled in equestrianship should be able to select a horse with the right temperament and training in the technique being used.

REFERENCES

Allen K, Shykoff BE, Izzo JL Jr: Pet ownership, but not ace inhibitor therapy, blunts home blood pressure responses to mental stress. Hypertension 38(4):815–820, 2001 11641292

Bonini L, Rotunno C, Arcuri E, et al: Mirror neurons 30 years later: implications and applications. Trends Cogn Sci 26(9):767–781, 2022 35803832

Carrillo M, Han Y, Migliorati F, et al: Emotional mirror neurons in the rat's anterior cingulate cortex. Curr Biol 29(8):1301–1312, 2019 30982647

Darwin C: The Expression of the Emotions in Man and Animals: With Photographic and Other Illustrations. New York, D. Appleton, 1897

Darwin C, Kebler L: On the Origin of Species by Means of Natural Selection, or, The Preservation of Favoured Races in the Struggle for Life. London, J Murray, 1859

Darwin E: Zoonomia; or The Laws of Organic Life: In Three Parts. Philadelphia, PA, Edward Earle, 1794

Friedmann E, Katcher AH, Lynch JJ, et al: Animal companions and one-year survival of patients after discharge from a coronary care unit. Public Health Rep 95(4):307–312, 1980 6999524

Friedmann E, Katcher AH, Thomas SA, et al: Social interaction and blood pressure: influence of animal companions. J Nerv Ment Dis 171(8):461–465, 1983 6875529

Handlin L, Hydbring-Sandberg E, Nilsson A, et al: Short-term interaction between dogs and their owners: effects on oxytocin, cortisol, insulin and heart rate—an exploratory study. Anthrozoos 24(3):301–315, 2011

Helmer A, Wechsler T, Gilboa Y: Equine-assisted services for children with attention-deficit/hyperactivity disorder: a systematic review. J Altern Complement Med 27(6):477–488, 2021 33835856

Kaminski M, Pellino T, Wish J: Play and pets: the physical and emotional impact of child-life and pet therapy on hospitalized children. Children's Health Care (Don Mills) 31(4):321–335, 2002

Kilner JM, Kraskov A, Lemon RN: Do monkey F5 mirror neurons show changes in firing rate during repeated observation of natural actions? J Neurophysiol 111(6):1214–1226, 2014 24371289

Kinney AR, Eakman AM, Lassell R, et al: Equine-assisted interventions for veterans with service-related health conditions: a systematic mapping review. Mil Med Res 6(1):28, 2019 31462305

Levinson BM: The dog as a "co-therapist." Ment Hyg 46:59–65, 1962 14464675

Lynch TR: The Skills Training Manual for Radically Open Dialectical Behavior Therapy: A Clinician's Guide for Treating Disorders of Overcontrol. Oakland, CA, New Harbinger, 2018

Muramatsu R, Thomas K, Leong S, et al: Service dogs, psychiatric hospitalization, and the ADA. Psychiatr Serv 66(1):87–89, 2015. Available at: https://ps.psychiatryonline.org/doi/10.1176/appi.ps.201400208. Accessed October 14, 2022.

Odendaal JS: Animal-assisted therapy—magic or medicine? J Psychosom Res 49(4):275–280, 2000 11119784

Odendaal JS, Meintjes RA: Neurophysiological correlates of affiliative behaviour between humans and dogs. Vet J 165(3):296–301, 2003 12672376

Ogechi I, Snook K, Davis BM, et al: Pet ownership and the risk of dying from cardiovascular disease among adults without major chronic medical conditions. High Blood Press Cardiovasc Prev 23(3):245–253, 2016 27174431

O'Haire ME, Rodriguez KE: Preliminary efficacy of service dogs as a complementary treatment for posttraumatic stress disorder in military members and veterans. J Consult Clin Psychol 86(2):179–188, 2018 29369663

Pérez-Gómez J, Amigo-Gamero H, Collado-Mateo D, et al: Equine-assisted activities and therapies in children with attention-deficit/hyperactivity disorder: a systematic review. J Psychiatr Ment Health Nurs 28(6):1079–1091, 2021 33171006

Polheber JP, Matchock RL: The presence of a dog attenuates cortisol and heart rate in the Trier Social Stress Test compared to human friends. J Behav Med 37(5):860–867, 2014 24170391

Schwartz J: Illuminating Charles Darwin's morality: slavery, humanity's origin and unity, and Darwin's evolutionary theory. Evo Edu Outreach 2:334–337, 2009

Somerville JW, Kruglikova YA, Robertson RL, et al: Physiological responses by college students to a dog and a cat: implications for pet therapy. N Am J Psychol 10(3):519–528, 2008

Stergiou A, Tzoufi M, Ntzani E, et al: Therapeutic effects of horseback riding interventions: a systematic review and meta-analysis. Am J Phys Med Rehabil 96(10):717–725, 2017 28252520

Trzmiel T, Purandare B, Michalak M, et al: Equine assisted activities and therapies in children with autism spectrum disorder: a systematic review and a meta-analysis. Complement Ther Med 42:104–113, 2019 30670226

Viau R, Arsenault-Lapierre G, Fecteau S, et al: Effect of service dogs on salivary cortisol secretion in autistic children. Psychoneuroendocrinology 35(8):1187–1193, 2010 20189722

Wu AS, Niedra R, Pendergast L, et al: Acceptability and impact of pet visitation on a pediatric cardiology inpatient unit. J Pediatr Nurs 17(5):354–362, 2002 12395303

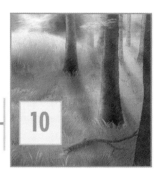

10

The Wondrous Outdoors

NATURE'S WINGED AMBASSADORS

Yonatan Kaplan, M.D.

Hope is the thing with feathers
That perches in the soul,
And sings the tune without the words,
And never stops at all

—Emily Dickinson (1891, p. 28), excerpt from "Hope"

Look outside and spend a moment in quiet observation. Use all of your senses to absorb the environment. See tree branches swaying gently in the wind, hear the Klaxon of a distant siren, and inhale the season's aroma. Unless you are in some remote, desolate landscape bereft of life, odds are that you noticed a bird. Congratulations, you have made your very first field observation and may now consider yourself an amateur naturalist. Birds are ubiquitous, and people have been noticing them since prehistory. They are taken for granted as defining features of our environments, such as ducks in a pond or pigeons in a city. Their comings and goings are associated with our calendar seasons, as with the American robin's song signifying the return of spring. They are insinuated into our language as idioms, metaphors, and character descriptions. They feature prominently in religion as omens, divine messengers, or even gods. We evoke their images as national symbols, sports team logos, and breakfast cereal mascots. We anthropomorphize them in televised media to educate and entertain. They inspire creative luminaries from every generation and are depicted in countless works of art, from Picasso's doves to Mozart's *Magic Flute*. Birds fill our skies, arts, and bellies. Domesticated fowl are some of the earliest farmed animals, and poultry meat and eggs are staples of modern industrial agriculture. Feathers, although largely replaced by synthetic fibers for mass consumption, still have a substantial luxury market as insulation for coats, blankets, and pillows. Even bird guano is so coveted as a natural resource that countries have gone to war over control of small islands with nitrogen-rich deposits (Archer 2009).

Birds provide valuable services in addition to the aforementioned goods. Birds living their best lives within their ecological niches save people millions of dollars in environmental stewardship. A few examples are insectivorous birds providing pest control, carrion eaters preventing the spread of disease, and frugivores pollinating plants and dispersing seeds (Wenny et al. 2011). Recognizing how prominently they feature in our daily lives, how might our feathered friends' presence or absence affect our mental health?

In this chapter, I focus on the psychological implications of human interactions with wild birds. I do not address farmed poultry or pet birds because the complex and rich interactions between people and their domesticated companions are better represented in Chapter 9, "The Friendly Outdoors." Previous chapters in this book cover the literature on forest bathing, urban green spaces, and the biophilia hypothesis. Although these themes describe the environments where people and birds meet, they do not account for the unique therapeutic potential of these interactions. People are invested in learning more about birds. Ornithology is an entire field of science dedicated to this study, and bird-watchers are a rapidly growing subculture of bird enthusiasts. Despite this demonstrated interest in bird biology and behavior, very little research has been done on what makes them such compelling subjects of study. Perhaps the answer to that question is so complex and multifactorial that designing a study to control for all the variables is too onerous to be feasible. Conversely, maybe the reason is so simple and obvious that there is no need to waste time and money on scientifically proving it. Birds are a diverse group of intelligent, charismatic, and aesthetically pleasing animals. Whatever the reasons, they have fascinated humankind for thousands of years and continue to inspire new avenues of investigation.

THE FIRST BIRD-WATCHERS

Three million years ago, a diminutive primate clambered down from the treetops and stepped into the African savanna. *Australopithecus afarensis*, also known as "Lucy's species" after the eponymous fossil, was a human ancestral species who lived in the African continent between 3 and 4 million years ago. Lucy and her kin were significant to the anthropological fossil record as one of the earliest hominins to demonstrate humanity's signature evolutionary trait of bipedalism.

With the benefit of hindsight, and through the lens of evolutionary biology, Lucy can be seen as belonging to a species in transition. She walked upright with the energy-efficient two-legged gait, covering long distances on the ground (Rodman and McHenry 1980), while retaining her long arms and curved fingers suitable for climbing trees (Schmid 2004). Modern humans outgrew Lucy's apelike proportions, but some of her other sylvan traits, which conferred a survival advantage on the ground, were preserved. Among these surviving traits were a suite of complex optic machinery and accompanying neural network.

A. afarensis had two forward-facing eyes with overlapping visual fields, or binocular vision. A strong primary visual cortex received input from both eyes to synthesize a fully three-dimensional visual landscape, a feat known as *stereoscopy* (Heesy 2009). Binocular stereoscopic vision added depth perception to the primate sensory toolbox.

Depth perception is the ability to recognize the relative positions of objects in space. Judging the distance to the next tree branch meant the difference between successful acrobatic travel of the forest canopy and a biological dead end on the forest floor. More than a navigational tool, binocular vision helped Lucy's species keep track of approaching dangers and spot promising opportunities (Changizi and Shimojo 2008).

A. afarensis were primarily fruit eaters, and their eyes were specially adapted to find their preferred foods. Their retinas had three types of color-sensitive cells to detect light in green, red, and blue wavelengths. This ability to see three wavelengths of light is called trichromatic vision. Trichromatic vision probably helped our frugivorous ancestors forage by distinguishing brightly colored ripening fruit from a background of green foliage (Gerl and Morris 2008).

Although the selective pressures that drove human visual adaptations are theorized to be directed toward survival, they are equally suitable for less vital pursuits. Birds famously sport some of the most vibrant and varied colors, shapes, and patterns in the animal kingdom. Trichromatic binocular vision allows people to follow the movements of a brightly colored bird as easily as triangulating the position of a ripe apple. Paying attention to birds' activities may confer an advantage beyond aesthetic appreciation.

Early hominin success is attributed largely to their social intelligence, which allowed them to learn from one another and pass down information iteratively through successive generations (Whiten and van Schaik 2007). Their adaptability led to a shift in their ecological niche from obligate frugivores to opportunistic generalists. Selective pressures favored traits that allowed them to recognize and benefit from multiple sources of nourishment. When early hominins expanded their habitat from the forests into the savanna, they also diversified their diets. Fruiting trees may have been less plentiful outside the treetops, but other food sources became available, including roots, tubers, and occasionally meat. Paleontological evidence from Dikika, Ethiopia, of 3-million-year-old fossil bones with cut marks suggests that *A. afarensis* was the earliest human species to butcher and eat meat (Morelli et al. 2015). Finding this protein-rich food source required new foraging habits suitable to wide expanses of grassland and open sky. Lucy's ancestors may have been accustomed to craning their necks up toward the treetops while patrolling the understory, hoping to spot the colorful signs of ripe fruit. The primate penchant for looking upward coupled with their problem-solving abilities may have led to the beginnings of human fascination with birds.

During the Pleistocene, 2–3 million years ago, early human species beginning with *A. afarensis*, then *Homo habilis*, and later *Homo erectus* developed the human survival strategies that eventually led to hominin dominion of the environment. Selective pressures favored strategies for obtaining food that maximized caloric return on energy investment. Large prey animals represented a high caloric reward, but hunting was risky and took energy. Scavenging a carcass had a more favorable cost/

benefit ratio, but unlike fruit, dead animals did not grow on trees. A hungry band of humans might occasionally chance on a meat-laden carcass of an animal that either died from natural causes or was already the meal of a large predator. Instead of relying on luck, early hominins may have combined their enhanced cognitive and observational abilities to recognize a reliable environmental signal of newly available carcasses within their vicinity. This signal was the activity of the scavenging family of birds known as vultures.

Vultures are a family of raptors that specialize in eating carrion. They soar high above the savanna and have keen senses of vision and smell. From their vantage, they can quickly zero in on dead animals and join great ominous flocks of other vultures circling down to feed on carrion. Present-day mammalian carnivores of the African plains such as lions, hyenas, and African wild dogs are known to follow vultures in pursuit of their next meal. It is very likely that prehistoric humans, who competed in the same ecological niche as the aforementioned predators, would have adopted this behavior. Although paleontological evidence of Pleistocene "vulture chasing" is speculative at best, the archeological record shows consistent incorporation of vulture body parts and motifs into human culture.

Vulture remains were found in European caves occupied by *Homo neanderthalensis* (Neanderthals) 40,000–60,000 years ago. The bones showed that Neanderthals skinned and plucked the large dark birds and probably used their feathers for rituals or symbolic adornment. *Homo sapiens*, or anatomically modern humans (AMHs), continued the tradition of cultural processing of vulture parts. The oldest known musical instrument is a 40,000-year-old flute made from the wing bone of a griffon vulture found at an AMH site in Hohle Fels, Germany (Conard et al. 2009). The vulture's importance in human cultural tradition was transmitted into the Holocene and followed AMH migration out of Africa across the globe and all the way to the New World. As the human lifestyle changed from hunter-gatherer to agrarian, the relationship with the vulture changed as well. The scavenging birds were no longer relied on to signal food but were indispensable for waste management, feeding on dead livestock and preventing the spread of disease. The vulture's association with positive and life-giving forces was conserved across even widely disparate civilizations, from the Mayans to the ancient Egyptians (Morelli et al. 2015).

A biological anthropology research team from the Czech University of Life Sciences in Prague, Czech Republic, and Poznań University of Life Sciences in Poland believe that the vulture's cultural impact goes beyond food beacon and waste management. The researchers suggested that humans may have learned how to cook with fire by watching vultures scavenge the charred remains of animals caught in brushfires. They also suggested that vultures following herds of ungulates northward may have led the human dispersal out of Africa (Morelli et al. 2015). Winged messengers from the heavens showed our ancestors where to find food, taught them the secret of fire, and led them to a global expansion, all in one species of bird!

THE VALUE OF BIRDS

Today there are more than 10,000 species of extant birds, each with their own level of abundance and human contact. Birds are perched prominently in the annals of human culture. Some of the oldest known examples of artwork from across the globe are depictions of birds. Chauvet Cave in present-day France has a 30,000-year-old painting of an owl (Clottes 2002), and the oldest known work of art from China is a 13,000-year-old carved bird figurine (Li et al. 2020). Birds have a firm hold on people's imaginations, as demonstrated by their ubiquitous appearances in visual, decorative, and literary arts.

People profit from their relationship to birds materially and artistically. Birds explicitly engage in mutually beneficial, or symbiotic, relationships with their human neighbors. The greater honeyguide (*Indicator indicator*) of East Africa lives up to its name by leading human honey-hunters to nearby bees' nests. Though neither captive nor domesticated, the birds learned to respond to a specific call from the endemic people in a practice dating back generations. People value honey as a delicious and marketable good, and the honeyguide relies on the hunters to break open the tough hive and expose the beeswax, which it eats. Both the Yao people of Mozambique and the Hadza people of northern Tanzania in East Africa have their own unique calls to signal the honeyguides. A 2016 study by the University of Cambridge and the Fitzpatrick Institute of African Ornithology found that honey-hunters who summoned the birds by using the traditional calls rather than a generic one were twice as likely to recruit a honeyguide and three times as likely to find a beehive (Spottiswoode et al. 2016).

The symbiosis with the honeyguide is another example of a survival advantage conferred by paying close attention to bird behavior. A loose application of evolutionary theory might speculate that the propensity to watch birds is a naturally selected adaptation, just like binocular vision. A more grounded analysis would probably recognize that the bird-watching behavior arises from a confluence of more generalizable cognitive traits such as curiosity, object relations, and theory of mind.

The genetic determinants of human psychology have yet to be fully characterized. Could there be a gene hidden somewhere in people's DNA that, when expressed by the right cells, in the right fold of the brain, pings its owner with a touch of delight when recognizing a bird? There may not be a single deterministic bird-watching gene, but people can still profit from their presence or lose out in their absence.

Wild birds enacting their natural behaviors within their ecological niches perform free environmental services with significant monetary value (Wenny et al. 2011). Calculating the exact global cost of those services is a challenge that interests economists, ecologists, agriculturalists, and conservationists. Estimating the dollar value that a single species provides requires an untangling of each of its economically relevant relationships within the web of life. One bird might eat a particular insect that is harmful to crops, or maybe it prefers seeds of a harmful weed. For example, one study of Jamaican coffee farms found that the black-throated-blue warbler (*Setophaga caerulescens*) provided pest-control services valued at more than $300 per hectare of farmland. Another bird may have no interaction with farmers' fields but is responsible for seed dispersal within its forest habitat. Clark's nutcracker (*Nucifraga columbiana*) is estimated to contribute more than $2,000 per hectare through its seed caching behavior, restoring the threatened white pine population. Unless they are intensively studied, many of these relationships will likely remain hidden unless the bird is removed and the downstream effect is seen. China felt the consequences of failing to consider trophic cascades during their 1958 campaign to exterminate the Eurasian tree sparrow (*Passer montanus*). The campaign's goal was to protect their rice fields from hungry sparrows. The campaign backfired when rice-eating insect populations ballooned in the absence of their natural predators, and the overall crop yield declined. Vultures' cultural, historical, and economic value was acutely appreciated in Southeast Asia after the local populations were devastated by diclofenac poisoning. Arthritic cattle that were treated with diclofenac and died in the field passed the toxic component on to vultures cleaning up their remains. As vultures disappeared, wild dogs filled the scavenging niche. Their population boomed and brought with it a widespread rabies outbreak. The overall cost in environmental and health services attributed to the loss of the vulture totaled more than $34 billion from 1993 to 2006 (Wenny et al. 2011). The case examples mentioned offer a glimpse into the economic implications of single bird species. More research is needed to account for the complex interdependencies of more than 10,000 bird species to accurately estimate the economic totality of environmental services rendered.

BIRD-WATCHERS TODAY

Despite wild birds' economic importance, their abundance and diversity are in precipitous decline, largely because of anthropogenic factors such as window strikes and habitat fragmentation. A study led by the Cornell Lab of Ornithology in 2019 reported that the North American total bird population has declined by 30% since 1970 (Rosenberg et al. 2019). Although bird populations plummeted in the last half-century, interest in recreational birding soared.

A Growing Population

A report from the U.S. Forest Service Southern Research Station compared survey data from 1983 to 2001 and estimated a 232% increase in the number of American bird-watchers, from 21 million in 1983 to 70 million in 2001 (Cordell et al. 2002). They defined *birding* as any outdoor activity where birds were seen. The report's authors caution interpretation of the 70 million figure, approximately one-third of the 2001 U.S. population, by admitting that their definition of birding was overly broad.

The U.S. Fish and Wildlife Service (USFWS) National Survey of Fishing, Hunting, and Wildlife-Associated Recreation is conducted every 5 years, and, since 2001, it has included an addendum specifically focused on birding. Their definition is stricter than the Forest Service's and includes a specific intent to observe wild birds, excluding those in captivity. The USFWS data from 2001 estimated 46 million birders. The explosive growth in the number of birders between the twentieth and twenty-first centuries seems to have leveled off around the turn of the millennium. The subsequent surveys from 2001 to 2016 each reported a total number of birders around the 46 million mark, with minor fluctuations that were not statistically significant. The most recent addendum on birding published in 2019, based on 2016 survey data, reported 45 million birders (Carver 2019).

The 2022 survey, which includes data from the coronavirus disease 2019 (COVID-19) pandemic era, estimated that the number of American birders has more than doubled since 2016 to a whopping 96 million (U.S. Department of Interior, U.S. Fish and Wildlife Service 2023). Although the report notes that significant methodological changes in data collection obfuscate direct comparison of the 2022 and 2016 numbers, the skyrocketing figure emerges from a background of pandemic-related societal trends. Headlines across media platforms from 2020 to 2022 declared burgeoning interest in birds and birding in reaction to pandemic-related lifestyle changes (Associated Press 2020; Fortin 2020;

Garrity 2022; MacLellan 2021). One study from the University of Vermont that surveyed 3,200 people found that 64% reported increased wildlife-watching activity since the beginning of the pandemic (Morse et al. 2020). Digital informatics showed that internet activity related to bird-watching also has increased since the beginning of the pandemic. Google search trends on birding-related terms such as *bird feeder*, *birdseed*, and *birdbath* increased by up to 10%, and spending on bird feeders increased by up to $116 million over previous years according to a 2021 study published in the *Ecological Economics: The Journal of the International Society for Ecological Economics* (Brock et al. 2021). Another measure of the birding activity is the growing number of downloads of mobile birding applications.

The Cornell Lab of Ornithology has developed and publishes two of the most popular birding applications: eBird and Merlin. From April 2019 to April 2020, eBird activity increased by 40%, more than twice its prior annual growth. The Merlin application also had 200,000 new downloads in February 2021, a 175% increase from the previous year (Harrison 2021). Although the current data suggest increasing interest in birding, the sampled populations number in the thousands for the Vermont study and the hundreds of thousands for Cornell's Merlin downloads. Both samples are orders of magnitude less than the 45 million bird-watchers reported by the USFWS. One critique of the USFWS number is that although 45 million people may have reported watching birds at some point in the 12 months preceding the survey, most may not self-identify as bird-watchers because of their lack of association with the hobby. More conservative estimates place the number of bird-watching hobbyists in the United States at closer to 1 million (Crotty 2020). Whether the trends from the data showing increased interest in birding reflect a significant addition of hundreds of thousands of new birders to a baseline of 1 million or simply greater electronic engagement from an existing population of 45 million birders remains to be seen.

Birding Motivations

Irrespective of how many more people are birding, the increased media attention to the hobby popularized it as a wellness activity (Associated Press 2020; Fortin 2020; Garrity 2022; Giordano 2020; MacLellan 2021). There are abundant anecdotal accounts of bird-watching for mental hygiene, a practice affectionately called "ornitherapy" (Merker et al. 2021). Some cases report reduced symptoms of psychiatric illnesses such as major depressive, generalized anxiety, and obsessive-compulsive disorders (Harkness 2021; Young 2022). Although birding as treatment for specific psychiatric diagnoses has not been scientifically studied, a growing body of literature supports a positive correlation between birding and happiness in the general population (Zarankin 2021). The bird-watching hobby predates these findings, and the pursuit of happiness does not fully describe its appeal. Researchers from a wide range of disciplines including city planners, environmental scientists, sociologists, and tourism managers are invested in better categorizing what motivates the growing population of birders.

One joint study (Eubanks et al. 2004) between the tourism consultancy Fermata Inc., the Department of Public and Environmental Affairs at the University of Wisconsin, and the Department of Wildlife and Fisheries Science at Texas A&M University surveyed participants of eight separate birding activities between 1998 and 2001. The 2,100 questionnaires returned identified a range of reported motivations and levels of commitment to the activity. Social factors such as "being with friends" and "family recreation" were equally important motivators across all levels of participation. Factors related to enjoying nature such as "being outdoors" and "enjoying the sights, smells, and sounds of nature" were also rated as highly important by most respondents. Birders participating in the activities who reported a higher level of birding skill or commitment were more likely to report achievement-related motivations such as "to see bird species that I had not seen before" and "to see as many bird species as possible" (Eubanks et al. 2004). Other studies from 2002 to 2022 identified more than a dozen motivating factors that are subdivided into four major categories, as described in Table 10–1 (Maake et al. 2022).

Participating in bird-watching as a motivator to participate in bird-watching presents a tautology without closer inspection of its components.

I Want to Be the Very Best

Bird-watching is a leisure activity with a low bar to entry and a high skill ceiling. Recreation specialization is a conceptual framework that describes leisure activity as a demographic trait. A population grouped by a shared activity is called its respective social world. The social world's members represent a continuum of engagement from the peripherally affiliated generalists to the most involved specialists (Eubanks et al. 2004). The social world of birding has three subdimensions of specialization. Birding knowledge is the cognitive subdimension, equipment and travel costs describe the behavior subdimension, and centrality to lifestyle is the affective subdimension. At the most generalist level, a birder might walk to a local park to see the ducks once a month. This birder may have no dedicated equipment other than eyes and ears and no knowledge of the species observed beyond ducks in a

Table 10-1.	Birding motivations		
Participate in bird-watching	**Relaxation and escape**	**Photography and nature appreciation**	**Social interaction**
Achievement	Exploration	Enjoying nature and solitude	Affiliation
Seeing as many bird species as possible	Escape	Conservation	Sharing knowledge
Appreciation of birds	Spirituality	Photography	Companionship
	Spiritual refreshment		Family recreation

pond. On the opposite extreme, a highly specialized birder might spend thousands of dollars each year on cameras, scopes, binoculars, and international travel to see wild birds. This birder might use extensive knowledge of species field marks, song, seasonality, and habitat to make identifications. The two illustrative examples bookend a full spectrum of birders' knowledge level, commitment, and investment.

A specialized birder is also more likely to achieve an optimal experience while birding, where time seems to speed up, worries are forgotten, and the sense of self is consumed by the task at hand. This experiential state, known as *flow*, increases leisure satisfaction and happiness. A flow experience is defined by eight conditions, the first of which is an alignment between an activity's challenge and the participants' skill. Birding as a flow experience is described in Table 10–2 (Dieser et al. 2015).

Acquiring flow experiences is a primary driver of participation in leisure activities. Insiders at the involved end of the social world of birding demonstrate psychological commitment, based on a continuity of participation and a low likelihood of losing interest. The depth of the psychological commitment determines the extent of that activity's incorporation into a person's self-image and value. Examples of psychological commitment include time invested in acquiring skills and knowledge related to birding and increased frequency of birding outings. In this way, anyone entering the birding social world as a novice can be drawn into specialization depending on their psychological commitment. A 2015 study from the National Chiayi University in Taiwan found a direct and positive relationship between recreation specialization and flow experience. The study also found that psychological commitment positively mediated the specialization-flow relationship (Cheng et al. 2016).

Commitment to bird-watching unlocks psychological benefits beyond access to flow. Birds live outside, and most species are found in naturalistic environs. Bird-watchers follow their quarries into forests, urban green spaces, and other settings described in previous chapters. The psychological restoration theories described in previous chapters also apply to bird-watching as a nature activity.

A 2022 joint study from the University of Tübingen Biology Department in Germany, the Centrum Medyczne Psychomedica Allenort in Poland, and the Poznań University of Life Sciences Zoology Department investigated psychological restoration in bird-watching (Randler et al. 2022). They surveyed 400 self-identified bird-watchers on indexes of bird-watching specialization and psychological restoration. Specialization was subdivided into three domains:

Table 10–2. **Flow in birding**

Flow characteristic	Example in birding
1. Alignment in skill and challenge	Greater birding skill increases awareness of bird species present and ability to identify them.
2. Clear goals with immediate feedback	*Goals:* See as many different bird species as possible.
	Feedback: Seeing a bird, and confidence in identifying it.
3. Merging action and awareness	Senses expand outward to find signs of birds: watching for movement, listening for singing, chirping, or wingbeats.
4. Intense concentration	Switching between the naked eye while searching to lifting binoculars for a closer look.
5. Loss of self-consciousness	Correlating birding knowledge with identifying features of the bird, often partially obstructed by foliage, to determine the species.
6. Sense of control	Choosing birding time and location, knowing likelihood of species to be seen based on habitat and seasonality.
7. Time moves faster	Taking 3 hours or more to complete a 1-mile hiking path.
8. Intrinsically rewarding	Birding is a recreational activity without external pressure or incentive to participate.

1. Behavior
2. Knowledge and skill (number of species able to identify by sight or sound)
3. Psychological commitment

Behavior was determined by total years of birding, number of days per year, and trips taken per year. Knowledge and skill were scored by the number of species a respondent could identify by sight or sound. Psychological commitment depended on how personally important birding was to respondents' lifestyle. An exploratory factor analysis found a significant relationship between psychological commitment and restoration in bird-watchers. The results suggested that recreation specialization in a nature activity enhances the psychological benefits described by restoration theories. The behavior and knowledge and skill domains had no significant relationship to restoration (Randler et al. 2022).

Bird-watching presents an opportunity for anybody, regardless of experience or resources, to readily access a flow activity and enhance the attention-restoring and stress-reducing properties of nature immersion. Birding trips or days spent birding require available time to spend on leisure or resources to travel. Knowledge and experience are limited by the time and effort they take to accrue. Psychological commitment is a state of mind that anyone with a passing interest can potentially lean into. In the birding social world, psychological commitment is metaphorized as a flame. The dry tinder of latent interest lies within every nonbirder, waiting to be ignited into a conflagration of enthusiasm for avifauna. Birders enjoy sharing their personal "spark bird" stories, the bird encounters that ignited their own passion for birding (Miller 2021).

The Birding List

To see as many bird species as possible is a motivation commonly reported in studies investigating why people go bird-watching (Maake et al. 2022). Birders motivated by this numbers game keep a running tally, or list, of species seen during their outings. An entire vocabulary has been developed for the listing approach to bird-watching, described in Table 10–3 (Saha 2015).

Although lists are an individual's personal journal of sightings, they contain useful data on the location and abundance of species. The Cornell Lab of Ornithology developed the eBird application to aggregate individual lists into one of the world's largest citizen science projects. Birders log their observations on the application as a list of distinct species found during their bird-watching effort. Additional data such as the number of individuals of each species and the location of the birding activity are also usually included. The lists are aggregated to an open access global dataset (McKee 2022).

The birding list is a collection of observations. Collecting as its own mode of recreation specialization can provide members of its social world with a sense of purpose and meaning in life. Birders whose engagement with the hobby revolves around the augmentation and embellishment of their life lists may be called *listers*. Pursuing acquisitions adds a layer of excitement that may otherwise be lacking in everyday life (Belk 2009).

A 2019 study from Radboud University, the Netherlands, conducted a thematic analysis of significant nature experiences reported by a cohort of Dutch volunteer biodiversity recorders (Ganzevoort and van den Born 2019). Of the 1,450 experiences analyzed, the most common theme described as significant was encountering a species new to the

Table 10–3.   Vocabulary for listing approach to bird-watching

Term	Definition
Big Year *(n)*	Competitive challenge to see the most birds in a given area within a year
Dip *(v)*	To arrive where a desirable species was reported after it left
Life list *(n)*	Living record of all species seen by an individual since beginning birding
Lifer *(n)*	A bird species never seen before by an individual birder
Nemesis-bird *(n)*	A species that a birder desires to list but has so far been elusive
Rarity *(n)*	A species reported in a location where it is not usually seen
Patch *(n)*	A personally frequented birding spot such as a backyard or local park
Twitch *(v)*	To go to extreme lengths to sight rare birds

observer or rediscovering one last seen in the distant past. The emotional response most associated with significant experiences was a sense of surprise. The results of the thematic analysis suggested that a thrill of discovery characterized the nature experiences that biodiversity citizen scientists remember as significant (Ganzevoort and van den Born 2019).

When a lister encounters a rare bird to add to their life list, they experience an analogous thrill of discovery. The collection serves as an external projection of their sense of self. Each addition to the collection incrementally strengthens the ego as a concrete signifier of the collector's mastery and expertise. A sense of the past that further supports the ego is built by reviewing entries in the collection, which cue favorable memories of the significant experience. Collectors gain a sense of accomplishment with each acquisition and an appreciation for their collection. Collectors aggregate around their common interest to share knowledge, compare collections, and socialize with like-minded peers (Belk 2009).

Bird-watchers bolster their self-esteem by practicing a socially condoned activity that encourages the development of specialized knowledge with the goal of amassing a large life list. Adding the birder identity to the self also improves self-esteem by providing multiple avenues for accomplishment that can buffer against ego injury. For example, a student who receives a poor grade on a test may be consoled by their confidence in their birding ability (McIntosh and Schmeichel 2004).

Hidden Truths

The unconscious motivations that lead people to bird-watch are highly individualized. The details of the unconscious vary from person to person, but a psychoanalytic approach can suggest some superficial commonalities. Psychoanalytic theory posits that nearly all conscious choices made in adulthood are steered by unconscious forces that developed in infancy. Emotional development begins with attachment to the parental figure and the instinctual defenses against distress. The emotional tools that the child learns during the progressive stages of development will carry forward to adulthood. Childhood motivations are transformed into socially acceptable adult behaviors. A Freudian model of the transmutation of developmental stages into aspects of birding is described in Table 10–4 (Clemens 2012).

The act of integrating unacceptable feelings or impulses into a socially condoned activity is called *sublimation*. Adults who use birding to manage internal conflicts and can do so without damaging their important relationships are said to sublimate successfully. An example would be a pathologist who became a prolific bird photographer after retirement. Both photography and pathology involve high-powered optics and reviewing minute details to identify what is in the image. He could manage his grief of leaving a beloved career by choosing a hobby in which he could practice similar skills (Clemens 2012).

Terror management theory proposes that a generalizable unconscious motivator to participate in socially sanctioned activities is to distract from awareness of mortality. The birder's collection of observations is a permanent extension of the self that will exist past a birder's life span. Imbuing the collection with a sense of legacy is a sublimation of the death anxiety (McIntosh and Schmeichel 2004).

Understanding what bird-watchers gain from identifying with the birding world resolves around the tautology of bird-watching for the sake of bird-watching. Seeing birds may draw a birder into a flow state, evoke a thrill of discovery, contribute to stress recovery and attention restoration, resolve an unconscious conflict, or stave off fear of death.

BIRDS IN NATURE

Wild birds are accessible to anyone regardless of affiliation with the bird-watching social world. Wherever people go, they are sure to meet the local birds. These highly adaptable descendants of dinosaurs are found on every continent, in every ocean, and at every extreme of the environment imaginable. They range in size from minuscule to gigantic

Table 10–4. **Freudian origins of birding behavior**

Freudian phase	Developmental pursuit	Analogous birding behavior
Oral	Trusting the caregiver	Love of nature embodied by Mother Earth
Anal	Bodily mastery	Counting and organizing observations
Phallic-oedipal	Curiosity in hidden parts Competition for love	Voyeurism of watching birds Comparing life lists or size of optic equipment

and sport a dazzling array of colors and shapes. Their acoustic repertoire is equally impressive, boasting melodious songs, inconspicuous chirps, guttural roars, and percussive feathers (BirdLife International 2013).

Birds invite interaction. Garden birds will nest outside people's windows and share their private lives, hatching a family in full view. Large geese tolerate proximity to people, subjecting themselves to being chased by bold toddlers or chasing them back. Turkeys imposingly stalk and terrorize neighborhoods in Massachusetts, demanding residents to confront the human intrusion into wild territory (Sullivan 2022). By inspiring pathos, curiosity, or terror, birds are charismatic reminders that nature still affects the human condition.

Nature Connectivity

Urban birds are the cultural ambassadors of the natural world. City dwellers' encounters with birds may account for most people's relationship to wildlife (Cox and Gaston 2015). More than 50% of the global population lives in urban areas, and this is predicted to increase to 70% by 2050. Urban environments are heavily modified biomes that displace animals and plants that are unable to adapt to those rapid ecosystem changes. Most people live and work in species-poor settings. Urbanization increases the physical and emotional distance between people and nature (Luck et al. 2011).

Nature connectedness is a personality trait that describes a person's affective identification with the natural world. People with greater nature connectedness tend to affiliate with environmental activism and have concern for the environmental consequences of human activity. Greater nature connectedness correlates with more time spent outside and personalities that are more open, conscientious, extroverted, and agreeable (Capaldi et al. 2014).

A meta-analysis from 2014 by the psychology department of Carleton University, Ottawa, Ontario, found a significant association between nature connectedness and happiness (Capaldi et al. 2014). A fixed effect size meta-analysis examined 30 papers that reported on a relationship between nature connectedness and happiness. The included studies represented a total sample of 8,523 subjects. Happiness was measured along three hedonistic dimensions.

1. Vitality: the state of feeling alive, alert, and energetic
2. Positive affect: a state of pleasant emotional experience lacking negative detractors
3. Life satisfaction: a favorable appraisal of the totality of personal experience up to and including the present

A statistically significant effect size ($r=0.19$) was found in the relationship between nature connectedness and the cumulative measures of happiness. This effect size is comparable to those found in studies associating happiness with other social factors such as personal income, education, religiosity, marital status, volunteering, and physical attractiveness. Because living in cities is associated with lower outdoor engagement and nature connectedness, interventions targeting these traits may increase happiness in urban populations (Capaldi et al. 2014).

Feeding wild birds is a popular activity that brings people closer to nature. About half of urban households in Australia, the United Kingdom, and the United States provide some kind of nourishment to their feathered neighbors (Cox and Gaston 2016). Bird feeding is a home-based activity where people lay out food for the express intent of attracting wild birds. U.S. households spend more than $100 million annually on bird food and feeding apparatus. A surge in interest during the 2020 COVID-19 pandemic is estimated to have increased expenditure on bird feeding by more than 30%. Government lockdown protocols led to a 15% increase in time spent at home (Brock et al. 2021).

Outdoor-based recreation and use of public parks increased in popularity during lockdowns as mental health refuges to escape pandemic-related anxiety (Grima et al. 2020). A 2020 analysis of internet data trends found that online interest in search terms related to bird feeding also increased during lockdown periods. Feeding birds offered people who were confined indoors a direct avenue to interact with wildlife for nature's restorative effects (Brock et al. 2021).

A 2016 study from the University of Exeter, United Kingdom, surveyed 330 English town dwellers on their bird-feeding attitudes and behaviors. Respondents rated, on a five-point scale, the extent to which they agreed with nine statements describing motivations for and approach to bird feeding. The results showed that subjects who fed birds regularly were largely motivated by psychological benefit. They related watching birds at their feeders to feelings of rest and relaxation in accordance with nature restoration theories. They also described feeling more connected to nature through observing the birds visiting their feeders (Cox and Gaston 2016).

Backyard bird-watching may ameliorate somatic and psychological distress. A 2021 study conducted by a research team from Michigan State and Duke Universities investigated how the COVID-19 pandemic influenced nature experiences among patients with breast cancer (Pearson et al. 2021). Fifty-six women with stage 2 or 3 breast cancer participated in a cross-sectional survey of habits of outdoor use and scales of distress. Patients reported decreased use of natural amenities and spaces outside the house since the beginning of the pandemic. Respondents reported a compensatory increase in home-based nature experiences such as watching wildlife through a window or listening to birdsong. Increased use of an outdoor space adjoining the home such as a backyard or porch was associated with decreases in overall stress, symptom-related stress, and symptom severity. Although the findings were not generalizable because the demographic scope was limited to women with breast cancer, future studies may continue to investigate indoor wildlife interactions as nonpharmaceutical adjuvants for pain management (Pearson et al. 2021).

The stress-reducing effects of nonthreatening wild animal encounters produce a measurable physiological response. A 2020 experiment from the University of Gloucester, United Kingdom, used a zoological lemur enclosure to simulate encounters with noncompanion wildlife (Sumner and Goodenough 2020). Eighty-six college students were guided along the lemur path and assessed for pre- and postencounter measures of mood, nature connectedness, and physiological markers of stress. Salivary cortisol, a steroid hormone associated with the sympathetic stress response, decreased after the lemur encounter. Research scales measuring emotional disturbance showed improved mood after participants met the lemurs. Nature connectedness was positively correlated with greater levels of stress reduction (Sumner and Goodenough 2020).

Biodiversity

Species richness, or biodiversity, is the number of different types of organisms living in a defined area. Biodiversity describes the variety but not the abundance of current species.

Whereas lemurs are range restricted to certain zoos or the island of Madagascar, birds are the appreciable wildlife most accepted by people. Not all birds are appreciated equally, and not all people are equally able to appreciate them. A 2015 study from the University of Exeter (Cox and Gaston 2015) compared the likability of 14 common garden bird species in southern England. A total of 330 people were surveyed on their preference of bird species, their knowledge of species, and their bird-feeding habits. Respondents with greater bird knowledge reported higher levels of nature connectedness and were more likely to feed birds regularly. When shown pictures of various combinations of birds at feeders, people overall preferred pictures that were richer in species over those that contained many images of just one species. People with less bird knowledge were unable to consistently differentiate species shown in the pictures. These findings suggest that stress reduction from feeding birds can be enhanced by improving the observer's ability to appreciate species richness. Bird identification is a teachable skill that offers a modifiable factor to augment nature connectedness (Cox and Gaston 2015).

In 2005, a research team from the University of Sheffield, United Kingdom, measured the biodiversity of 15 different local parks by tallying all the different plant, bird, and butterfly species seen over a 2-hour period. Park goers were asked to rate statements relating measures of psychological well-being to their park visits on 5-point Likert scales from "agree" to "disagree." The researchers found that parks with greater biodiversity elicited higher attributed levels of personal well-being. This correlation was statistically significant for bird but not butterfly species richness (Fuller et al. 2007).

Bird species richness was also used as a proxy measure for neighborhood biodiversity in a 2011 study from Charles Sturt University, Bathurst, Australia. The research team conducted field observations in 35 neighborhoods to measure bird species richness. Surveys assessing neighborhood satisfaction were collected from 1,100 respondents. Neighborhood well-being was positively correlated with bird biodiversity (Luck et al. 2011).

The finding that neighborhood bird biodiversity contributes to quality of life was further supported by a research project conducted by a multidisciplinary team from several German academic institutions (Methorst et al. 2021). The team collected measurements of life satisfaction, demographics, and socioeconomic factors from the 2012 European Quality of Life Survey. Data from 26,000 Europeans from 26 countries were included in the analysis. Data on the geographic distribution of biodiversity of birds were adapted from *The EBCC Atlas of European*

Breeding Birds (Hagemeijer and Blair 1997). Biodiversity information on mammals and plants was also retrieved from other publicly accessible datasets. An econometric model was used to calculate the effect of local species richness on life satisfaction while the study controlled for socioeconomic and geographic variables. A statistically significant positive relationship was found between bird biodiversity and life satisfaction. The other biodiversity measures did not show this relationship. Life satisfaction's association with bird biodiversity was similar in strength to its association with income level (Methorst et al. 2021).

Song

Species richness may not buy happiness any more than money can, but mounting evidence suggests a generalizable association between bird biodiversity and measures of well-being. Birds are appreciated in human encounters not just for their appearance but also for their acoustic contributions. Bird sounds are iconic symbols of the human imagination. They evoke joy, optimism, and new beginnings. The rooster's crow heralds the dawn, the robin's song is a sign of spring, and the bluebird's trill is synonymous with happiness. Mounting evidence suggests that birdsong and mood are more than metaphorically related. A study from the University of Gothenburg, Sweden, found that college students preferred both being in environments where birds were singing and listening to multiple species singing rather than a single bird (Hedblom et al. 2014).

The restorative ambience generated by natural spaces includes an auditory component. The acoustic environment, known as the *soundscape*, is the collection of audible features observed in a given location. Qualitative explorations show birdsong to be commonly identified as the most restorative element of a natural soundscape (Ratcliffe et al. 2013).

Natural soundscapes composed of birdsong and rustling leaves were quantitatively shown to facilitate mood recovery in a 2014 experiment at Pennsylvania State University. One hundred thirty college students were shown an upsetting video to induce a dysphoric mood state. They were then randomly assigned to four soundscape conditions: natural sounds, natural sounds with voices, natural sounds with motorized noise, and a control condition with no sound. Mood states were measured by the Brief Mood Introspection Scale at baseline, after the distressing stimulus, and after the experimental sound condition. The experiment was conducted indoors in the absence of visual natural elements. Although Brief Mood Introspection Scale scores for all participants were negatively affected by the distressing video, only the group exposed to the purely natural soundscape showed subsequent score improvement to baseline levels (Benfield et al. 2014).

The contribution of birdsong to the restorative properties of nature in situ was investigated in 2020 by a team of researchers from several U.S. universities, led by California Polytechnic State University. They manipulated ambient sound along two hiking trails by placing hidden speakers that played a "phantom chorus" of several species of birdsong. The phantom chorus artificially enhanced the biodiversity of the hiking trail soundscape. Hikers who completed the trail were surveyed on their perceptions of the trail's biodiversity and its soundscape's contribution to their well-being. Psychological restorativeness scores were higher when the phantom chorus was played on the trail (Ferraro et al. 2020).

CONCLUSION

Biodiversity, nature connectedness, and psychological well-being show a clear association with one another, as validated by the studies reviewed in this chapter. From actively forming friendships by offering food to unconsciously receiving their background noise and everything in between, people's relationships to birds lie at the heart of this association. Limitations of these studies include reliance on self-report in surveys, selection bias for subjects already involved in nature activities, and use of nonclinical measures of well-being.

To quote a famed British naturalist, Sir David Attenborough, "Everyone likes birds. What wild creature is more accessible to our eyes and ears, as close to us and everyone in the world, as *universal* as a bird?" (Davies 2014).

How might clinicians leverage this common fascination to their patients' advantage? Can patients with mental illness benefit from birding interventions? What does a birding intervention look like, and for whom is it appropriate? These questions are fertile ground for future research. Until empirical evidence catches up to popular interest, ornitherapy will remain more a clinical art than a science.

CLINICAL GUIDELINES

The available evidence suggests that wild birds' therapeutic potential is linked to nature restoration theories. Human-bird interactions thus can be viewed from a positive psychiatry perspective as a therapy that confers a benefit in contrast to medication, for example, which is used to negate a symptom. Positive psychiatry helps patients identify and support areas in their lives that are enjoyable and meaningful and helps patients focus on strengths rather than deficits (Messias 2020).

Biodiversity and nature connectedness are both independently associated with psychological well-being. In positive psychiatry, well-being can be built along three pathways.

1. Pleasure: seeking positive emotions, avoiding negative emotions, reducing stress
2. Engagement: participating in flow activities, making close relationships
3. Meaning: feeling a sense of belonging, believing in a greater good

Pleasure in birding might come from seeing or hearing a bird and experiencing attention restoration and stress reduction. Biodiversity is an external environmental trait, whereas nature connectedness is an internal personality trait. Nature connectedness can positively mediate the restorative effects of nature through several means, one of which is by enhancing the detection of biodiversity. However, the hedonistic pathway to well-being is the most fleeting. Engagement and meaning are more likely to lead to lasting well-being (Buijs and Jacobs 2021).

Patients who identify nature connectedness as a strength may be open to clinical guidance toward the meaning pathway. Nature connectedness is reinforced by repeated positive experiences with nature. Bird feeding presents an opportunity for patients to experience the hedonistic joy of watching the birds while cultivating the eudaemonic meaning of providing for another creature. The association between nature connectedness and proenvironmental behaviors also may help a patient find belonging by identifying with an ecologically minded movement (Cox and Gaston 2016).

Patients who affiliate with the birding social world invite the clinician to explore well-being through their engagement. The clinician may ask about the patient's birding habits, what role birding plays in their life, and how involved they are in the birding community. Changes in birding habits may indicate a change in clinical status, especially if the patient uses birding to manage symptoms.

Positive psychiatry emphasizes a patient-centered approach to determining treatment. A detailed clinical interview can help identify patients who are appropriate for bird-related plans. Assessing for nature connectedness and birding activity can be incorporated into the social history portion of the psychiatric evaluation. A sample line of questioning might begin as open ended ("What do you do for fun?") and become progressively more direct ("How often do you go outside?"). Clinicians also may ask about a patient's accessibility to and sense of safety in nature and outdoor spaces. Patients who express interest in and comfort with nature may be considered candidates for further conversations on incorporating birds into their wellness practice.

Contraindications to birding therapy include specific phobia of birds and paranoid delusions involving birds. For appropriate patients, a birding plan can be designed to meet their needs. A bird-feeding plan can improve nature connectedness and provide meaning for patients at home. An outdoor birding plan is behaviorally activating and adds a physical activity component. Encouraging patients to join local birding clubs can deepen their social engagement and broaden their support networks. Clinical judgment and creativity can offer patients a unique adjuvant to treatment as usual.

SPECIAL CONSIDERATIONS

People With Disabilities

Knowledge of the accessibility of nearby natural spaces can help in planning birding interventions. The following list describes examples of considerations for several patient categories. This list is not exhaustive and intends to direct attention toward barriers to care. Advocacy groups, such as Birdability, provide resources, guidelines, and information on improving inclusivity in nature for people with disabilities (Gilger and Campbell 2021).

- People who have mobility challenges: Search for local trails that, at a minimum, conform to the Americans With Disabilities Act.
- People who have physical challenges: Consider consultation with occupational therapy to assess for appropriateness of adaptive equipment to improve birding comfort and experience.
- People who are blind or have low vision: Place microphones at a bird feeder connected to an indoor speaker system to allow auditory appreciation of backyard birds.
- People who are Deaf or hearing impaired: Convert birdsong to a visual spectrogram in real time by certain smartphone applications.

Older Adults

Although many older adults remain fully functional and independent into late age, some need higher levels of care. Patients with functional and cognitive decline who are in residential care are at greater risk for developing depression and anxiety because of inactivity. Introducing birding programs into nursing homes can engage sedentary residents in meaningful activity. Two case examples of birding programs for older adults are described below.

Goldielea Care Home, Scotland

Goldielea Care Home provides nursing and residential care to 48 residents. In 2012, it implemented a birding program based on the Royal Society for Protection of Birds Big Garden Birdwatch. Residents were accompanied outside to observe the wildlife at a bird feeder on the care home grounds. Residents ranged in cognitive ability and participation from simply watching the birds to writing down observations and field notes. A whiteboard in the common area was a social focal point that allowed residents to post comments and observations from the field. Residents were oriented to changes in the seasons by care home staff describing what to expect at the feeders each day. The program also provided community connection through invited guest speakers who taught residents about their local wildlife. Residents channeled their nature experiences into creative expressions of poetry and art. The British Broadcasting Company filmed a segment on the program, much to the residents' delight. Goldielea reports that residents frequently request to rewatch a recording of the segment to relive fond memories (Wilkie 2013).

Bird Tales

Bird Tales is an indoor birding program designed in 2013 for use in dementia care. In 2022, a research team from the University of Texas at Arlington conducted a qualitative analysis of responses to Bird Tales participation by adults in assisted living. The program consists of multimedia and multisensory group activities intended to drive social engagement between patients with dementia. Activities include watching videos, listening to recordings, and handling three-dimensional models of birds. Participants overall reported enjoying the activities and felt cognitively stimulated, spiritually refreshed, and socially closer to one another (Lee et al. 2022).

Doctors, Medical Students, and Allied Health Professionals

Burnout, the antithesis of well-being, is emotional exhaustion that leads to loss of energy, enjoyment, and efficacy in patient care. More than half of the doctors in the United States experience some level of burnout, and this can start as early as during training in medical school. Burnout is multifactorial, but some commonly named culprits are increased administrative burden, loss of work-life balance, and decreased sense of autonomy (Karacic et al. 2021).

Carving out time for self-care by reconnecting with nature offers physicians an avenue to reassert control, decompress from monotonous administrative tasks, and introduce recreation to balance out professional duty. A 2021 pilot program in Poland invited five mental health professionals with no birding experience on an ornithological outing. They were asked to reflect on their emotional states and responses to nature before and after the outing and 1 week later. The experience continued to resound after 1 week, with responses describing sustained restorative aspects of the outing (Murawiec et al. 2021).

Ornithological outings can be as brief as a 10-minute "sunshine rounds," weather permitting, where hospital-based teams and trainees can search the courtyard for signs of life before returning indoors, or as extensive as a weekend birding getaway, and everything in between.

Clinical Translation: Case Example

Ms. M, a 23-year-old woman, has a history of major depressive disorder with anxious distress. She is seen on a biweekly basis for medication management and psychotherapy. Her presenting symptoms include depressed mood, difficulty falling asleep, difficulty concentrating, and feelings of guilt and helplessness. She endorses anxious symptoms related to a difficult relationship with her father, whom she is currently living with and financially dependent on. She also has a history of panic attacks that occur three times per week, managed with hydroxyzine, 50 mg as needed. She began taking mirtazapine, 15 mg at bedtime, for depression and anxiety. She reports that she illustrates as a hobby and for stress relief. Ms. M stated that her goal was to gain financial independence, but she felt inhibited by low self-esteem of "I'm not good enough" and "I'm too shy."

In addition to cognitive-behavioral therapy, Ms. M was encouraged to explore her connection to nature. She mentioned that she often went to the park as a refuge from her father's house, which she described as "stifling and judgmental." Ms. M reported that she enjoyed the chirping of "little brown birds" and was curious to learn more about what she was hearing.

Ms. M was encouraged to combine her existing talent for drawing with her frequent outings. She began drawing the birds she saw each week. She described that concentrating on drawing the birds helped her relax and offered temporary relief from her anxiety.

When she brought her observations home, she tried to look up the birds she saw, and she connected with an online bird identification group. As Ms. M continued to share the birds she drew, her illustrations became more detailed and diverse in plumage. She was able to name them by species, no longer as generic "little brown birds." Ms. M was able to recognize and appreciate her competence in learning a new skill and felt more confident in her self-efficacy. After 9 months of treatment, Ms. M was no longer having panic attacks, and hydroxyzine was discontinued. She applied for a job in retail and started working. She was able to find a roommate to rent an apartment and moved out of her father's house.

KEY POINTS

- The human-bird relationship spans millions of years of planetary cohabitation, during which they influenced each other's behavioral evolution, and birds ensconced themselves as human cultural symbols.

- Bird-watching is a hobby with growing popularity that offers a social world for engaging in recreational specialization, obtaining flow state, and expanding social networks.

- Interactions with birds are the most common wildlife interactions and connect people to nature.

- Bird biodiversity is an environmental trait with a similar level of effect to income level on population well-being.

- Birdsong facilitates mood recovery and enhances the restorative effects of natural settings.

QUESTIONS

1. A patient seen for psychotherapy reports that their last child just left for college. The patient reports feeling surprisingly content considering that they were initially saddened by the prospect of an empty house. The patient explains, "Now that I'm not cooking and doing groceries for everyone, I have much more time to relax." The patient proudly shows a picture of a brand-new bird feeder they installed. Which psychological defense did this patient deploy?

    A. Denial.
    B. Humor.
    C. Repression.
    D. Sublimation.
    E. Dissociation.

Correct answer: D. Sublimation.

This patient is coping with the grief of empty nest syndrome by redirecting their nurturing instinct toward feeding the local birds. The act of integrating unacceptable feelings or impulses into a socially condoned activity is called *sublimation*. The patient accepts that they initially had apprehensions about their child leaving (A), the patient is not making a joke (B), the patient is transforming their grief rather than constraining it (C), and the patient remains present and connected to their internal emotional world (E).

2. Which of the following nature encounters would most commonly be ascribed emotional significance?

    A. Seeing a blue jay for the first time in 10 years.
    B. Hearing a chorus of various birds on a hike.
    C. Going to the zoo to see the exotic birds.
    D. Counting pigeons on the way to work.
    E. Chasing a squirrel away from a bird feeder.

Correct answer: A. Seeing a blue jay for the first time in 10 years.

According to a Dutch thematic analysis of 1,450 accounts of nature experiences, the most common theme described as significant was encountering a species new to the observer or rediscovering one last seen in the distant past. Surprise was the most described emotion. The chorus is not identified, so no new species can be inferred (B), going to the zoo removes the emotional impact of surprise (C), pigeons are common and described here as a routine encounter (D), and the squirrel is an expected pest rather than a cherished new guest (E).

3. A security guard at an art museum complains that the new exhibit gives them "the heebie jeebies." It is a multimedia exhibit of a looping video clip portraying graphic imagery. The guard feels unsettled at the end of each day. Which birding intervention would probably help this guard?

    A. Take a week-long birding vacation to Panama.
    B. Bring headphones and listen to birdsong on breaks.
    C. Draw birds on a notepad to distract from the video.
    D. Join the local Audubon society to improve social well-being.
    E. Bring binoculars to work and look out the windows instead of at the art.

Correct answer: B. Bring headphones to work and listen to birdsong on breaks.

> Birdsong has been shown to facilitate affective recovery after exposure to a distressing video. This guard can take advantage of the restorative properties of birdsong to unobtrusively take audio breaks from the art exhibit. A vacation would be a temporary removal from the situation but would not alter the work environment (A). Drawing has not been associated with the restorative effects that birdsong has (C). The patient made no complaint about social connectedness (D). Looking out the windows would interfere with performing the guard's job (E).

REFERENCES

Archer CI: Review of Andean tragedy: fighting the war of the Pacific, 1879–1884. Journal of Military History 73(4):1346–1347, 2009

Associated Press: Bird-watching takes flight amid coronavirus outbreak as Americans head back outdoors. Los Angeles Times, May 3, 2020. Available at: https://www.latimes.com/world-nation/story/2020-05-03/bird-watching-soars-amid-covid-19-as-americans-head-outdoors. Accessed June 6, 2022.

Belk RW: Collecting as luxury consumption: effects on individuals and households, in Collectible Investments for the High Net Worth Investor. Edited by Satchell S. Cambridge, MA, Academic Press, 2009, pp 73–84

Benfield JA, Taff BD, Newman P, et al: Natural sound facilitates mood recovery. Ecopsychology 6(3):183–188, 2014

BirdLife International: Birds are found almost everywhere in the world, from the poles to the equator. 2013. Available at: http://www.birdlife.org. Accessed October 15, 2022.

Brock M, Doremus J, Li L: Birds of a feather lockdown together: mutual bird-human benefits during a global pandemic. Ecol Econ 189:107174, 2021

Buijs A, Jacobs M: Avoiding negativity bias: towards a positive psychology of human-wildlife relationships. Ambio 50(2):281–288, 2021 33026581

Capaldi CA, Dopko RL, Zelenski JM: The relationship between nature connectedness and happiness: a meta-analysis. Front Psychol 5:976, 2014 25249992

Carver E: Birding in the United States: A Demographic and Economic Analysis: Addendum to the 2016 National Survey of Fishing, Hunting, and Wildlife-Associated Recreation. Arlington, VA, U.S. Fish and Wildlife Service, 2019. Available at: https://digitalmedia.fws.gov/digital/collection/document/id/2252. Accessed October 14, 2022.

Changizi MA, Shimojo S: "X-ray vision" and the evolution of forward-facing eyes. J Theor Biol 254(4):756–767, 2008

Cheng TM, Hung SH, Chen MT: The influence of leisure involvement on flow experience during hiking activity: using psychological commitment as a mediate variable. Asia Pac J Tour Res 21(1):1–19, 2016

Clemens NA: Psychotherapy: sublimation and the psychodynamics of birding. J Psychiatr Pract 18(4):287–290, 2012 22805903

Clottes J: Chauvet Cave (ca. 30,000 B.C.). Heilbrunn Timeline of Art History. New York, Metropolitan Museum of Art, 2002. Available at: http://www.metmuseum.org/toah/hd/chav/hd_chav.htm. Accessed October 14, 2022.

Conard NJ, Malina M, Münzel SC: New flutes document the earliest musical tradition in southwestern Germany. Nature 460(7256):737–740, 2009 19553935

Cordell H, Herbert K, Nancy G: The popularity of birding is still growing. Birding February 2002:54–61, 2002

Cox DT, Gaston KJ: Likeability of garden birds: importance of species knowledge and richness in connecting people to nature. PLoS One 10(11):e0141505, 2015 26560968

Cox DT, Gaston KJ: Urban bird feeding: connecting people with nature. PLoS One 11(7):e0158717, 2016 27427988

Crotty J: How many birders are there, really? (updated). 10,000 Birds—Birding, Blogging, Conservation, and Commentary, May 12, 2020. Available at: https://www.10000birds.com/how-many-birders-are-there-really-updated.htm. Accessed October 14, 2022.

Davies GH: Meet Sir David, in The Life of Birds by David Attenborough. PBS online staff, December 22, 2014. Available at: https://www.pbs.org/lifeofbirds/sirdavid/index.html. Accessed May 21, 2024.

Dickinson E: Poems: 2nd Series. Boston, MA, Roberts Brothers, 1891

Dieser RB, Christenson J, Davis-Gage D: Integrating flow theory and the serious leisure perspective into mental health counseling. Couns Psychol Q 28(1):97–111, 2015

Eubanks Jr TL, Stoll JR, Ditton RB: Understanding the diversity of eight birder sub-populations: socio-demographic characteristics, motivations, expenditures and net benefits. Journal of Ecotourism 3(3):151–172, 2004

Ferraro DM, Miller ZD, Ferguson LA, et al: The phantom chorus: birdsong boosts human well-being in protected areas. Proc Biol Sci 287(1941):20210037, 2020 33499796

Fortin J: The birds are not on lockdown, and more people are watching them. New York Times, May 29, 2020. Available at: https://www.nytimes.com/2020/05/29/science/bird-watching-coronavirus.html. Accessed June 6, 2022.

Fuller RA, Irvine KN, Devine-Wright P, et al: Psychological benefits of greenspace increase with biodiversity. Biol Lett 3(4):390–394, 2007 17504734

Ganzevoort W, van den Born R: The thrill of discovery: significant nature experiences among biodiversity citizen scientists. Ecopsychology 11(1):22–32, 2019

Garrity T: America's youth have a new favorite activity. it's more wholesome than you think. InsideHook, March 18, 2022. Available at: https://www.insidehook.com/wellness/birding-popular-social-media. Accessed October 14, 2022.

Gerl EJ, Morris MR: The causes and consequences of color vision. Evo Edu Outreach 1:476–486, 2008

Gilger L, Campbell K: Audubon Society's Birdability program helps spread joy of birding to people with disabilities. KJZZ, March 16, 2021. Available at: https://kjzz.org/content/1631576/audubon-societys-birdability-program-helps-spread-joy-birding-people-disabilities. Accessed October 14, 2022.

Giordano M: A bird feeder will bring you joy. Wired, Conde Nast, June 14, 2020. Available at: https://www.wired.com/story/own-a-bird-feeder-rave. Accessed October 14, 2022.

Grima N, Corcoran W, Hill-James C, et al: The importance of urban natural areas and urban ecosystem services during the COVID-19 pandemic. PLoS One 15(12):e0243344, 2020 33332364

Hagemeijer EJM, Blair MJ (eds): The EBCC Atlas of European Breeding Birds: Their Distribution and Abundance. London, T & A.D. Poyser, 1997

Harkness J: The therapeutic benefits of birding. Bird Spot, January 25, 2021. Available at: https://www.birdspot.co.uk/bird-chat/joe-harkness-the-therapeutic-benefits-of-birding. Accessed October 14, 2022.

Harrison S: Pandemic bird-watching created a data boom—and a conundrum. Wired, September 30, 2021. Available at: https://www.wired.com/story/pandemic-bird-watching-created-a-data-boom-and-a-conundrum. Accessed October 14, 2022.

Hedblom M, Heyman E, Antonsson H, et al: Bird song diversity influences young people's appreciation of urban landscapes. Urban for Urban Green 13(3):469–474, 2014

Heesy CP: Seeing in stereo: the ecology and evolution of primate binocular vision and stereopsis. Evol Anthropol 18:21–35, 2009

Karacic J, Bursztajn HJ, Arvanitakis M: Who cares what the doctor feels: the responsibility of health politics for burnout in the pandemic. Healthcare 9(11):1550, 2021

Lee K, Cassidy J, Tang W, et al: Older adults' responses to a meaningful activity using indoor-based nature experiences: Bird Tales. Clin Gerontol 45(2):301–311, 2022 32799781

Li Z, Doyon L, Fang H, et al: A Paleolithic bird figurine from the Lingjing site, Henan, China. PLoS One 15(6):e0233370, 2020 32520932

Luck GW, Davidson P, Boxall D, et al: Relations between urban bird and plant communities and human well-being and connection to nature. Conserv Biol 25(4):816–826, 2011 21535147

Maake LA, Hermann UP, Tshipala NN: Is it all about twitching? A descriptive attendee motivational profile to a birding event in Gauteng. Afr J Hosp Tour Leis 11(3):1288–1300, 2022

MacLellan L: New data show that birding mania isn't just a lockdown fad. Quartz, June 25, 2021. Available at: https://qz.com. Accessed October 14, 2022.

McIntosh WD, Schmeichel B: Collectors and collecting: a social psychological perspective. Leis Sci 26(1):85–97, 2004

McKee J: A beginner's guide to using eBird. Audubon Magazine, October 7, 2022. Available at: https://www.audubon.org/news/a-beginners-guide-using-ebird. Accessed October 14, 2022.

Merker H, Crossley R, Crossley S: Ornitherapy. Crossley Bird ID Guides, July 1, 2021. Available at: https://crossleybooks.com/book/ornitherapy. Accessed October 14, 2022.

Messias E: Positive psychiatry: an introduction, in Positive Psychiatry, Psychotherapy and Psychology. Edited by Messias E, Peseschkian H, Cagande C. Cham, Switzerland, Springer, 2020, pp 3–9

Methorst J, Rehdanz K, Mueller T, et al: The importance of species diversity for human well-being in Europe. Ecol Econ 181:106917, 2021

Miller JG: Avian obsession. National Wildlife Federation, August 1, 2021. Available at: https://www.nwf.org/Home/Magazines/National-Wildlife/2021/Aug-Sept/Conservation/Spark-Birds. Accessed October 14, 2022.

Morelli F, Kubicka AM, Tryjanowski P, et al: The vulture in the sky and the hominin on the land: three million years of human–vulture interaction. Anthrozoos 28(3):449–468, 2015

Morse JW, Gladkikh TM, Hackenburg DM, et al: COVID-19 and human-nature relationships: Vermonters' activities in nature and associated nonmaterial values during the pandemic. PLoS One 15(12):e0243697, 2020 33306716

Murawiec S, Tryjanowski P, Nita A: An ornithological walk to improve the well-being of mental health professionals during the COVID-19 pandemic: a pilot study. Psychiatria 18(3):190–195, 2021

Pearson AL, Breeze V, Reuben A, et al: Increased use of porch or backyard nature during COVID-19 associated with lower stress and better symptom experience among breast cancer patients. Int J Environ Res Public Health 18(17):9102, 2021 34501691

Randler C, Murawiec S, Tryjanowski P: Committed bird-watchers gain greater psychological restorative benefits compared to those less committed regardless of expertise. Ecopsychology 14(2):101–110, 2022

Ratcliffe E, Gatersleben B, Sowden PT: Bird sounds and their contributions to perceived attention restoration and stress recovery. J Environ Psychol 36:221–222, 2013

Rodman PS, McHenry HM: Bioenergetics and the origin of hominid bipedalism. Am J Phys Anthropol 52(1):103–106, 1980 6768300

Rosenberg KV, Dokter AM, Blancher PJ, et al: Decline of the North American avifauna. Science 366(6461):120–124, 2019 31604313

Saha P: The Audubon Dictionary for Birders. New York, National Audubon Society, January 13, 2015. Available at: https://www.audubon.org/news/the-audubon-dictionary-birders. Accessed October 14, 2022.

Schmid P: Functional interpretation of the Laetoli footprints, in From Biped to Strider: The Emergence of Modern Human Walking, Running, and Resource Transport. Edited by Meldrum DJ, Hilton CE. New York, Kluwer Academic/Plenum, 2004, pp 50–52

Spottiswoode CN, Begg KS, Begg CM: Reciprocal signaling in honeyguide-human mutualism. Science 353(6297):387–389, 2016 27463674

Sullivan M: Aggressive turkeys take over Woburn neighborhood. CBS News, September 19, 2022. Available at: https://www.cbsnews.com/boston/news/aggressive-turkeys-take-over-woburn-neighborhood. Accessed October 14, 2022.

Sumner RC, Goodenough AE: A walk on the wild side: how interactions with non-companion animals might help reduce human stress. People Nat 2(2):395–405, 2020

U.S. Department of Interior, U.S. Fish and Wildlife Service: 2022 National Survey of Fishing, Hunting, and Wildlife-Associated Recreation. Washington, DC, U.S. Fish and Wildlife Service, 2023. Available at: https://digitalmedia.fws.gov/digital/collection/document/id/2321/rec/1. Accessed May 20, 2024.

Wenny DG, Devault TL, Johnson MD, et al: The need to quantify ecosystem services provided by birds. Auk 128(1):1–14, 2011

Whiten A, van Schaik CP: The evolution of animal "cultures" and social intelligence. Philos Trans R Soc Lond B Biol Sci 362(1480):603–620, 2007 17255007

Wilkie C: Studying the outdoors to stimulate mental health. Nurs Res Care 15(4):223–224, 2013

Young I: Anxious birding (blog), 2022. Available at: https://anxiousbirding.wordpress.com. Accessed October 14, 2022.

Zarankin J: More birds bring more happiness, according to science. Audubon, January 5, 2021. Available at: https://www.audubon.org/news/more-birds-bring-more-happiness-according-science. Accessed October 14, 2022.

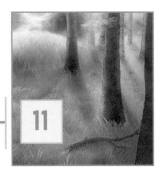

11

Nature Activism

FIND YOUR ACTIVISM BLISS!

H. Steven Moffic, M.D.

Everybody needs beauty as well as bread,
places to play in and pray in,
where nature may heal and give strength to body and soul.
—John Muir (1912, p. 256)

Illustrations by Barry Marcus, M.S.W.

Inadvertently, after I retired from clinical and administrative work in 2012, I started to spend more time, weather allowing, on our open porch swing. Soon, I was aware that I was among friends. Right in front of me were several clusters of towering birch trees (Figure 11–1). Whenever I looked at them for a while, I felt calmer and even joyous. Sometimes, sound was added as the strong wind rustled the leaves and branches. That sound was so very different from the lionlike roar of the hurricanes we experienced in Houston, Texas. I try to take care of the trees as they take care of me. My wife and I even decided to wash them in a kind of tree bathing to remove the accumulated dirt from their bark, at least as far as we could reach, for these trees had grown to towering heights over the 31 years we lived in our Milwaukee, Wisconsin, suburb. I love the bark, which sometimes looks like abstract art, and the leaves glisten when the sun is out and move like a Calder mobile when the breezes are gentle. Not long ago, we planted a young birch tree on the other side of the house for the next owners to watch as it grows.

Unfortunately, another psychiatrist and climate activist (Pollack 2021) recently lost a beloved tree in the Oregon ice storm of February 2021, probably at least in part due to climate instability. He said that the worst aspect was the damage to many mature trees around his house. One in particular, a walnut tree planted 44 years earlier, provided a family welcoming place but was destroyed when another falling tree struck it, and it fell apart.

Yet another psychiatrist, Carl Hammerschlag (2011), an activist for Indigenous Americans and for adapting their wisdom to the rest of us, connected the trees to his house with a treehouse. In his Schlagbytes blog entry on July 19, 2021, he began by describing a recent storm in Arizona where the wind had blown down trees, structures, and power lines. When he woke up the next morning, he discovered that half of a beloved giant cedar tree next to their house had fallen over. Their pets had been buried under it. They had also built that treehouse, which was accessible only to grandchildren who knew the secret handshake and password. It was there that they hid from enemies and plotted revolutions. The half of the tree that survived was still connected to the treehouse. Hammerschlag could only reach the hiding place, where he recalled the magical times that occurred there. He knew that this was a metaphor for himself in his late life, as he still stands very tall but with some physical damage.

How different it has been for the Black residents who have been living in the historic Hillcrest neighborhood of Corpus Christi, Texas, as they have become boxed in by refineries, oil tanks, an interstate highway, and a bridge under construction. As ironically reported on July 4, 2021 (Azhar 2021), our national holiday of independence that origi-

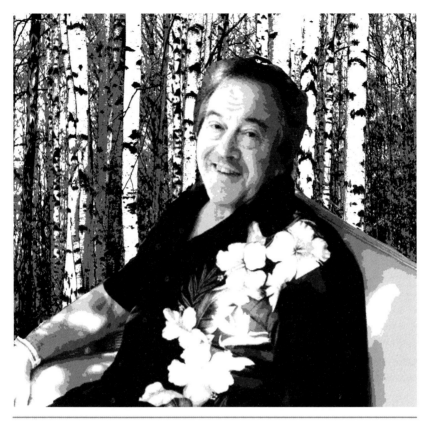

Figure 11–1. My point of view.
The author at home in his backyard. Beloved birch trees bring joy and peace.

nated when African Americans were not counted as a full person, the area is now a wasteland, barren of trees. Instead, there is traffic noise and pollution from vehicular exhaust. As the late Rev. Adam Carrington conveyed in the Azhar (2021) article, those who have stayed in this neighborhood fight for the basic necessities that such a city usually provides. Instead of trees growing, Justine Knox, a Corpus Christi resident quoted in the July 4 report, sees untended grass, probably 10 feet tall, and overgrown shrubs. Clearly, this is a socially determined adverse humanmade alteration to nature and mental health.

It has been said that when Albert Einstein was stuck on a problem, he would go to a small patch of forest on the Princeton University campus (Ferguson 2019). Looking all around, he would try to imagine the workings of all he saw. He wanted to feel somewhat disoriented because that could lead to freer associations and thinking, not unlike free associating on a couch during Freudian psychoanalysis.

The examples so far suggest that tree lovers who are social activists are mainly men, but of course, that is not true. Take nature activist and primatologist Jane Goodall. She has led conservation efforts for nearly 50 years. Motivated by caring passionately for nature and children, she feels that she cannot stop and retire. How does she cope with the demands on her and her desire to help? She takes time to sit where she grew up, "looking out the window at my favorite tree" (Marchese 2021).

THERAPEUTIC NATURE OF TREES

Trees have long been known to provide literal and figurative benefits to humans (Simard 2021). Besides beauty, they produce shade and lumber, and they sequester carbon, among other beneficial things.

Like humans, trees have social networks through their interconnected root systems (Wohlleben 2016). I am not trying to anthropomorphize, but they seem to be able to count, learn, and remember. They are masters of resilience, being able to endure fallow periods in winter. They are generous, sharing nutrients with other trees; they know how to age well unless vitally infected; and they can provide awe in just a few minutes of view. Therapeutically, they can nurse their ill tree neighbors and warn each other of danger. In fact, they can give us advice, too! I have a t-shirt that is titled "Advice From a Tree" and includes the following:

> Stand tall and proud.
> Sink your roots into the earth.
> Be content with your natural beauty.
> Go out on a limb.
> Drink plenty of water.
> Remember your roots.
> Enjoy the view!

Trees can enhance human father and son relationships. The final book of the Greek mythical classic *The Odyssey* brings together a father and son after 10 years of war and travel for Odysseus. To convince his father, Laertes, that he is his son, Odysseus points to the trees in their orchard and starts to recount their numbers, names, and stories that Laertes taught him.

Symbolically, the Tree of Life (Figure 11–2) is used as a diagram in various mystical traditions (Parpola 1993). The Tree of Life represents the interconnected nature of all things. It is a symbol of rebirth, of personal individual growth. The family tree, which often becomes important in a psychiatric evaluation, links past and future generations. Some

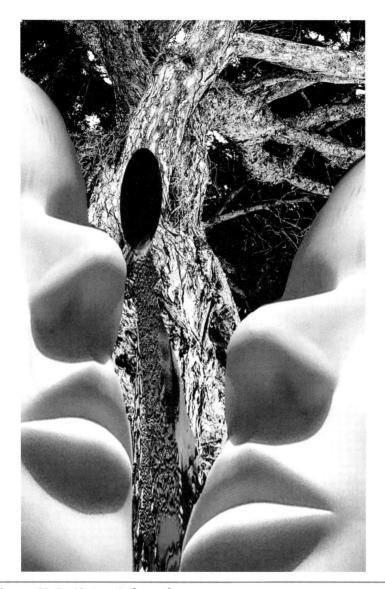

Figure 11-2. Nature's breath.
Everything is in relationship, if you notice. The Tree of Life is a reminder of our connection
to nature and to one another.

kinds of birch trees, in particular, are characterized by smooth white
bark that peels into thin paper strips. When the huge glaciers of the last
Ice Age receded, birch trees were one of the first types of trees to recol-
onize the landscape. No wonder, then, that they are a Celtic symbol of
renewal and purification.

However, as seen not only in the tree storm in Pollack's Oregon, and their increased forest fires (Figure 11–3), but also in the long-running drought in the West, the United States may be headed for a tree shortage. Science fiction recognized that risk decades ago and takes it into the future (Moreno-Garcia 2021). The popular novel *Dune* portrays a desert planet called Arrakis, where war is fought over the precious water (Herbert 1965).

THE NATURE OF NATURE

If truth be told, there really is no such thing as a stand-alone tree. It is interconnected to the fungi that nitrify the soil, which helps the trees grow and exhale the oxygen that we breathe. Indeed, nature is hard to define and often thought to be the natural world outside of ourselves. Yet, especially as Indigenous people believe, humans are nature too, not separated. Nature has always been there, over billions of years, and will be there, although the specifics can change. However, humans can survive only with certain conditions of the Earth's nature.

Humans are not all alike in our relationship to the rest of nature. Indigenous people seem to have a different relationship to nature than do those who came to America over the last 500 years and who conquered, displaced, and eventually came to ignore these natives and their knowledge. It is the difference between living in harmony with nature and trying to control nature, as conveyed in the two different creation stories in the Old Testament (Torah). Although there is no single Indigenous view of nature, there seem to be these commonalities:

- We live within and are part of nature.
- Nature is the location of spiritual reality and a sense of the sacred.
- The spiritual value of nature calls for reverence, respect, and humility toward nature.
- Nature can be used but in a sense of sustainability, not superiority.

We can learn lessons from nature, which are so important in the changing climate and release of toxins to the environment. One journalist (Ferguson 2019, pp. ix, x) made a list of eight master lessons of nature:

1. Wisdom begins with the mystery when we embrace all that we don't know.
2. Life on Earth can thrive with a thriving garden of connections.
3. The more kinds of life in the forest, the stronger that life can become.

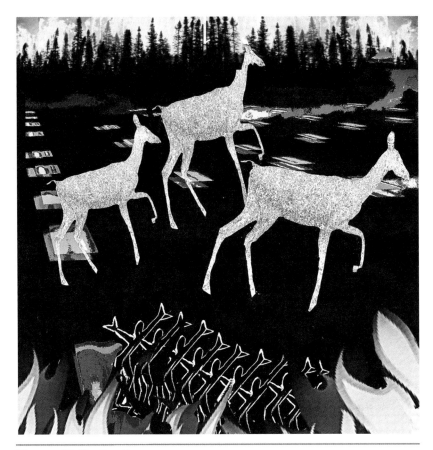

Figure 11-3. On the run.

Climate instability is expressed in extreme weather with blazing fires that destroy forests and towns. The life of the landscape, of the creatures who lose homes and lives, is entwined with human loss and tragedy.

4. Healing the planet and ourselves may mean to recover and use the Jungian archetype of the feminine caring.
5. Other animals can make us happier and smarter.
6. Our planet is full of energy, yet it shouldn't be wasted.
7. After disasters and disruption, nature shows us how to rise again even stronger and more resilient.
8. Like old forest growth, elders can help us be better at life.

Trees are the source of just one therapeutic modality of nature (Kellert 2012). Other nature therapeutic activities include walking, running, swimming, bird-watching, sports, hiking, painting, and mountain climbing. Besides trees, mountains, water, animals, birds, and even deserts or glaciers can be the site of therapeutic experiences.

Gardening can provide nature therapy to the gardener, and the flowers can be therapeutic for the community. If that happens in a geographic area that has gone through a brutal winter, the flowers will be all the more uplifting. Gardening may even be part of political dissent. The courtyard of the Robben Island prison, where Nelson Mandela was incarcerated for 18 years, had a small, scruffy-looking garden. Despite the size, this garden was a mighty nature accomplice to social activism because Mandela hid his political writings in that garden, which were smuggled out. Along another wall was a struggling apple tree marked by a sign commemorating Nelson Mandela Day on July 18, 2013, which said, "Symbolism of the tree to the learners: 'Your circumstances do not define who you are; it is your actions that define your destiny.' As the apple tree grows, it emulates its environment, so did Nelson Mandela use his circumstances to mould the person he became" (Brettschneider 2017).

There must be an extra value in doing these activities outside in nature rather than indoors. The everyday benefits can include better focus and decreased anxiety. Occasionally, a feeling of awe will emerge, and awe is associated with improved health and mental health. Although such activities can be done alone, doing them with others can add value and strengthen friendships.

Ironically, the coronavirus disease 2019 (COVID-19) pandemic has clearly shown that both the benefits and the adverse effects on some aspects of nature, such as carbon emissions and animal behavior, can change. Carbon emissions decreased as less fossil fuel was used during the lockdowns. Many people turned to outdoor activities in nature as a coping mechanism for being more safely separated from people. However, the pandemic made live activism more difficult.

Unfortunately, children now spend much less time playing in nature, enough that the prevalence of what has been called "nature-deficit disorder" is increasing (Louv 2008). Instead, they stay indoors using social media, along with more parent-planned activities for safety. Part of the deficit also comes from our increasing urbanization. These children are growing up with more anxiety for their future (Aylward et al. 2021). Environmental toxins, especially lead poisoning, remain a significant risk for children.

In addition, access to green spaces is unequal across socioeconomic and racial/ethnic lines. Time availability is also a potential limitation to nature access, especially for parents whose time is further limited by responsibilities toward children.

That is why nature availability right at home can be so important. As our tree examples indicate, sociocultural and health status may influence the availability of these nature therapies. Poor, disabled, and more physically vulnerable individuals are all likely to have less access to everyday nature and our national parks. Safety is paramount, especially for women and older adults. The U.S. National Recreation and Park Association (2018) has recognized this problem and developed a formal inclusion policy. In particular, culturally congruent programming for members of the LGBTQ and refugee communities is needed and planned. The U.S. National Recreation and Park Association's website offers comprehensive guides for municipal and state park authorities to implement inclusive programming. In 2021, Union County, New Jersey, broke ground on an LGBTQ+ affirming park (Union County 2021). In 2024, the National Park Foundation launched a program to showcase underrepresented narratives including immigrants and refugees within the park system (National Park Foundation 2024). Another endeavor geared for the underserved began after Hurricane Katrina in 2005 and is now led by a Black psychiatrist (Annelle B. Primm, M.D., M.P.H.). The All Healers Mental Health Alliance (2018) consists of a unique coalition of mental health professionals, faith leaders, first responders, and public health advocates, with the goal of responding to the mental health needs of marginalized communities who have experienced environmental disasters.

OUR ETHICAL RESPONSIBILITIES TOWARD NATURE AND PROFESSIONALISM

Focusing specifically on organized psychiatry, *The Principles of Medical Ethics, With Annotations Especially Applicable to Psychiatry* (American Psychiatric Association 2013), includes at least three sections that are particularly relevant to nature therapy. Actually, that is implied in the Preamble (from the American Medical Association's *Principles of Medical Ethics*): "As a member of this profession, a physician must recognize responsibility to patients first and foremost, as well as to society, to other health professionals, and to self" (American Psychiatric Association 2013, p. 2).

Societal obligations would include community matters that adversely influence mental health. That is why, for a weekly video series I did for *Psychiatric Times* during the COVID-19 pandemic, I chose the title "Psychiatry and Society." That weekly video series has expanded to a daily news column titled "Psychiatric Views on the Daily News." Both cover the climate and nature intermittently.

The following sections of *The Principles of Medical Ethics* seem to be relevant in regard to nature therapy.

> Section 1: "A physician shall be dedicated to providing competent medical care with compassion and respect for human dignity and rights." (p. 3)
> Annotation 2: "A psychiatrist should not be a party to any type of policy that excludes, segregates, or demeans the dignity of any patient because of ethnic origin, race, sex, creed, age, socioeconomic status, or sexual orientation." (p. 3)

The most nature-relevant aspect of this principle and annotation is the greater risk to poor individuals during natural disasters.

> Section 3: "A physician shall respect the law and also recognize a responsibility to seek changes in those requirements which are contrary to the best interests of the patient." (p. 5)
> Annotation 1: "It would seem self-evident that a psychiatrist who is a law-breaker might be ethically unsuited to practice his or her profession. When such illegal activities bear directly upon his or her practice, this would obviously be the case. However, in other instances, illegal activities such as those concerning the right to protest social injustices might not bear on either the image of the psychiatrist or the ability of the specific psychiatrist to treat his or her patient ethically and well. While no committee or board could offer prior assurance that any illegal activity would not be considered unethical, it is conceivable that an individual could violate a law without being guilty of professionally unethical behavior. Physicians lose no right of citizenship on entry into the profession of medicine." (pp. 5–6)

This annotation seems to clear the way for one type of activism, that of civil disobedience. In the case of the climate and nature, if less extreme actions such as protests are not effective, law-breaking may be the ethical response. An earlier example occurred when psychiatrist Robert Jay Lifton (2011) was jailed for his civil disobedience in protesting the Vietnam War.

> Section 7: "A physician shall recognize a responsibility to participate in activities contributing to the improvement of the community and the betterment of public health." (p. 9)
> Annotation 2: "Psychiatrists may interpret and share with the public their expertise in the various psychosocial issues that may affect mental health and illness." (p. 9)

The social determinants of mental health have been receiving increased attention, and although generally not mentioned specifically, those social determinants can impede receiving the benefits of nature. Two community issues related to nature are impairing mental health.

The first issue is the adverse changes in nature that are at least partially caused by humanmade climate change. What we see so far is increased climate instability in terms of wildfires, storms (Figure 11–4), and heat records. Acute and slowly developing disasters can result in trauma and PTSD. Climate refugees are emerging in some parts of the world. Children are more anxious about their future. If one cannot leave a beloved but changed home environment, a syndrome called *solastalgia* (Albrecht et al. 2007) can emerge.

Second, the groups most adversely affected tend to be those from poor and minority communities. Any devastating weather event tends to cause more destruction to less prepared communities with fewer resources to recover and achieve resilience. Toxic chemical exposure such as lead poisoning is much more common in poor communities. These same communities often have less exposure to the benefits of nature. If one lives in the inner city with more asphalt and fewer trees, temperatures tend to be higher, which is especially risky in the summer. Uncomfortably hot temperatures increase irritability and violence.

Corresponding to our professional ethical principles as they might relate to nature and activism are the ethical principles in regard to nature itself. The challenge is to make our ethical principles toward professionalism and nature go hand in hand.

Various ethical principles have been suggested over time in regard to nature and our natural environment (Gardiner et al. 2010). The following are some examples:

1. Anthropocentrism: This nature principle puts humans as the most important beings and holds that nature should be used first and foremost for our benefit.
2. Nonanthropocentrism: This principle gives value to every object and living thing in nature because they all help sustain nature.
3. Psychocentrism: Although everything in nature is important, this principle gives human beings more value because our mental capabilities are better and more complex.
4. Biocentrism: This principle emphasizes the proper balance of ecology on the planet.
5. Holism: This principle considers nature and environmental systems as a whole rather than just individual parts of something.
6. Resourcism: This principle considers nature valuable mainly because of its resources, which can be exploited.
7. Speciesism: This principle considers the human race to be superior and thereby justifies the exploitation and maltreatment of animals and other living things.

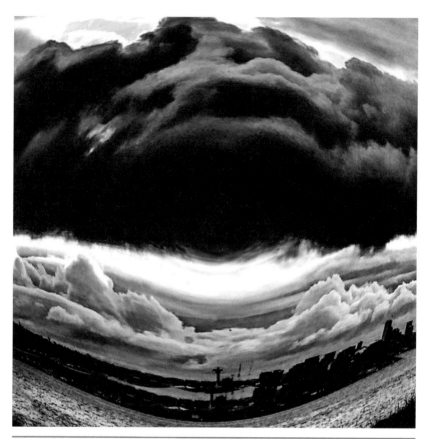

Figure 11–4. There will be a change in the weather. A change in the sea. From now on, what will the changes be?
The storm is surging; the waters rise as the city skyline changes shape and begins to crumble. A tall and prominent Space Needle gives way like an uprooted tree.

At first glance, the first nature ethical principle, anthropocentrism, seems to best fit psychiatric ethics because they seem to solely pay attention to other human beings, especially those with mental health problems. Moreover, the deterioration and destruction of nature and our climate are harmful to human beings. Human beings also have the capability to adapt to—and mitigate—the natural disasters that nature produces from its own natural systems. Yet the same is more or less true of other living things: the loss of species, the restorative aspects of natural fires, and the general systems that tie all together. Therefore, what is likely to protect humans, other living things, and nature is biocentrism. Finding the proper balances in ecology (Figure 11–5), in the relationship of humans and the environment, seems to be the most encompassing

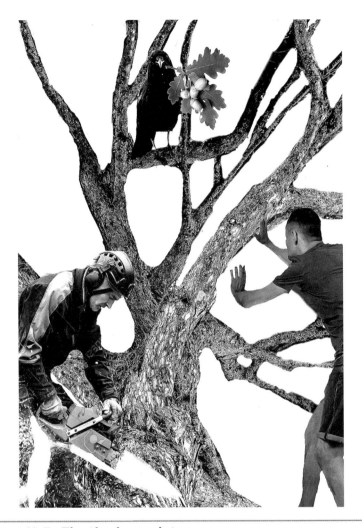

Figure 11–5. The tipping point.
Are we stewards of this Earth, or is it ours to make use of? Ethical choices determine the outcome of the push and pull of human will.

ethical principle for nature therapy and psychiatric professional ethical principles.

NATURE ACTIVISM

Fulfilling the ethical responsibilities to improve the mental health of a community can take many forms. Such activism in medicine has a long history. Two well-known physician activists are celebrating their anniversaries (Mangione and Tykocinski 2021). It is the 200th anniversary of the birth of German physician Rudolf Virchow (1848/1983a, 1848/1983b). He was certain of the social determinants of health and illness, claiming that "medicine is a social science" (p. 125) and that physicians should be "natural attorneys of the poor" (p. 2). When he took his medical students to the barricades of the Märzrevolution in 1848, he was fired from his job. He then turned to politics and helped pass laws that made Berlin a model city of the time for health and hygiene.

Dr. Bernard Lown would have turned 100 in June 2021. For his career activism, he accepted the Nobel Peace Prize on behalf of the organization he cofounded, the International Physicians for the Prevention of Nuclear War. Certainly, nuclear war would have devastating consequences for nature and its support for humans. He concluded that "you cannot be committed to health without being engaged in social struggle for health" (Feeney 2021). In the last year of his life, Lown focused on the climate crisis, concluding that it probably contributed to the emergence of the COVID-19 pandemic.

Both Virchow and Lown can be ideal role models for psychiatrists. Despite the data indicating that the social determinants of health play a significant role in 80% of health outcomes, education about them remains spotty in medical schools.

Given that psychiatry is a relatively new specialty, it has a more limited activist history. In 1964, psychoanalyst and philosopher Erich Fromm (1973, p. 366) laid the groundwork for the behavioral framework of *biophilia*, that is, "the passionate love of life and all that is alive." The term expanded and became popularized with the work of evolutionary biologist Edward O. Wilson (1984), which put humankind's connection with nature in a larger historical arc of adaptive evolutionary behaviors critical for survival and health. Wilson hypothesized that being in nature makes us feel good because the environment in which humans evolved influenced their brains to respond positively to cues that enhanced their ancestors' survival, including trees, savannas, lakes, and waterways. Twenty or so years later, this morphed into the concept of *biophilic design* (Kellert 2012), which tries to use the premise of incorporating nature into the built environment so that people are regularly in contact with nature in some way, thereby aiding health and well-being. Less prominent and less researched, but important psychologically, is the apparent opposite of biophilia, which is biophobia. *Biophobia* includes fear-related responses to nature and nature triggers, such as danger from snakes, spiders, and predators, as well as distress such as noise and images of extreme weather. When too strong, these fears must be mitigated through programs and education.

In the 1960s, many psychiatrists became involved in other kinds of societal activism, particularly civil rights, including disobedience leading to personal incarceration (Lifton 2011). The effect of racism leading to misdiagnosis and inappropriate treatment of Black patients became a cause, especially for the growing numbers of Black psychiatrists.

The range of potential activism is broad. It can range from academic investigation to letter writing to protests to civil disobedience. It can try to prevent further damage to nature or to adapt to the adverse changes with resilience (Doppelt 2016). The more extensive and riskier the activism, the more personal risk there is, whether that is burnout or job loss. Realistic, but not reckless, courage is necessary. For example, a social worker, Michael Foster, who had participated in the Keystone pipeline protests, was arrested for turning off and damaging the valve to the pipeline. A lawyer committed suicide in 2018 to protest climate change. The further an activist goes, the more likely it is that collegial supporters will be lost.

How best to react to those who are not activists but bystanders? Although Dante relegated bystanders to the worst part of his hell, the Ante-Inferno, and the ancient Greeks called such people "idiots," mental health professionals tend to be more empathetic and understanding of such behavior and work to change it (Geiger et al. 2017). Some may even experience learned helplessness after having been more active (Landry et al. 2018). Bystanders, despite their passive role, stand to benefit from activists' efforts to address climate change and can be grateful for them. Climate scientists, even when they intend not to be activists but rather straightforward and unbiased scientists, risk their mental health from facing intense criticism and being immersed in depressing information, which tends to worsen over time.

In terms of psychiatric social activism and nature in particular, that seemed to emerge only over the past decade. As an early example, psychologist and author Mary Pipher (2013, p. 169) became one of the leaders of a grassroots organization fighting energy company Trans-Canada's proposal to install an oil pipeline across the Midwest and beloved environments in her home state of Nebraska. Disparate citizens of various values found common cause and moved from despair to determination. Popular slogans helped rally the troops, such as

Tar sands oil

Thick and gooey

Pipeline promises

A bunch of hooey.

A dramatic therapeutic moment came for Pipher when, after encountering political obstacles, weary and imagining feeling like a wild turkey running in circles when caught in the middle of a busy highway, she happened to glance up and see a half-moon seemingly caught in the branches of an ancient oak tree. Her breathing changed, and she felt intensely and perfectly present, with a sense of bliss and wonder.

As her example illustrates, a personal moral imagination can arise to complement professional ethics. That can take people beyond empathy and Buber's (1971) I-it and I-thou relationships to sense that all relationships to people, animals, and plants can be sacred.

One group that joined the Nebraska cause was refugees from Nigeria, Africa, where protesters of an oil company risked their lives. Indeed, as seen in such examples, becoming significantly involved in activism often carries great personal risk and stress.

In psychiatry specifically, the emergence of nature activism started slowly. An early coalition was the informal Psychiatrists for Environmental Action and Knowledge, which later morphed into the formal Climate Psychiatry Alliance (Moffic 2021). The alliance has written and presented extensively, with increasing numbers of psychiatrists joining it and the related Climate Caucus and the new Committee on Climate Change and Mental Health of the American Psychiatric Association.

Increasing appreciation of the psychosocial harm being done has led to advances in addressing psychological problems related to nature. A recommendation to add ecology and have a biopsychosocial-ecology model has been suggested (Moffic 2019).

At least two community-wide psychiatric movements have emerged to address the adverse repercussions of natural disasters and disruptions. One is called *transformational resilience*, which consists of developing programs to proactively build mental health systems to prepare for upcoming challenges and to build resilience (Doppelt 2016). In particular, and once again, poor communities with fewer resources need such planning to avoid severe mental health adverse consequences. Goals of such transformational resilience initiatives included empowering adults and youths to

- Practice healthy behavior in both good and poor conditions.
- React to adversity with meaning, direction, and hope to achieve more resilience and posttraumatic growth.
- Be active in addressing adverse environmental nature changes.
- Collaborate at various community levels.
- Consult with mental health experts to prevent and reduce psychological problems.

Resilience building can have drawbacks, however. It can lead to ignoring the prevention of future traumas or, as in the case of burnout, plowing ahead and ignoring that the mental health provider or the organization is burning out (LoboPrabhu et al. 2019).

Integrative community therapy is a related endeavor for poor neighborhoods that was created by Brazilian psychiatrist and anthropologist Alberto Barreto. Its essence is community building led by small trained groups to

- Promote a sense of "shared suffering."
- Provide an atmosphere of inclusiveness and diversity.
- Promote healthy coping strategies.
- Enhance social support networks.

Tens of thousands of community therapists are said to have been trained in Brazil and elsewhere. Although little has been published in English, preliminary research has been promising. Integrative community therapy is being brought to the United States to help working-class Americans with inadequate formal and traditional mental health services (Silva 2019). The Visible Hands Collaborative (2024) is a Pittsburgh, Pennsylvania, based nonprofit organization that offers free integrative community therapy facilitator training and hosts weekly integrative community therapy sessions open to the public via Zoom.

Many more nature intervention models could be mentioned, but there is also a need for a more structured approach. To begin that process, as reported in a special issue of *Sports* devoted to health and well-being in an outdoor and adventure sports context, Shanahan et al. (2019) conducted a Delphi expert elicitation process with 19 experts from 7 countries to identify the common forms that such interventions could take, the potential health outcomes, and the target beneficiaries. They identified 27 nature-based health and mental health interventions, which could be broadly categorized into those that try to change the environment and those that try to change behavior (Figure 11–6). Caution was expressed about the socioeconomic variation that can influence outcomes.

The specific and general programs discussed reflect increasing psychiatric attention to social injustice and mental health (Shim 2021). The *American Journal of Psychiatry* recently published an unprecedented issue focusing on structural racism in psychiatry and psychiatric illnesses (Kalin 2021). Even so, such social injustice has rarely been applied to nature and ecology.

The adverse influence of racism and nature therapy even extends to a more experimental process. As the psychedelic drugs are being re-

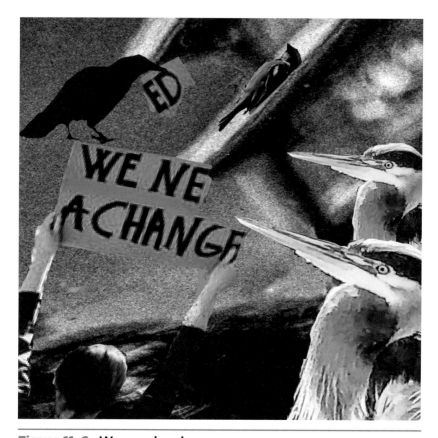

Figure 11–6. We need a change.
A battered house begins to topple within the chaos of destructive natural and social forces. A bird lies lifeless at the window. Two great blue herons stand together in solidarity with a human protester who holds a ripped sign demanding change.

searched more carefully and extensively, there are indications that they could jump-start increased attention to—and connection with—nature. With the right setting, psychedelics can inspire a sense of deep connection with nature (Kettner et al. 2019). Yet if this becomes better verified and available, Black people tend to have a strong distrust of such research, given that they were used as guinea pigs for the early Central Intelligence Agency research on whether lysergic acid diethylamide could be a valuable truth serum (Strauss et al. 2021).

Within community mental health systems, therapists have the challenge to recognize and appropriately treat nature-related psychological problems. As a new concept and consideration for the public and patients, it often puts the onus on clinicians to recognize the nature-related problems, conscious or otherwise, of relevance for the patient while avoiding countertransference and reductionism. In addition, this global problem implies that psychiatrists who are nature activists can be considered therapists for the Earth. Thus, Earth's condition can be called ecocide or ecosuicidal, as compared with an individual's suicide risk. To do all that well necessitates some soul searching on the part of the nature therapy activist. Despite the apparent ethical goodness of the work, one can be motivated by other issues that need their own attention via collegial discussion, the input of loved ones, and personal therapy. Without that, the activist may be more prone to frustration and single-mindedness. As Pipher found, it also helps to keep a sense of humor and have some fun in the face of life-and-death challenges.

Although being a nature activist has psychological risks, it also has psychological benefits. Taking any steps today to address climate challenges can be satisfying (Eichacker 2021), as can reducing any conscious or unconscious guilt about having contributed in the first place over many years of fossil fuel energy use (Weintrobe 2012).

Clinical Translation: Case Example

Although the range of nature climate activism can be so wide, thereby making an average example impossible, consider psychiatrist Mark A. Haven.

Although he had long been concerned with the underserved in psychiatry, he had not been much concerned with nature and the environment. In fact, he was personally pretty wasteful. Then, a granddaughter was born a few years back. On a visit to his home, Mark was asked to go to the store to buy a few things. At the counter, he was asked, as usual, "Paper or plastic?" But this time he froze and could not answer, so he just grabbed the few items in his hands and left. Driving home, he had the epiphany that his anxiety came from what those choices meant for the future of his granddaughter. He investigated the options and found out that the correct answer was neither, but to bring your own bag so as not to pollute nature with substances that are hard to break down.

Afterward, he found some other psychiatrists interested in climate change and the environment, and he started to become an activist by speaking and writing about the apparent challenges for our future health and mental health. When he was frustrated, he found that going out into nature was relaxing and restorative. That was no surprise to him, for when he was younger, he loved to play sports outdoors. But was that enough to explain his later love of trees? His answer came when his best friend from childhood recalled their nature forays. He reminded Mark that they used to ride their bikes to what they called "Bicycle Paradise," which was a wooded area behind one of the early McDonald's restaurants. They went to golf courses, not to play golf but to lie against trees lining the course. Near his friend's house was a small undeveloped area that the friend called "The Woods," which became a refuge for their friends to play. But one day, his friend's father said that it would be paved over with an asphalt parking lot. The friend was dismayed, but his father recommended that they rescue one tree, and they planted it in the backyard of their house. The friend protected it as only a child would imagine he could. Sixty years later, they visited, and that oak tree had grown to fill the backyard and had become a sacred tree to the young Indian American boy of the house (Marcus 2021). These childhood experiences must have been part of the basis for Mark's activist concerns. Although he had forgotten them, his best friend recalled all, speaking as if this were a therapeutic exploration. This insight inspired him to try to protect any and all trees.

However, as time went on and the crisis did not abate, there seemed to be more and more to do: sign petitions, read more articles, listen to presentations, attend meetings, and so on. Finally, he realized that he needed to pull back and try to find what in particular the expertise of being a psychiatrist could add to the struggle and to let go of activities that just added names and numbers to the general cause. His role model was psychiatrist Robert Jay Lifton (2011), who not only was an incarcerated activist during the Vietnam War era but also is a climate activist more than 50 years later.

Now Mark is trying to determine what psychiatric interventions might work and ensuring that he will not burn out along the way. Mark wondered about climate reparations (Moffic 2021). Climate and environmental disruptions are producing climate refugees, who tend to have trauma as a result of their losses and situation. Does their psychological suffering call for reparations from the countries with the greatest responsibility? Clearly, however, his long-term interest in the underserved could be transferred here because, as in so many other matters, in regard to nature and the environment, the underserved are being underserved.

CONCLUSION

At first glance, the task of activism for nature therapy appears simple and straightforward: just do what is possible to increase therapeutic opportunities in nature for all (Figure 11–7). However, it is much more complex and challenging than that.

Clearly, nature influences the mental well-being of humans, and human behavior influences the processes of nature. Myths tell us that. History tells us that. Psychiatric ethics tell us that. Science tells us that. In either direction, there can be benefits and risks. Climate change and other environmental changes in nature are associated with threats to mental health such as PTSD, undue anxiety, grief, and depression. Conversely, nature is a therapeutic resource for mental changes such as poor focus and anxiety. In other words, nature can be both a source of and a solution for mental distress. Moreover, people and communities differ

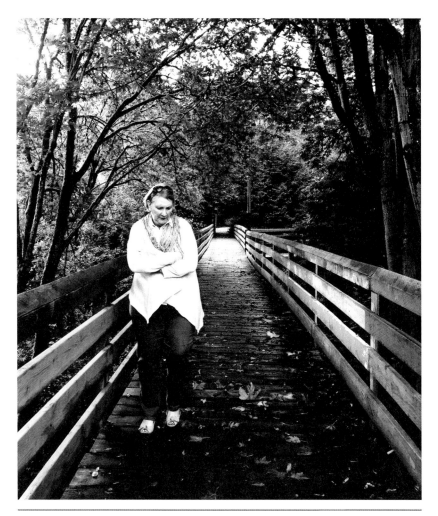

Figure 11-7. In my solitude.
There is nothing as refreshing as a walk in nature. It is a chance for reflection and repose, a way to restore harmony within the chaos of modern life.

in their exposure to nature benefits and risks. Poorer communities and people with limitations or those subject to discrimination need special social justice attention in order to increase opportunities to experience the therapeutic aspects of nature. These interactions necessitate pairing our professional ethics with corresponding nature ethics, such as psychiatric ethics with biocentrism. Biocentrism extends our activist concerns not only to the mental well-being of people but also to the needs of other living things. Some would add a spiritual or religious component to the ethics and morality.

At their worst, these interactions can result in a vicious psychological circle. As nature and the environment are harmed by people, their mental health tends to worsen. We need more nature therapy, but the opportunities to incorporate this therapy may be lessening, especially for certain cultural groups. If our collective mental health worsens, then we are less likely to be successful activists. Perhaps the psychedelics being researched once again can help some break through the obstacles to identifying with nature.

Psychiatric professionals can contribute at various levels. As an individual, clinicians should become involved in nature for their own mental health, obtaining at least brief exposure daily. They should fill their office and home with plants. In turn, clinicians must recognize the importance of nature in their patients, especially those of lower socioeconomic status who may have become accustomed to their circumstances. Individual modeling of the importance of nature can have social contagion spreading and rippling out to others just by talking about it. Becoming a nature activist can be rewarding but also dangerous to one's mental health and well-being. Activists can be working against very powerful corporate and political forces and must watch out for one another. Psychiatric help must be available when needed. A cadre of readily available psychotherapists expert in this area is of the essence. We probably will need subspecialty training in nature psychiatry.

On another level, psychiatric professionals should join a small group of like-minded colleagues. Whether famous cultural anthropologist Margaret Mead actually said this or not, there seems to be historical truth in this quote: "Never doubt that a small group of thoughtful, committed citizens can change the world; indeed, it's the only thing that ever has."

Perhaps such a small group example would include the original group called Psychiatrists for Environmental Action and Knowledge, because that has morphed into much larger groups of climate-concerned psychiatrists and a recommendation to add ecology to the traditional biopsychosocial model.

The larger groups concerned with nature and nature therapy also have been slowly evolving. Such groups may include mental health professionals, general health professionals, politicians, and the public (Pipher 2013). Especially complementary could be those who work in environmental biology, artists, and Indigenous people. Education about nature and nature therapy must become much more widespread. Press releases can become potent nature prescriptions. More mass organizing to combat organized financial support of fossil fuels may be necessary.

We need to address and pay attention to many things in nature, but as one example, growing more trees is an attainable goal for all levels of intervention: individual, small group, and larger populations. Trees can lower air temperatures in neighborhoods, which is so crucial in the hotter neighborhoods in poor communities. Taking care of them and exposing oneself to them, daily if possible, may help prevent the burnout that is so common in activism of any sort. Trees will save energy costs. Advocating for reforestation is a matter of professional ethics and environmental justice. Research indicates that green is good for mental health (Barton and Rogerson 2017). Planting trees and using ultrawhite paint seem to temper dangerous heat islands. Some cities are deploying millions of trees to fight against climate change. If any city could be at risk for being a "concrete jungle" (Figure 11–8), it is New York, and they recently planted a million more trees (Rogers 2019) to supplement those already in Central Park and other parks. A study in Toronto, Ontario, found that adding just 10 trees to a city block had a major effect on people's perceptions of their health and well-being. Perhaps this urban tree planting is a complement to the forest bathing therapeutic opportunities. We also need to plant more trees to help make up for those consumed by the increasing climate-fueled wildfires. As trees grow, they pull more and more carbon out of the atmosphere, but if the trees burn, they release massive amounts of that carbon into the atmosphere.

Well-known mythologist Joseph Campbell's advice was "follow your bliss" for a fulfilling life (Campbell and Moyers 1991, p. 113). For a mentally healthy life, I would add only one word to that: follow your nature bliss. A nature activist might add one more word: follow your nature activist bliss (trees or whatever that may be), as long as it is ethical. What is your bliss?

KEY POINTS

- Individuals should find an aspect of nature that they love, such as trees, and use it for their own mental well-being.

- Various cultural groups have more limited access to the benefits of nature therapy.

- Activism has multiple psychiatric ethical roots.

- Psychiatric professionals should find models of psychiatric activism and join a small group of like-minded colleagues.

- Nature therapists should learn and incorporate the knowledge of nature of the Indigenous people.

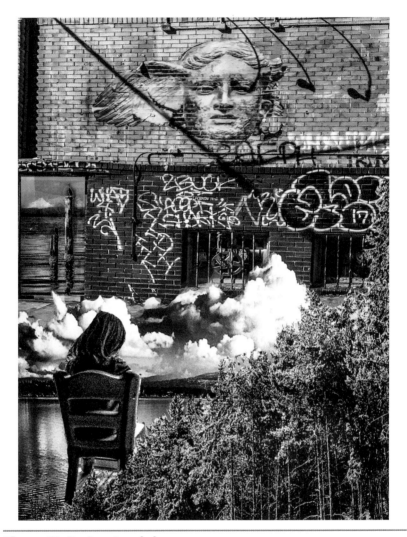

Figure 11-8. A natural dream.

A child sits facing an urban landscape devoid of natural light. It is marked by bricks and barred windows, bare of trees and other signs of nature. The child is not looking at the walled barrier. He is looking inside himself, imaginatively transforming the world into a living landscape.

QUESTIONS

1. Activism in nature therapy is best characterized as

    A. A psychologically safe activity.

    B. Producing better contact with nature.

C. Applicable only in direct patient care.
D. A professional ethical principle.
E. Applicable mainly to certain cultural groups.

Correct answer: D. A professional ethical principle.

Although all the answers have some truth to them, the most comprehensive answer is that activism in nature therapy is best characterized as a professional psychiatric ethical principle (D). Although activism in nature therapy is a psychologically safe activity (A) for the most part, there are also risks of activism burnout, facing criticism and depressing information, and frustration, which worsen over time. Producing better contact with nature (B) is an outcome of activism in nature therapy but does not describe the term itself. A large part of activism in nature therapy happens outside of direct patient care (C), including community organizing, peer interactions, and governmental lobbying efforts. Participation in nature therapy activism is nondiscriminatory with respect to cultural identity (E).

2. Psychiatrists can best become nature activists by

A. Joining activist groups.
B. Signing petitions.
C. Applying the unique expertise of psychiatry.
D. Bringing up nature therapy with all patients.
E. Ignoring personal motivation to be an activist.

Correct answer: C. Applying the unique expertise of psychiatry.

Clearly, psychiatrists and other mental health professionals have the most potential to contribute to nature therapy by using the biopsychosocial-ecology model of understanding and care, which points to applying the unique expertise of psychiatry (C). Joining activist groups (A) and signing petitions (B) are both forms of nature activism available to the layperson that are not as specifically targeted as actions guided by professional expertise. Not every patient is a candidate for nature therapy, so bringing up nature therapy with all patients (D) would not be appropriate. Ignoring personal motivation to be an activist (E) is the opposite action of best becoming a nature activist.

3. The most desired outcome in psychiatric nature activism is

A. Personal satisfaction.
B. Increased availability of nature therapy.
C. New collegial relationships.
D. Better reputation of psychiatry.
E. Record-setting mountain climbing.

Correct answer: B. Increased availability of nature therapy.

Given that our foremost ethical value is the needs and care of the patient, increased availability of nature therapy (B) is the best answer, although all the other answers, except possibly (E), have some value too.

REFERENCES

Albrecht G, Sartore GM, Connor L, et al: Solastalgia: the distress caused by environmental change. Australas Psychiatry 15(Suppl 1):S95–S98, 2007 18027145

All Healers Mental Health Alliance: Welcome to All Healers Mental Health Alliance: About us. 2018. Available at: https://allhealersmha.com/about-us. Accessed May 17, 2024.

American Psychiatric Association: The Principles of Medical Ethics, With Annotations Especially Applicable to Psychiatry. Washington, DC, American Psychiatric Association, 2013

Aylward B, Cooper M, Cunsolo A: Generation climate change: growing up with ecological grief and anxiety. Psychiatric News, May 27, 2021. Available at: https://psychnews.psychiatryonline.org/doi/full/10.1176/appi.pn.2021.6.20. Accessed May 16, 2024.

Azhar A: In Corpus Christi's Hillcrest neighborhood, Black residents feel like they are living in a "sacrifice zone." Inside Climate News, July 4, 2021. Available at: https://insideclimatenews.org/news/04072021/corpus-christi-texas-highway-infrastructure-justice. Accessed May 16, 2024.

Barton J, Rogerson M: The importance of greenspace for mental health. BJPsych Int 14(4):79–81, 2017 29093955

Brettschneider M: Nelson Mandela's political dissident garden. Damselwings, LLC (blog), April 29, 2017. Available at: https://damselwings.com/2017/04/29/nelson-mandelas-political-dissident-garden. Accessed May 16, 2024.

Buber M: I and Thou. Nashville, TN, Touchstone, 1971

Campbell J, Moyers G: The Power of Myth. New York, Anchor, 1991

Doppelt B: Transformational Resilience: How Building Human Resilience to Climate Disruption Can Safeguard Society and Increase Wellbeing. Sheffield, UK, Greenleaf, 2016

Eichacker C: Feeling anxious about the climate emergency? Experts say small steps can help. Maine Public Radio, August 10, 2021. Available at: https://www.mainepublic.org/environment-and-outdoors/2021-08-10/feeling-anxious-about-the-climate-emergency-experts-say-small-steps-can-help. Accessed May 16, 2024.

Feeney M: Bernard Lown, doctor at the vanguard of cardiac care, antiwar activist who shared Nobel Peace Prize, dies at 99. Boston Globe, February 16, 2021. Available at: https://www.bostonglobe.com/2021/02/16/metro/bernard-lown-doctor-vanguard-cardiac-care-antiwar-activist-who-shared-nobel-peace-prize-dies-99/?camp=bg%3Abrief%3Arss%3Afeedly&rss_id=feedly_rss_brief&s_campaign=bostonglobe%3Asocialflow%3Atwitter. Accessed May 17, 2024.

Ferguson G: The Eight Master Lessons of Nature: What Nature Teaches Us About Living Well in the World. New York, Penguin, 2019

Fromm E: The Anatomy of Human Destructiveness. New York, Holt, Rinehart & Winston, 1973

Gardiner S, Caney S, Jamieson D, et al (eds): Climate Ethics: Essential Readings. New York, Oxford University Press, 2010

Geiger N, Swim J, Fraser J: Creating a climate for change: interventions, efficacy and public discussion about climate change. J Environ Psychol 51(August):104–116, 2017

Hammerschlag C: Kindling Spirit: Healing From Within. New York, Turtle Island, 2011

Herbert F: Dune. New York, Ace, 1965

Kalin NH: Impacts of structural racism, socioeconomic deprivation, and stigmatization on mental health. Am J Psychiatry 178(7):575–578, 2021 34270339

Kellert S: Birthright: People and Nature in the Modern World. New Haven, CT, Yale University Press, 2012

Kettner H, Gandy S, Haijen ECHM, et al: From egoism to ecoism: psychedelics increase nature relatedness in a state-mediated and context-dependent manner. Int J Environ Res Public Health 16(24):5147, 2019

Landry N, Gifford T, Milfont T, et al: Learned helplessness moderates the relationship between environmental concern and behavior. J Environ Psychol 55(February):18–22, 2018

Lifton RJ: Witness to an Extreme Century: A Memoir. New York, Free Press, 2011

LoboPrabhu S, Summers R, Moffic HS: Combating Physician Burnout: A Guide for Psychiatrists. Washington, DC, American Psychiatric Association Publishing, 2019

Louv R: Last Child in the Woods: Saving Our Children From Nature-Deficit Disorder, Updated and Expanded Edition. Chapel Hill, NC, Algonquin, 2008

Luke D: Ecopsychology and the psychedelic experience. European Journal of Ecopsychology 4:1–8, 2013

Mangione S, Tykocinski M: Virchow at 200 and Lown at 100—physicians as activists. N Engl J Med 385:291–293, 2021

Marchese D: Why Jane Goodall still has hope for us humans. The New York Times Magazine, July 12, 2021. Available at: https://www.nytimes.com/interactive/2021/07/12/magazine/jane-goodall-interview.html. Accessed May 16, 2024.

Marcus B: Our trees of life. Psychiatric Times, April 16, 2021. Available at: https://www.psychiatrictimes.com/view/our-trees-of-life. Accessed May 16, 2024.

Moffic HS: Toward a bio-psycho-social-eco model of psychiatry. Psychiatric Times, December 30, 2019. Available at: https://www.psychiatrictimes.com/view/toward-bio-psycho-social-eco-model-psychiatry. Accessed May 16, 2024.

Moffic HS: Psychiatry has opened its eyes and seen our environmental issues. Psychiatric News, June 30, 2021. Available at: https://psychnews.psychiatryonline.org/doi/full/10.1176/appi.pn.2021.4.10#:~:text=Now%20there%20are%20even%20more,or%20alter%20the%20immediate%20climate. Accessed May 16, 2024.

Moreno-Garcia S: Beyond Dune: fiction and fantasy novels about ecology and climate change. The Washington Post, July 12, 2021. Available at: https://www.washingtonpost.com/entertainment/books/beyond-dune-lets-talk-about-science-fiction-and-fantasy-novels-about-ecology-and-climate-change/2021/07/10/95103d72-b904-11eb-a5fe-bb49dc89a248_story.html. Accessed May 18, 2024.

Muir J: The Yosemite. New York, Century, 1912

National Park Foundation: NPF launches new round of funding for inclusive storytelling program. May 8, 2024. Available at: https://www.national-parks.org/news-and-updates/updates/npf-launches-new-round-funding-inclusive-storytelling-program. Accessed May 17, 2024.

National Recreation and Park Association. Park and Recreation Inclusion Report. Ashburn, VA, National Recreation and Park Association, 2018

Parpola S: The Assyrian tree of life: tracing the origins of Jewish monotheism and Greek philosophy. J Near East Stud 52(3):161–208, 1993

Paterson JM: Tree Wisdom. London, Thomson's, 1996

Pipher M: The Green Boat: Reviving Ourselves in Our Capsized Culture. New York, Riverhead, 2013

Pollack D: Whither the weather, whether we wither. Psychiatric News, March 31, 2021. Available at: https://psychnews.psychiatryonline.org/doi/full/10.1176/appi.pn.2021.4.20. Accessed May 18, 2024.

Rogers J: Urban roots. Nature Conservancy Magazine, May 31, 2019, pp 42–51

Shanahan DF, Astell-Burt T, Barber EA, et al: Nature-based interventions for improving health and wellbeing: the purpose, the people and the outcomes. Sports (Basel) 7(6):141, 2019 31185675

Shim RS: Dismantling structural racism in psychiatry: a path to mental health equity. Am J Psychiatry 178(7):592–598, 2021 34270343

Silva J: We're Still Here: Pain and Politics in the Heart of America. New York, Oxford University Press, 2019

Simard S: Finding the Mother Tree: Discovering the Wisdom of the Forest. New York, Knopf, 2021

Strauss D, de la Salle S, Sloshower J, et al: Research abuses against people of colour and other vulnerable groups in early psychedelic research. J Med Ethics July 12, 2021 34253622 Epub ahead of print

Union County: County commissioners break ground on inclusive affirmative park space in Plainfield. June 29, 2021. Available at: https://ucnj.org/press-releases/public-info/2021/06/29/county-commissioners-break-ground-on-inclusive-affirmative-park-space-in-plainfield. Accessed May 17, 2024.

Virchow R: 'Der Armenarzt,' Die Medizinische Reform (1848), in Die medicinische Reform 52 volumes. Collected by Christa Kirsten and Kurt Zeisler. Berlin, Germany, Akademie-Verlag, 1983a, p 125

Virchow R: 'Was die "medicinische Reform" will' (1848), in Die medicinische Reform 52 volumes. Collected by Christa Kirsten and Kurt Zeisler. Berlin, Germany, Akademie-Verlag, 1983b, p 2

Visible Hands Collaborative: Become a facilitator for your community or organization: about ICT. Available at: https://www.visiblehandscollaborative.org/about-ict. Accessed May 18, 2024.

Weintrobe S (ed): Engaging With Climate Change: Psychoanalytic and Interdisciplinary Perspectives. London, Routledge, 2012

Wilson E: Biophilia. Cambridge, MA, Harvard University Press, 1984

Wohlleben P: The Hidden Life of Trees: What They Feel, How They Communicate—Discoveries From a Secret World. Vancouver, BC, Greystone, 2016

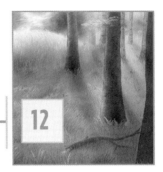

12

The Outdoor Classroom

Grace S. Ro, M.D.
Leia Chemmacheril, M.D., M.B.A.

> *Earth and sky, woods and fields, lakes and rivers, the moun-*
> *tain and the sea, are excellent schoolmasters, and teach some*
> *of us more than we can ever learn from books.*
> —John Lubbock (1894, p. 70), 1st Baron Avebury

In this chapter, we explore nature therapy in the classroom setting for the child and adolescent population and how such interventions are relevant to their mental and physical health and wellness. The
concept of a classroom also can be applied to later stages in life—
namely, the geriatric population—less so as a structured environment
to learn basic concepts but rather to restore and maintain mental health
in the context of aging and medical comorbidities.

CHILDREN AND ADOLESCENTS

The American Academy of Pediatrics has clinical reports on the value of unstructured play and recommends at least 60 minutes of daily physical activity (Lobelo et al. 2020; Yogman et al. 2018). From outdoor recess to visits to the park to walks to the grocery store, the outdoors can be a versatile environment for physical activity and exploration. Studies have shown that several positive outcomes are associated with physical activity, such as strength building, decreased cardiovascular risk factors, and improved cognition (Landry and Driscoll 2012). Inconclusive evidence indicates a significant difference in the outcomes of physical activity in nature and physical activity indoors (Lahart et al. 2019). However, it is worth exploring and placing more emphasis on the specific setting and therapeutic effects that nature and the outdoors can have from an early age. Outdoor, "green" exposure also has had positive effects on mental health and self-regulation (Beute and de Kort 2014; Christian et al. 2015; Raney et al. 2019). For example, forest bathing by South Korean elementary school students has been explored as a form of nature therapy, with a significant improvement in self-esteem and a significant decrease in depressive symptoms (Bang et al. 2018).

The Centers for Disease Control and Prevention has published resources for educators to encourage outdoor play because it can be a powerful tool not only for children to learn but also for caregivers to observe childhood development through social, emotional, and cognitive milestones. Free, unstructured play is essential for brain development in children because they can learn to interact with others, explore, resolve conflicts, and use their imaginations while being physically active. Several studies have aimed to explore the potential correlation between nature exposure and its positive effects, but research is limited on the effects in the child and adolescent population (Weeland et al. 2019). The literature also varies in how nature therapy or exposure is defined, which presents challenges in comparing various studies and outcomes.

Many schools include outdoor recess, gym class, and field trips as part of a child's educational experience. The available outdoor exposure may depend on the setting of various school districts, from more to less urban, which may offer different levels of outdoor opportunities and exposure (Kellert 2002). This brings into question the disparities in childhood experiences, education, and development, because limited access to safe green spaces may reduce the potential for nature therapy's positive effects. One study found that increased green space reduces the risk of behaviors associated with conduct disorders at age

7 years and reduces the risk of behaviors associated with mood disorders such as anxiety and depression at age 12 years (Madzia et al. 2019). Other studies have reported lower incidence rates of mood disorders such as depression and anxiety in adults living in urban areas with more green space availability (Astell-Burt et al. 2014; White et al. 2013). Further studies are needed to explore the correlation between increasing green spaces and enhanced mental health and behaviors.

Autism Spectrum Disorder and Nature Therapy

About 1 in 36 children has autism spectrum disorder, with 3.1 times more boys affected than girls (Maenner et al. 2023; Shaw et al. 2023). Risk factors include genetic predisposition, prenatal risks including maternal age and metabolic conditions, in utero risks, and other potential causes for neurodevelopmental injury (Mandy and Lai 2016). Children with autism spectrum disorder have deficits in engaging in social interactions, language delays, and sensitivity to changes in their environment. They can also present with repetitive actions or rituals, limited attention, restricted interests, or rigid routines. Other medical conditions such as motor abnormalities, seizures, and sleep disorders often co-occur with autism spectrum disorder (Lai et al. 2014). Often, these children can show impairments in social play behaviors, which can ultimately affect their ability to build relationships with their peers (Tanner et al. 2015).

Nature therapy can be used as a powerful tool to provide diversity in structure, sensation, and experience. It has the potential to provide cognitive, mental, and physical benefits in children with autism spectrum disorder (Barakat et al. 2019; Table 12–1). Therapeutic gardens have been explored and studied for children with autism spectrum disorder, given the versatility in their design to cater to people who may be over- or understimulated. For example, a monochromatic color scheme can have a calming effect, whereas vivid, contrasting shades can have a stimulating effect. Smooth leaves and finely textured plants could be relieving, whereas coarse bark and coarsely textured walkways could be more captivating. It is important to consider that autism spectrum disorder may present differently; for example, one child may be hypersensitive to overstimulation, and another may be hyposensitive, which may result in opposing effects of the same stimulus. Nevertheless, the flexibility and creativity in designing a therapeutic garden are endless. More research should be done to explore the efficacy of these types of interventions, with hopes of designing a replicable curriculum for widespread use by youths who may benefit from it.

Table 12–1.   Benefits of outdoor learning

Cognitive benefits	Mental benefits	Physical benefits
Creativity, observation	Stress reduction	Coordination, balance
Collaboration, imagination	Positive emotions	
Intrapersonal skills	Concentration	
Learning, curiosity	Privacy, intimacy	

Source.   Adapted from Barakat et al. 2019.

Although nature can be a powerful tool for children with autism spectrum disorder, important barriers and caveats must be considered. Safety is a major concern that was reported by caregivers of children with autism spectrum disorder, because they may be easily distracted (Ayvazoglu et al. 2015). A higher incidence of injuries is also seen in those with autism spectrum disorder because of common co-occurring medical conditions such as seizures and visual impairment, so appropriate preventive interventions should be explored and established (Jain et al. 2014). Other factors to consider are associated behaviors, core symptoms of autism spectrum disorder, and unintentional injuries resulting from inadequate supervision (Lee et al. 2008). Thus, further studies to explore risk factors for potential harm and necessary support are crucial for nature therapy models to be beneficial, feasible, and safe. This information also may encourage caregivers to support and implement interventions such as therapeutic gardens.

Nature therapy also has been explored in youths with disabilities. A day school for children with special needs in Israel explored the use of nature as a vessel for improved communication, teamwork, and self-esteem (Berger 2006). This was inspired by the observation that classic psychotherapeutic interventions may be less efficacious for those with lower IQ and abstract skills (Butz et al. 2000; Nezu and Nezu 1994). Berger (2006) found that nature served as a space that was ever changing yet provided an opportunity to encourage flexibility in responding and adapting to these changes. Direct experiential interactions with nature allowed for the progression of fear and alienation into familiarity, belonging, and caring. This study suggested that nature can be a powerful vessel to use for those who rely on fewer verbal and cognitive cues.

ADHD and Nature Therapy

In the classroom setting, young students are constantly stimulated by their peers, teachers, and environment. Children are expected to maintain directed attention to focus on tasks and remain engaged in the learning process. However, such high levels of stimulation can lead to a phenomenon called *cognitive fatigue*. This has been conceptualized as an inability to maintain optimal performance over an acute period (Holtzer et al. 2011). Although cognitive fatigue may be a result of excessive stimulation, some people experience fatigue more readily or have reduced productivity, resulting in suboptimal outcomes.

ADHD is a neurodevelopmental disorder that is becoming increasingly common, with significant effects on children's learning, mood, and interpersonal relationships (Wolraich et al. 2019). Symptoms of inattention, hyperactivity, and impulsivity must be present in at least two social settings (e.g., home, school, church) for at least 6 months before age 12 years (American Psychiatric Association 2013). The neurobiology of ADHD is not fully understood; however, structural differences in various brain regions have been proposed (Tripp and Wickens 2009). When dysfunctional, the frontal lobe, which includes the motor cortex, can result in disinhibited motor activity and disturbed attention (Niedermeyer and Naidu 1997). The anterior cingulate cortex has associated mesolimbic dopamine circuitry, which may be deficient in ADHD, resulting in motivational deficits and behavioral dysfunction (Silvetti et al. 2013).

Early diagnosis and treatment are thought to prevent worsening symptoms and comorbid conditions in adulthood (Magnus et al. 2021). Medications (stimulants, nonstimulants) are more effective when provided in combination with therapy and environmental modification strategies (Brown et al. 2018). Stimulants such as methylphenidate and amphetamine increase the availability of norepinephrine and dopamine in the prefrontal cortex. Nonstimulants such as atomoxetine target the same neurotransmitters but without abuse potential (Brown et al. 2018). Although pharmacological agents can reduce distractibility, improve sustained attention, and reduce impulsivity, ways to augment these effects can be explored through nature therapy. Medications approved for ADHD, though effective for many, can have side effects such as mood changes, personality changes, and decreased appetite (Charach and Fernandez 2013). The stigmatization of ADHD diagnosis and treatment can also reduce adherence to pharmacological interventions (Mueller et al. 2012). Although the medications have been shown to increase academic productivity, the evidence that they improve long-term social and academic outcomes is limited (Hinshaw 1994). Thus, alternative supplemental treatment modalities continue to be explored.

From a genetic perspective, ADHD has been associated with the allele of the *DRD4* gene (Tovo-Rodrigues et al. 2013). Researchers have explored possible evolutionary advantages of ADHD, given its current existence (Williams and Taylor 2006). To appreciate this, it is important to consider the context and societal norms that have also evolved through time. In the past, humans were nomad hunters and gatherers, learning through experience without the pressures or structure of modern education. Some propose that those with ADHD tendencies may have freely sought ways to adapt to challenges, even if it meant exploring different places to survive. Although today's education system is more regimented, there may be value in providing individualized support, especially for children who may not succeed in that setting. This brings in the potential for nature and outdoor therapy to provide an alternative learning space as an adjunct to the traditional classroom setting.

According to attention restoration theory (Kaplan 1995), attention fatigue should be restored to regain optimal functioning, and nature therapy is one way to provide this restoration (Kaplan and Kaplan 1989). This is broken down into voluntary and involuntary forms of attention (Hartig et al. 1991). Daily activities require voluntary attention, with competing stimuli or thoughts that must be inhibited to get certain tasks done. In contrast, involuntary attention is driven by interest, curiosity, and fascination. One such medium would be exposure to natural environments, which invites attention and focus that may be less mentally demanding. Some propose that removing oneself from a setting of voluntary attention and focusing on a new environment necessitating involuntary attention may ultimately allow the restoration process to occur (Kaplan and Talbot 1983).

Data are limited on how exactly nature exposure affects attention (Ohly et al. 2016). One review suggested that there may be differences between the effects of real environments and those of virtual exposure (Stevenson et al. 2018). However, as explored in previous chapters, *nature therapy* is a broad term that can target virtually any of the human senses. Whether it be through auditory or visual stimulation or full immersion in a natural environment, nature therapy has been shown to have the potential for positive effects (Gamble et al. 2014; Zhang et al. 2017). One study found that attentional functioning in children with severe ADHD improved during and after activities in greener spaces, as observed by parents (Taylor et al. 2001). The findings further support exploring how these effects can be used in various settings such as home and school so that children with ADHD can benefit from enhanced attention and complete tasks more efficiently. However, in 2002 the U.S. Food and Drug Administration approved stimulants to treat ADHD, which may have placed a greater emphasis on pharmacological treatment than on nature therapy. The recent global coronavirus disease

2019 (COVID-19) pandemic, which brought about extended periods of isolation, inevitably reintroduced the value of open, green spaces (Davies and Sanesi 2022).

Although emotional dysregulation is not included in the DSM-5 (American Psychiatric Association 2013) diagnostic criteria for ADHD, studies have shown that youths with an ADHD diagnosis are at higher risk for developing depression later in life (Seymour et al. 2012). Adult ADHD is often comorbid with depressive disorder, anxiety disorder, and substance use. Thus, early interventions to promote mood stability could improve outcomes longitudinally. As the sources of stress increase through adolescence, the time and value placed on outdoor excursions decrease. Outdoor field trips and recess time are replaced with study hall periods, standardized testing, and online assignments. Technology is constantly advancing, and the evolution of daily living is thought to further disconnect people from natural unstructured play. Some studies have shown that children with ADHD have greater difficulty maintaining behavioral control in an industrialized environment than in a green space (van den Berg and van den Berg 2011).

Although proving a correlation between nature therapy and improving mental health is challenging, researchers, clinicians, and educators continue to explore ways in which to do so. Increasing numbers of studies are exploring the effects of outdoor educational programs, which encompass teaching, learning, or experiencing in an outdoor setting, beyond the classroom. Active, experiential, guided learning can improve the physical, psychological, and social aspects of education (Quinn and Russo 2022). A survey of undergraduate students found that early nature exposure can increase engagement in wellness initiatives in higher-level education (Sachs et al. 2020). This is further evidence that engaging youths in nature-based activities and learning can have long-lasting benefits. Especially in an age of urbanization and technological advancement, the outdoors can be a source of relief. Thus, creatively applying nature as a medium for learning and growth from an early age may establish long-term benefits and continued engagement with nature as a beneficial tool (Table 12–2).

The discussion does not end with children and adolescents but extends to include the family and community. The concept of multifamily therapy has been studied and used for schizophrenia, relapse prevention, and vocational and social skill rehabilitation, with an emphasis placed on the family and community network (Stuart and Schlosser 2009). A study done in Hong Kong suggested that multifamily therapy can also be applied to families with children who have ADHD (Ma et al. 2019). In this study, children were able to display creativity and risk-

Table 12–2.   Ideas to implement nature in the educational setting

Educational approach	Connectivity with others	Learning environment
Nature-based field trips	Group-based nature activities	Classrooms with windows
Nature-based homework assignments	Family-based nature activities	Dorm room windows facing nature
Nature-based classroom design Encouragement of exploration, fascination, and curiosity through nature	Meditation and mindfulness in the outdoors	Early introduction of nature as source of wellness

taking behaviors in the natural environment, leading to a shift in the parents' perception of their behaviors. The green space was a change in environment and an opportunity for the families to engage in a different, more enriching way. Children who participated in this study reported narrative themes of positive time with family, safe space, entertainment, and enhanced communication with parents.

OLDER ADULTS

Aging Population and Demographics

The world's population is aging. A 2022 report from the Department of Economic and Social Affairs of the United Nations, Population Division, predicted that the proportion of people age 65 years and older in the United States will increase from 9.7% of the global population in 2022 to 16.4% by 2050. In the United States and Europe, the population age 65 years and older was 18.7% in 2022 and is predicted to increase to 26.9% by 2050 (United Nations Department of Economic and Social Affairs, Population Division 2022). South Korea is predicted to have an even greater jump, from a 15.7% geriatric population in 2020 to 40.1% in 2050, with 16.1% of South Korean adults being 80 years or older (Statistics Korea 2021). Aging can lead to cognitive and functional decline, and a significant portion of the population is going through this change at this time (Detweiler et al. 2012).

According to the *2020 Profile of Older Americans* (Figure 12–1), 61% of older adults lived in the community with their partners, 27% lived alone in the community, and a small number lived in nursing homes. Furthermore, 1% of people between ages 65 and 74, 2% of people between ages 75 and 84, and 8% of people older than 85 lived in nursing homes. In 2019, 51% of people age 65 and older lived in nine U.S. states: California, Florida, Texas, New York, Pennsylvania, Ohio, Illinois, Michigan, and North Carolina. Older adults are dispersed in terms of geography and living arrangements (Administration for Community Living 2021).

Urbanization

Another factor that plays a key role in changes in overall population health, especially for older adults, is urbanization. *Urbanization* refers to population growth and increase in population density. The process results in increased traffic, air and noise pollution, and heat island effects and loss of open green and blue spaces (Kabisch et al. 2017; see Chapter 8, "The Wet Outdoors"). These changes have negative health effects on people of all ages but especially older adults. For instance, outdoor air pollutants have been associated with increased hospitalizations due to respiratory complaints, such as chronic obstructive pulmonary disease, asthma, and pneumonia, with higher risks in older adults than in the rest of the population (Simoni et al. 2015). Urbanization is also associated with lower levels of physical activity, particularly for low- and middle-income households (Boakye et al. 2023). Sedentary lifestyles are a risk factor for long-term illness such as diabetes, obesity, and depression. This affects the vulnerable populations more, which includes older adults (Kabisch et al. 2017).

Physical Activity and Aging

Physical activity helps with the process of healthy aging. Urbanization often results in difficulty finding the appropriate environment for physical activity. Takano et al. (2002) conducted a study to determine whether walkable green spaces affect the longevity of older adults in cities. The study analyzed the 5-year survival of 2,211 senior citizens with respect to residential environmental characteristics. The physical environments near residences were characterized as having spaces for strolling, tree-lined streets, more hours of sunlight, and less noise from automobiles and factories. The results showed that walkable green streets and spaces near residences were significantly associated with increased 5-year survival of senior citizens, irrespective of age, sex, marital status, attitude toward community, and socioeconomic status. This study was conducted between 1992 and 1997 and published in 2002. Even at

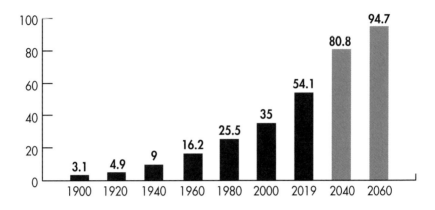

Figure 12–1. Number of U.S. persons age 65 years and older, 1900–2060 (numbers in millions).
Increments in years are uneven. Lighter bars (2040 and 2060) indicate projections.
Source.   Reprinted from Administration for Community Living: *2020 Profile of Older Americans.* May 2021. Available at: https://acl.gov/sites/default/files/Profile%20of%20OA/2020ProfileOlderAmericans_RevisedFinal.pdf.

that time, evidence indicated that nature therapy can improve the health of the aging population, and the study called for changes in urban planning policy for the better health of residents (Takano et al. 2002).

Inactivity in Long-Term-Care Facilities

Physical activity by older adults has been associated with decreased functional decline, lower risk of obesity and hypertension, and decreased risk of falls. High levels of inactivity can also lead to higher levels of depression and anxiety (Leung et al. 2017). Thus, physical activity should be an essential part of older adults' routines, but this population is one of the least physically active parts of society (Cvecka et al. 2015). Many older adults are moving into assisted living and nursing homes. These facilities provide older adults with more care than they would typically receive if they lived in the general community. Assisted living homes, as compared with nursing homes, provide tenants with more independent living and self-directed care. However, the level of physical and cognitive impairment in assisted living residents is still greater than in older adults living in the community. A study by Leung et al. (2017) screened 114 residents from assisted living facilities across British Columbia for daily levels of physical activity. The study showed that residents spent 87% of their awake hours in sedentary behavior. The increased sedentary time was associated with significantly worse scores on the Modified Falls Efficacy Scale and Timed Up and Go scale. The

Timed Up and Go scale is used to assess physical function, and the Modified Falls Efficacy Scale measures the confidence of participants to partake in activities without falling. This study indicated that older adults in care facilities have more sedentary lifestyles, and this can affect their health status (Leung et al. 2017).

Evidently, the general population is aging at a rapid rate. This, combined with external factors, such as urbanization and the reduction in overall physical activity, puts the aging population at risk for significant cognitive and physical health problems. As discussed in previous chapters of this book, evidence suggests that exposure to natural environments can improve overall human health and well-being at all ages. Therefore, it is certainly worthwhile to explore nature therapy to better the physical, emotional, and cognitive health specifically in the aging population.

Possible Benefits of Nature Therapy for Older Adults

Agricultural activity, which is a form of horticultural therapy, is part of many psychiatric hospital settings because of the well-established mental health benefits of such activity (Detweiler et al. 2012). Similarly, horticultural therapy has been shown to have positive effects on older adults by increasing positive affect and decreasing anger (Chan et al. 2017). Another way to incorporate nature into the lives of older adults is through therapeutic gardens. Therapeutic gardens provide sensory stimulation and a safe environment for exercise and spending time in assisted living facilities and nursing homes. These gardens stimulate the senses by including various plants to promote visual, tactile, and olfactory stimulation; leaves to produce sound when ruffling in the wind; and trees to provide color and shade. They can also include vegetables and herbs that residents can harvest themselves. Studies have shown overall health benefits from nature therapy, including pain reduction, improved attention, and stress reduction. It is thought that these positive effects can extend specifically to older adults (Detweiler et al. 2012).

Dementia

Nature therapy has been studied in older patients with dementia. A 2018 article in the *American Journal of Medicine* defined dementia as "any decline in cognition that is significant enough to interfere with independent, daily functioning" (Gale et al. 2018, p. 1161). The root cause of the onset of dementia can be neurological, psychiatric, or secondary to other medical conditions. Dementia is more common in older adults, with the leading causes being neurocognitive disorders such as Alzheimer's disease and dementia with Lewy bodies (Gale et al. 2018). In 2010, 4.4 million American adults had dementia, which included 14.7% of adults older than 70 years. The total population with dementia is expected to triple by 2050 if no advancements are made in the prevention and treatment of the disease. The treatment and care of patients with dementia would benefit from more attention, given the lack of disease-modifying treatments. However, interventions affect different aspects of dementia, and these therapies combined can make a substantial difference in the quality of life for patients (Tisher and Salardini 2019). Behavior therapy is at the forefront of dementia treatment, with the aim of extinguishing difficult learned behaviors. However, only a few studies support the efficacy of this type of therapy, and this form of treatment must be tailored to specific behaviors (Douglas et al. 2004). This certainly leaves room for investigation into other forms of nonpharmacological therapies for dementia, especially those that can be used more broadly and in group settings, such as nature therapy.

Depression is a risk factor for developing Alzheimer's disease, a form of dementia that is most common in the older population. Rates of mood disorders are high in patients with dementia; 50% of patients with diagnosed Alzheimer's disease also have diagnosed depression. Mood disorders and dementia both affect attention, memory, motivation, processing speed, and organization. Thus, mood disorders in patients who have dementia can significantly affect their quality of life. Medications such as selective serotonin reuptake inhibitors and talking therapy are used to treat depression in dementia (Tisher and Salardini 2019). However, nature therapy also has been shown to improve mood in patients with dementia. A 2017 study by White et al. assessed changes in mood of residents in a dementia facility in the United Kingdom with mid- to late-stage dementia after being exposed to a nature garden (White et al. 2018). The outdoor areas of the facility had been renovated to encourage activity, by including various plants such as fruit trees and vegetable beds. Qualitative data on the outdoor experiences of residents were collected in 2012 from primary caregivers and activity coordinators. The study showed that significant improvement in mood occurred with exposure to nature. This association was not linear, with 80–90 minutes of exposure leading to maximal benefits (White et al. 2018). This is simply one study showing the benefit of nature therapy for mood improvement in dementia. These results should prompt more studies to be done on this topic, especially in multiple settings, such as the residential home, and with various forms of nature therapy (Table 12–3).

Sleep deprivation is also a risk factor for dementia, especially Alzheimer's disease. Sleep deprivation also leads to delirium and affects

Table 12–3. **Ideas to implement nature therapy in dementia facilities**

Intervention	Benefits
Addition of wander gardens to facility	Decreased inappropriate behaviors and improved mood (Detweiler et al. 2008)
Increase in time spent outdoors and addition of courtyards	Improved sleep (Calkins et al. 2007)
Implementation of community-based horticultural program	Decreased agitation, increased time spent engaging in activity (Lu et al. 2020), and improved sleep (Lee and Kim 2008)

cognition, particularly in patients with dementia (Tisher and Salardini 2019). Sleep disturbance and behavioral symptoms are two primary burdens on caregivers that lead to the institutionalization of patients (Phillips and Diwan 2003). Current treatment for sleep disorders in dementia is the same as in older adults without dementia, including maintaining sleep hygiene, assessing comorbidities, and taking medications such as high-risk sedative-hypnotics and neuroleptics (Tisher and Salardini 2019). However, studies have shown that nature therapy can influence sleep in patients with dementia. A study by Lee and Kim in 2008 examined gardening as a physical activity in institutionalized patients with dementia. The study included 23 institutionalized patients with dementia and sleep disturbances or agitation. The subjects selected their own plants and grew them for 28 days, tending to them twice a day, in the morning and afternoon. The study found that indoor gardening led to significant increases in nocturnal sleep time efficacy, decreases in awakening after sleep onset, and decreases in nap times. In the same study, Lee and Kim (2008) also found that agitation was significantly decreased, and cognition was significantly improved in patients with dementia after exposure to indoor gardening. This study suggested that nature therapy is associated with improvement in several facets of dementia that affect quality of life, and this tool should be used as an adjunct in the treatment of the disease (Lee and Kim 2008).

Clinical Translation: Case Example

A therapeutic high school arranged a field trip to a state park. The park's interpretive staff taught the students about the local ecosystems and led a hike over a short trail. When they returned to the visitor center, they learned how to make collage art from fallen leaves. The students provided positive feedback about the trip and requested more such experiences.

Students are enrolled in both classrooms and group therapy as part of their daily schedule. The social skills group leader decided to take inspiration from the student feedback and arranged an outing for the group that week.

Students were brought to a local park down the block from the school. They were encouraged to forage for fallen plant materials on the ground to use in collaging back at the school. They were given strict guidelines on weeds that were permissible to pick and instructed to avoid disrupting other park vegetation. They were encouraged to share their observations as part of the social skills component while foraging. The students expressed surprise and wonder at the number and variety of leaves and flowers in the park. They reported that they had not looked that closely at the ground before, despite walking past the park to get to school every day.

Although many of the students in the group had a history of poor frustration tolerance and low threshold for emotional dysregulation, they showed resilience in the face of the activity's minor discomforts. From tolerating soiled hands sticky with sap to recoiling in disgust from insects in the vicinity, the students encouraged one another to persevere.

The students practiced reframing their negative automatic thoughts. For example, the group leader modeled enthusiasm for observing insect behavior in its natural habitat. The students learned that the insects they initially feared were not dangerous and could be intrinsically rewarding to see. With the group's support, they cautiously overcame their initial repulsion.

The group leaders began a group discussion in which each student explained how they picked the various elements of their collection. The discussion encouraged curiosity and allowed the students to demonstrate mastery by sharing their acquired knowledge of the natural world.

The group session ended with a return to the classroom and the students assembling collage artwork from their trimmings. While working on their art, they informally continued the discussion about their natural discoveries, their reignited excitement about the natural world, and their plans to explore the outdoors in their own backyards.

CONCLUSION

Nature therapy provides benefits to physical and mental health, especially in special vulnerable populations, children, and older adults. Nature therapy has been shown to have a positive effect on conditions such as autism, ADHD, and dementia. This supports the idea that nature therapy should be implemented in places such as schools, assisted living facilities, and nursing homes, and there are several ways to incorporate nature into these settings. It would certainly be worthwhile to do further research on how nature therapy can affect other illnesses in these special populations.

KEY POINTS

- Nature therapy has the potential to provide cognitive, mental, and physical benefits in children with autism spectrum disorder and ADHD.

- According to attention restoration theory, attention fatigue should be restored to regain optimal functioning, and nature therapy is one way to provide this restoration.

- Involving caregivers and family members in the nature therapy interventions can be beneficial for children and adolescents and their families.

- The rapidly aging population combined with urbanization, as well as the reduction in overall physical activity, puts older adults at risk for significant cognitive and physical health concerns.

- Nature therapy has been shown to provide therapeutic effects in older adults with dementia, and this form of treatment should be further explored for other conditions that affect older adults.

QUESTIONS

1. Which of the following best describes the versatility of a therapeutic garden specifically for children with autism spectrum disorder?

    A. Open space for large groups to congregate.
    B. Plants with finely textured leaves.
    C. An audible speaker for constant communication.
    D. Easily accessible laptops to research nature-based concepts.
    E. Limited space to ensure constant supervision.

Correct answer: B. Plants with finely textured leaves.

The use of therapeutic gardens has been explored and studied for children with autism spectrum disorder, specifically catering to their individual needs. Color schemes, contrasting shades, and various textures in nature are examples of ways to provide either stimulating or calming effects. Of the choices available, plants with finely textured leaves (B) are the best option. The therapeutic garden should not be designed for the purpose of congregating large groups (A). Access to electronic devices should be

limited (C, D), and the overall space should be open for exploration rather than restricted (E).

2. According to the attention restoration theory, how would nature therapy be beneficial?

    A. For effective nature therapy, one must have intense mental fo-
cus to increase productivity.
    B. Being in a quieter environment can allow effective meditation
and reflection.
    C. Nature therapy can allow a transition from voluntary atten-
tion to involuntary attention.
    D. Nature therapy provides a distraction from everyday tasks,
which can provide mental and emotional restoration.
    E. In the outdoor setting, there is unfamiliarity and the unknown,
which relieves the stress caused by attending to voluntary tasks.

**Correct answer: C. Nature therapy can allow a transition from volun-
tary attention to involuntary attention.**

According to the attention restoration theory, there are two forms of
attention: voluntary and involuntary. Daily activities require voluntary attention, which may lead to fatigue. Nature therapy may provide a transition from voluntary to involuntary attention, driven by
interest, curiosity, and fascination (C). This allows a restorative process to occur, rather than further burdening the mind (A, D, E). Although a quieter environment could improve focus (B), the best
answer according to the attention restoration theory is choice C.

3. Indoor gardening has been associated with which of the following effects on sleep patterns for people with dementia?

    A. Increase in nocturnal sleep efficacy.
    B. Decrease in awakening after sleep onset.
    C. Decrease in nap times.
    D. All of the above.
    E. A and B only.

Correct answer: D. All of the above.

A study by Lee and Kim in 2008 found that indoor gardening led
to significant increases in nocturnal sleep time efficacy, decreases
in awakening after sleep onset, and decreases in nap times for pa-

tients with dementia (D). This study also showed that cognition and agitation were significantly improved, further supporting the potential benefits of nature therapy for the geriatric population.

REFERENCES

Administration for Community Living: 2020 Profile of Older Americans. Administration for Community Living, May 2021. Available at: https://acl.gov/sites/default/files/Aging%20and%20Disability%20in%20America/2020ProfileOlderAmericans.Final_.pdf. Accessed May 19, 2024.

American Psychiatric Association: Diagnostic and Statistical Manual of Mental Disorders, 5th Edition. Arlington, VA, American Psychiatric Association, 2013

Astell-Burt T, Mitchell R, Hartig T: The association between green space and mental health varies across the lifecourse: a longitudinal study. J Epidemiol Community Health 6(1):578–583, 2014 24604596

Ayvazoglu NR, Kozub FM, Butera G, et al: Determinants and challenges in physical activity participation in families with children with high functioning autism spectrum disorders from a family systems perspective. Res Dev Disabil 47:93–105, 2015 26368652

Bang KS, Kim S, Song MK, et al: The effects of a health promotion program using urban forests and nursing student mentors on the perceived and psychological health of elementary school children in vulnerable populations. Int J Environ Res Public Health 15(9):1977, 2018 30208583

Barakat HA, Bakr A, El-Sayad Z: Nature as a healer for autistic children. Alexandria Engineering Journal 58(1):353–366, 2019

Berger R: Using contact with nature, creativity and rituals as a therapeutic medium with children with learning difficulties: a case study. Emot Behav Diffic 11(2):135–146, 2006

Beute F, de Kort YA: Salutogenic effects of the environment: review of health protective effects of nature and daylight. Appl Psychol Health Well Being 6(1):67–95, 2014 24259414

Boakye K, Bovbjerg M, Schuna J Jr, et al: Urbanization and physical activity in the global Prospective Urban and Rural Epidemiology study. Sci Rep 13(1):290, 2023

Brown KA, Samuel S, Patel DR: Pharmacologic management of attention deficit hyperactivity disorder in children and adolescents: a review for practitioners. Transl Pediatr 7(1):36–47, 2018 29441281

Butz MR, Bowling JB, Bliss CA: Psychotherapy with the mentally retarded: a review of the literature and the implications. Prof Psychol Res Pr 31(1):42–47, 2000

Calkins M, Szmerekovsky JG, Biddle S: Effect of increased time spent outdoors on individuals with dementia residing in nursing homes. J Hous Elderly 21(3–4):211–228, 2007

Chan HY, Ho RC, Mahendran R, et al: Effects of horticultural therapy on elderly' health: protocol of a randomized controlled trial. BMC Geriatr 17(1):192, 2017 28851276

Charach A, Fernandez R: Enhancing ADHD medication adherence: challenges and opportunities. Curr Psychiatry Rep 15(7):371, 2013 23712722

Christian H, Zubrick SR, Foster S, et al: The influence of the neighborhood physical environment on early child health and development: a review and call for research. Health Place 33:25–36, 2015 25744220

Cvecka J, Tirpakova V, Sedliak M, et al: Physical activity in elderly. Eur J Transl Myol 25(4):249–252, 2015 26913164

Davies C, Sanesi G: COVID-19 and the importance of urban green spaces. Urban for Urban Green 74:127654, 2022 35754930

Detweiler MB, Murphy PF, Myers LC, et al: Does a wander garden influence inappropriate behaviors in dementia residents? Am J Alzheimers Dis Other Demen 23(1):31–45, 2008 18276956

Detweiler MB, Sharma T, Detweiler JG, et al: What is the evidence to support the use of therapeutic gardens for the elderly? Psychiatry Investig 9(2):100–110, 2012 22707959

Douglas S, James I, Ballard C: Non-pharmacological interventions in dementia. Adv Psychiatr Treat 10(3):171–177, 2004

Gale SA, Acar D, Daffner KR: Dementia. Am J Med 131(10):1161–1169, 2018 29425707

Gamble KR, Howard JH Jr, Howard DV: Not just scenery: viewing nature pictures improves executive attention in older adults. Exp Aging Res 40(5):513–530, 2014 25321942

Hartig T, Mang M, Evans GW: Restorative effects of natural environment experiences. Environ Behav 23(1):3–26, 1991

Hinshaw SP: Attention Deficits and Hyperactivity in Children. Thousand Oaks, CA, Sage, 1994

Holtzer R, Shuman M, Mahoney JR, et al: Cognitive fatigue defined in the context of attention networks. Neuropsychol Dev Cogn B Aging Neuropsychol Cogn 18(1):108–128, 2011 21128132

Jain A, Spencer D, Yang W, et al: Injuries among children with autism spectrum disorder. Acad Pediatr 14(4):390–397, 2014 24976351

Kabisch N, van den Bosch M, Lafortezza R: The health benefits of nature-based solutions to urbanization challenges for children and the elderly—a systematic review. Environ Res 159:362–373, 2017 28843167

Kaplan R, Kaplan S: The Experience of Nature: A Psychological Perspective. New York, University Press, 1989

Kaplan S: The restorative benefits of nature: toward an integrative framework. J Environ Psychol 15:169–182, 1995

Kaplan S, Talbot JF: Psychological benefits of a wilderness experience, in Behavior and the Natural Environment. Edited by Altman I, Wohlwil JF. New York, Plenum, 1983, pp 163–203

Kellert SR: Experiencing nature: affective, cognitive, and evaluative development in children, in Children and Nature: Psychological, Sociocultural, and Evolutionary Investigations. Edited by Kahn PH Jr, Kellert SR. Cambridge, MA, MIT Press, 2002, pp 117–151

Lahart I, Darcy P, Gidlow C, et al: The effects of green exercise on physical and mental wellbeing: a systematic review. Int J Environ Res Public Health 16(8):1352, 2019 30991724

Lai MC, Lombardo MV, Baron-Cohen S: Autism. Lancet 383(9920):896–910, 2014 24074734

Landry BW, Driscoll SW: Physical activity in children and adolescents. PM R 4(11):826–832, 2012 23174545

Lee LC, Harrington RA, Chang JJ, et al: Increased risk of injury in children with developmental disabilities. Res Dev Disabil 29(3):247–255, 2008 17582739

Lee Y, Kim S: Effects of indoor gardening on sleep, agitation, and cognition in dementia patients—a pilot study. Int J Geriatr Psychiatry 23(5):485–489, 2008 17918774

Leung PM, Ejupi A, van Schooten KS, et al: Association between sedentary behaviour and physical, cognitive, and psychosocial status among older adults in assisted living. BioMed Res Int 2017:9160504, 2017 28913360

Lobelo F, Muth ND, Hanson S, et al: Physical activity assessment and counseling in pediatric clinical settings. Pediatrics 145(3):e20193992, 2020 32094289

Lu LC, Lan SH, Hsieh YP, et al: Horticultural therapy in patients with dementia: a systematic review and meta-analysis. Am J Alzheimers Dis Other Demen 35:1533317519883498, 2020 31690084

Lubbock J: The Use of Life. New York, Macmillan, 1894

Ma JLC, Lai KYC, Wan ESF, et al: Multiple family therapy for Chinese families of children with attention hyperactivity disorder (ADHD): treatment efficacy from the children's perspective and their subjective experiences. J Fam Ther 41:599–619, 2019

Madzia J, Ryan P, Yolton K, et al: Residential greenspace association with childhood behavioral outcomes. J Pediatr 207:233–240, 2019 30545565

Maenner MJ, Shaw KA, Baio J, et al: Prevalence of autism spectrum disorder among children aged 8 years—Autism and Developmental Disabilities Monitoring Network, 11 sites, United States, 2016. MMWR Surveill Summ 69(4):1–12, 2020

Maenner MJ, Warren Z, Williams AR, et al: Prevalence and characteristics of autism spectrum disorder among children aged 8 years - Autism and Developmental Disabilities Monitoring Network, 11 Sites, United States, 2020. MMWR Surveill Summ 72(2):1–14, 2023

Magnus W, Nazir S, Anilkumar AC, et al: Attention deficit hyperactivity disorder. StatPearls. Bethesda, MD, National Center for Biotechnology Information, 2021. Available at: https://www.ncbi.nlm.nih.gov/books/NBK441838. Accessed May 19, 2024.

Mandy W, Lai MC: Annual research review: the role of the environment in the developmental psychopathology of autism spectrum condition. J Child Psychol Psychiatry 57(3):271–292, 2016 26782158

Mueller AK, Fuermaier AB, Koerts J, et al: Stigma in attention deficit hyperactivity disorder. Atten Defic Hyperact Disord 4(3):101–114, 2012 22773377

Nezu CM, Nezu AM: Outpatient psychotherapy for adults with mental retardation and concomitant psychopathology: research and clinical imperatives. J Consult Clin Psychol 62(1):34–42, 1994 8034826

Niedermeyer E, Naidu SB: Attention-deficit hyperactivity disorder (ADHD) and frontal-motor cortex disconnection (electroencephalography). Clin Electroencephalogr 28(3):130–136, 1997 9241465

Ohly H, White MP, Wheeler BW, et al: Attention restoration theory: a systematic review of the attention restoration potential of exposure to natural environments. J Toxicol Environ Health B Crit Rev 19(7):305–343, 2016 27668460

Phillips VL, Diwan S: The incremental effect of dementia-related problem behaviors on the time to nursing home placement in poor, frail, demented older people. J Am Geriatr Soc 51(2):188–193, 2003 12558715

Quinn A, Russo A: Adaptive school grounds design in response to COVID-19: findings from six primary schools in South East England. Build Environ 215:108946, 2022 35250152

Raney MA, Hendry CF, Yee SA: Physical activity and social behaviors of urban children in green playgrounds. Am J Prev Med 56(4):522–529, 2019 30772148

Sachs NA, Rakow DA, Shepley MM, et al: The potential correlation between nature engagement in middle childhood years and college undergraduates' nature engagement, proenvironmental attitudes, and stress. Front Psychol 11:540872, 2020 33192785

Seymour KE, Chronis-Tuscano A, Halldorsdottir T, et al: Emotion regulation mediates the relationship between ADHD and depressive symptoms in youth. J Abnorm Child Psychol 40(4):595–606, 2012 22113705

Shaw KA, Bilder DA, McArthur D, et al: Early identification of autism spectrum disorder among children aged 4 years - Autism and Developmental Disabilities Monitoring Network, 11 Sites, United States, 2020. MMWR Surveill Summ 72(1):1–15, 2023

Silvetti M, Wiersema JR, Sonuga-Barke E, et al: Deficient reinforcement learning in medial frontal cortex as a model of dopamine-related motivational deficits in ADHD. Neural Networks 46:199–209, 2013

Simoni M, Baldacci S, Maio S, et al: Adverse effects of outdoor pollution in the elderly. J Thorac DiStatisticss 7(1):34–45, 2015 25694816

Statistics Korea: Statistics Korea; Daejeon: 2021. Population projections and summary indicators by scenarios (Korea): 2020–2070. 2021

Stevenson MP, Schilhab T, Bentsen P: Attention restoration theory II: a systematic review to clarify attention processes affected by exposure to natural environments. J Toxicol Environ Health B Crit Rev 21(4):227–268, 2018 30130463

Stuart BK, Schlosser DA: Multifamily group treatment for schizophrenia. Int J Group Psychother 59(3):435–440, 2009 19548790

Takano T, Nakamura K, Watanabe M: Urban residential environments and senior citizens' longevity in megacity areas: the importance of walkable green spaces. J Epidemiol Community Health 56(12):913–918, 2002 12461111

Tanner K, Hand BN, O'Toole G, et al: Effectiveness of interventions to improve social participation, play, leisure, and restricted and repetitive behaviors in people with autism spectrum disorder: a systematic review. Am J Occup Ther 69(5):6905180010p1–6905180010p12, 2015 26356653

Taylor AF, Kuo FE, Sullivan WC: Coping with ADD: the surprising connection to green play settings. Environ Behav 33(1):54–77, 2001

Tisher A, Salardini A: A comprehensive update on treatment of dementia. Semin Neurol 39(2):167–178, 2019 30925610

Tovo-Rodrigues L, Rohde LA, Menezes AM, et al: DRD4 rare variants in attention-deficit/hyperactivity disorder (ADHD): further evidence from a birth cohort study. PLoS One 8(12):e85164, 2013 24391992

Tripp G, Wickens JR: Neurobiology of ADHD. Neuropharmacology 57(7–8):579–589, 2009 19627998

United Nations Department of Economic and Social Affairs, Population Division: World Population Prospects 2022: Summary of Results. UN DESA/POP/2022/TR/NO. 3. 2022. Available at: https://population.un.org/wpp/Publications. Accessed May 19, 2024.

van den Berg AE, van den Berg CG: A comparison of children with ADHD in a natural and built setting. Child Care Health Dev 37(3):430–439, 2011 21143265

Weeland J, Moens MA, Beute F, et al: A dose of nature: two three-level meta-analyses of the beneficial effects of exposure to nature on children's self-regulation. J Environ Psychol 65:101326, 2019

White MP, Alcock I, Wheeler BW, et al: Would you be happier living in a greener urban area? A fixed-effects analysis of panel data. Psychol Sci 24(6):920–928, 2013 23613211

White PC, Wyatt J, Chalfont G, et al: Exposure to nature gardens has time-dependent associations with mood improvements for people with mid- and late-stage dementia: innovative practice. Dementia (London) 17(5):627–634, 2018 28835119

Williams J, Taylor E: The evolution of hyperactivity, impulsivity and cognitive diversity. J R Soc Interface 3(8):399–413, 2006 16849269

Wolraich ML, Hagan JF Jr, Allan C, et al: Clinical practice guideline for the diagnosis, evaluation, and treatment of attention-deficit/hyperactivity disorder in children and adolescents. Pediatrics 144(4):e20192528, 2019 31570648

Yogman M, Garner A, Hutchinson J, et al: The power of play: a pediatric role in enhancing development in young children. Pediatrics 142(3):e20182058, 2018 30126932

Zhang Y, Kang J, Kang J: Effects of soundscape on the environmental restoration in urban natural environments. Noise Health 19(87):65–72, 2017 29192615

Index

Page numbers printed in **boldface** type refer to tables or figures.